ADVANCE PRAISE FOR
CANCER CAREGIVERS

"Family caregivers do a lot more than simply support their loved ones with cancer, they are our greatest over-tapped, yet under-appreciated, societal resource. In *Cancer Caregivers*, Dr. Allison Applebaum has brought together a stellar group of diverse, internationally recognized, leaders in clinical care, research and program development. The authors share their data and experiences in a manner that is sharply focused, practical and ready to be put into practice. *Cancer Caregivers* is the new Gold Standard and must have reference for any professional interested in being on the cutting edge of cancer care."

—**Matthew J. Loscalzo, LCSW,**
APOS Fellow, Liliane Elkins Professor in Supportive Care Programs,
Professor, Department of Population Sciences, Executive Director,
Department of Supportive Care Medicine, Administrative Director,
Sheri & Les Biller Patient and Family Resource Center,
City of Hope-National Medical Center,
Duarte, CA

"This comprehensive text unites the work of the leaders of the field into a single accessible resource on cancer caregiving."

—**William Pirl, MD, MPH,**
Vice Chair for Psychosocial Oncology,
Dana-Farber Cancer Institute,
Harvard Medical School,
Boston, MA

"Cancer Caregivers is a landmark publication that elucidates the burgeoning science of caregiving. The information provided by pioneers and leaders in this field is enlightening; the writing is crisp throughout with thoughtful editing by Dr. Applebaum, and the message is clear: care for caregivers cannot be overlooked. Oncology treatment providers, patients and caregivers will all benefit by this timely volume."

—**Andrew J. Roth, MD,**
Attending Psychiatrist, Memorial Sloan Kettering Cancer Center,
Professor of Clinical Psychiatry, Weill Cornell Medical College,
New York, NY

Cancer Caregivers

Edited by
Allison J. Applebaum, PhD

Assistant Attending Psychologist
Director, Caregivers Clinic
Memorial Sloan Kettering Cancer Center
Assistant Professor of Psychology in Psychiatry
Weill Cornell Medical College
New York, NY

OXFORD
UNIVERSITY PRESS

Oxford University Press is a department of the University of Oxford. It furthers
the University's objective of excellence in research, scholarship, and education
by publishing worldwide. Oxford is a registered trade mark of Oxford University
Press in the UK and certain other countries.

Published in the United States of America by Oxford University Press
198 Madison Avenue, New York, NY 10016, United States of America.

Library of Congress Cataloging-in-Publication Data
Names: Applebaum, Allison, editor.
Title: Cancer caregivers / edited by Allison Applebaum.
Description: New York, NY : Oxford University Press, [2019] |
Includes bibliographical references and index.
Identifiers: LCCN 2018031707 | ISBN 9780190868567 (alk. paper)
Subjects: | MESH: Caregivers—psychology | Neoplasms—psychology |
Psychosocial Support Systems | Cognitive Therapy
Classification: LCC RC263 | NLM QZ 260 | DDC 616.99/4—dc23
LC record available at https://lccn.loc.gov/2018031707

9 8 7 6 5 4 3 2 1

Printed by WebCom, Inc., Canada

For my Father, who has taught me the deepest meaning
of what it means to be a caregiver.

And to truly love.

CONTENTS

FOREWORD

This book on informal caregivers is timely and needed. It addresses our current need for direction and information to educate caregivers, patients, providers, administrators, researchers, and policymakers to meet the increasing demands of providing adequate resources for patients with cancer and their families. It was during our first randomized clinical trial in the mid-1980s that Jeanne Benoliel and I recognized the critical role the spouse assumed in the care of patients with lung cancer.[1]

At that time, the word *caregiver* was not a part of our vocabulary to describe the spouse's role. We secured funding through a supplement attached to our patient trial. The purposes of this landmark study were to describe spouses' psychological distress associated with the patients' cancer from diagnosis until 2 years after the patients' death and to test the effects of our oncology nursing intervention on patient and caregiver outcomes. Of the subsample of patients with spouses, 100 of the 127 eligible spouses agreed to participate. The final sample was limited to 46 spouses who had baseline data and whose loved one had died during the study. Spouses randomized to the oncology home care group were taught to help care for their loved one during the loved one's illness and reported significantly less depression and paranoid ideation during bereavement than spouses who were not taught these skills. We concluded that our findings demonstrated that spouses' psychological distress can be positively influenced after the patients' death by the caregivers' involvement in providing care during the patients' terminal phase of illness.[2]

Informal caregiving by families and friends has been an essential part of patients' experiences of living with cancer, but it was not until the last decade of the twentieth century that we documented how important caregiving is to the patients' well-being and the caregivers' health.[3] This book describes much needed evidence-based interventions targeted at caregivers' well-being.

With the increasing complexities of new advances in cancer diagnostic workups and treatments, caregivers are assuming a heavy burden of assisting patients with not only their physical and emotional care, but also the logistics and financial demands of care. We now know that caregiving influences patient outcomes and requires coordinated efforts at multiple levels: the patient level (making sure the patient has his or her medications and gets to appointments); the system level (providing support groups for caregivers of disease-specific types of cancer); and the policy level (advocating for funding for local and state laws, including funds for family members who must leave their jobs to care for a loved one).

The demands of caregiving vary across the cancer trajectory, with patients requiring more caregiving at different critical times throughout the illness. With people living longer with cancer and the number of people diagnosed increasing, resources to help them manage their disease and its effects are limited or nonexistent. The evidence to direct practice is increasing, but much more research is needed. This book helps to fill some of the gaps in our understanding of the growing responsibilities of caregivers and offers answers and some possible solutions to help caregivers provide care and take care of themselves.

The book is presented in five sections. The first section describes who caregivers are, what they do, and their burden and health consequences of caregiving. The challenges of measuring caregiver burden are discussed, along with the current state of the science. The section includes a thorough description of the burden of caregiving and singles out three special vulnerable populations: those caring for patients with brain tumors, caregivers of patients undergoing stem cell transplant, and caregivers of patients with comorbid conditions, including psychiatric disorders. Insights are included by the authors regarding the special needs of these caregivers. The chapter by Litzelman is a welcome addition, describing the experience of caregiving based on life stage. The author discusses the unique challenges of caregiving through three time periods: early adulthood (18 to 44 years); middle age (45 to 64 years); and older age (adults over 65 years). The section also includes a chapter by Pedreira, Mitchell, Ting, and Kim, who describe the sociocultural factors of cancer caregiving and their consequences. The authors recommend that taking these factors into account helps to identify subgroups of caregivers who are vulnerable to the adverse effects of caregiving so evidenced-based interventions can be developed and tested.

The second section of the book includes five evidence-based interventions that have been proven to help caregivers of patients with cancer. These interventions are well established with caregivers and have been proven to be significant in affecting both patient and caregiver outcomes. Each chapter includes a case example to illustrate how the intervention is used and results expected. Dionne-Odom and colleagues describe their psychoeducation intervention, which includes telehealth palliative care as the first treatment. They emphasize the importance of the caregiver being an informed participant in the care of the patient. Northouse and her colleagues describe their FOCUS (family involvement, optimistic attitude, coping effectiveness, uncertainty reduction, symptom management) intervention. Jacobs and colleagues present an overview of Cognitive Behavioral Therapy, while Nezu and colleagues present their well-established Problem-Solving Therapy and skills training. The fifth intervention is presented by Schuler and colleagues on Family-Focused Grief Therapy. These interventions have been tested by disciplines that primarily provide the services, such as psychologists coaching caregivers on cognitive behavioral techniques and nurses providing education on how to manage patients' symptoms. The FOCUS intervention by Northouse et al. represents a comprehensive approach to helping caregivers and is modified so social workers can administer it rather than nurses. The fundamental principle of palliative care applies to caregiving in that caregivers must be recognized in the management of patients' cancer, preferably at the time of diagnosis and included early as essential members of the patients' team.

The third section of the book describes interventions that have shown promise to be effective with caregivers of cancer patients, but the editor cautions us that additional research is needed. Shaffer and colleagues present their results of working with caregivers who have difficulty sleeping and the potential value of Cognitive Behavioral Therapy for Insomnia among caregivers. Panjwani and colleagues present Emotion Regulation Therapy and their promising results with caregivers. Applebaum discusses the impact of existential distress experienced by caregivers and the importance of helping them find meaning in their experiences with the help of Meaning-Centered Psychotherapy for Cancer Caregivers.

The fourth section of the book focuses on the delivery of support to caregivers in the community. This section will be invaluable to providers in planning resources for caregivers. Three well-established community organizations are described. Buzaglo and colleagues describe the services of the Cancer Support Community. Cannady and Sharpe describe the mission, integration, and dissemination of services of the American Cancer Society. Kelly and Goeren describe CancerCare. These three organizations provide a range of free services and resources for patients with cancer and their caregivers, including direct care, support groups, education materials, and advocacy efforts to effect policy. They play a critical role in helping to meet the needs of caregivers and providing practical and emotional support services.

In the fifth section of the book, Wolf and Pejoves Gorman describe the legal and ethical issues faced by cancer caregivers, including the need to take time off from work to provide care and their role in decision-making and potential conflicts that can occur when families do not agree. Applebaum concludes the book by providing an overview of future research directions and gaps in our current evidence-based practice.

This book represents the current state of the science on caregiving of patients with cancer. With the explosion of new targeted therapies to treat cancer within the last few years, there is a critical need for our research efforts to keep pace with designing and testing new interventions to help caregivers in their role of caregiving and to adopt strategies to keep themselves healthy to maintain their role. This book is a welcome addition to our understanding of the complexity of caregiving and the importance caregivers serve in the care of patients with cancer; it also illustrates that caregivers are a limited resource and should be recognized and nurtured to ensure their involvement and longevity. Professionals who care for patients with cancer, including physicians, nurses, social workers, psychologists, psychiatrists, and chaplains will find this book useful and filled with practical advice to help improve caregivers' experiences with caring for their loved one and, most importantly, helping caregivers care for themselves.

Ruth McCorkle
Yale University

REFERENCES

1. McCorkle, R., Benoliel, J. Q., Donaldson, G., Georgiadou, F., Moinpour, C., Goodell, B. A randomized clinical trial of home nursing care of lung cancer patients. *Cancer.* 1989;6(4):199–206.
2. McCorkle, R., Robinson, L., Nuamah, I., Lev, E., Benoliel, J. The effects of home nursing care for patients during terminal illness on the bereaved's psychological distress. *Nurs Res.* 1998;47(1):2–10.
3. Williams, A. L., McCorkle, R. Cancer family caregiver during the palliative, hospice, and bereavement phases: a review of descriptive psychosocial literature. *Palliat Support Care.* 2011;9:315–325.

PREFACE

Over the past decade, improved long-term cancer survivorship has coupled with increasingly complicated cancer treatment courses. This trend has coincided with a shift in the general population to older cancer survivors and a movement toward outpatient rather than inpatient care. Collectively, such factors have greatly expanded the number of tasks and time required for the management of patient needs, as well as the associated economic burden enveloping caregivers.

These enormous responsibilities placed on caregivers have come into increasing focus. In 1996, the National Alliance for Caregiving was founded as a nonprofit coalition of national organizations to advance family caregiving through research, innovation, and advocacy, with the goal of increasing public awareness of family caregiving issues. In 2012, the first academic textbook on this topic, *Cancer Caregiving in the United States: Research, Practice, Policy* (Talley, McCorkle, and Baile, 2012), was published. However, most of the caregiving research available for review primarily focused on the needs of caregivers of patients with neurodegenerative illnesses, such as Alzheimer's and Parkinson's diseases. At that time, it seemed that psychosocial oncology—and the world—had just begun to recognize the specific needs of the incredibly vulnerable population of cancer caregivers, and the research summarized therein revealed the tip of an iceberg.

It is remarkable how far our field of psychosocial oncology has come in the years since the first textbook's publication when one considers some of the key challenges Talley, McCorkle, and Baile highlighted. For example, the authors called for an increase in our understanding of the unique experience of caregivers across genders, race, and life span and to understand the vast economic costs of caregiving. Investigations of interventions for cancer caregivers lacked methodological rigor; the majority of studies did not use randomized designs and frequently relied on small convenience samples. Indeed, the authors highlighted the need to document the efficacy of standardized intervention strategies and to define distinct windows of opportunity for specific interventions to be used across the care trajectory. Moreover, those interventions that had demonstrated efficacy were generally intended to increase caregivers' proficiency in addressing the physical and psychological needs of the patient, not specifically to improve the well-being of the caregiver. Finally, there was a call to understand the legal and ethical implications of assuming the caregiving role and the recognition of caregivers as key members of the healthcare team. Our scientific agenda was indeed vast.

The contents of this first edition of our present volume, *Cancer Caregivers*, is responsive to many of the core issues highlighted by Talley, McCorkle, and Baile and is reflective of the extensive work conducted with cancer caregivers since 2012. The first section is devoted to describing the characteristics and experiences of cancer caregivers based on caregivers' life stage, relationship to the patient, and ethnic group membership, as well as patients' disease and treatment type. The second and third sections highlight significant progress in research focused on the development and dissemination of interventions for cancer caregivers. This includes empirically supported interventions, as well as those currently being developed. Importantly, the majority of these interventions focus on addressing the varying needs of cancer caregivers as their primary outcome, a relatively new target of intervention research. The fourth section focuses on the delivery of support to caregivers in the community and highlights community-based organizations that devote resources to addressing the needs of cancer caregivers and their care recipients. *Cancer Caregivers* concludes with a crucial chapter for all readers that focuses on many of the legal and ethical concerns faced by caregivers, including an overview of relatively new legislation that has the potential to significantly impact the ways in which the US government and healthcare system view and interface with cancer caregivers.

The magnitude of growth in our field over the past decade is in great part a reflection of the increasing recognition by governing and funding bodies of the critical need to move cancer caregiving research forward in a timely fashion. In the past 5 years alone, there have been several joint meetings by the National Cancer Institute and National Institute of Nursing Research, convening leaders in the field to examine the state of the science of informal cancer caregiving and set priorities for future research. One of these meetings (May 2015) was soon followed with Funding Opportunity Announcements from the National Institutes of Health aimed at advancing caregiver-focused interventions to improve caregiver and patient quality of life and healthcare utilization. There has also been an increase in supportive services for caregivers in comprehensive cancer centers and a parallel response from community-based organizations and providers to address their needs. Indeed, there has been a shift across the United States from patient-centered to family-centered cancer care that places caregivers in a bright spotlight.

Cancer Caregivers reveals the depth of complexities in caregiving experiences that our field has been tirelessly exploring for the past decade and the vast expanses we have left to understand. The first chapter in this textbook alone—in its presentation of data from the 2016 National Alliance for Caregiving report "Cancer Caregiving in the US"—documents the enormous and growing number of caregivers who are in continued need of support. It is our responsibility as individuals, as colleagues, and as a field to support caregivers in this important role, to prevent the adverse outcomes that are so well documented in the following chapters, and to assist caregivers in enhancing and sustaining well-being, resilience, and growth.

Allison J. Applebaum, PhD
Assistant Attending Psychologist
Director, Caregivers Clinic
Memorial Sloan Kettering Cancer Center
Assistant Professor of Psychology in Psychiatry
Weill Cornell Medical College
New York, NY
June 2018

ACKNOWLEDGMENTS

I am indebted to my family and friends for their love and support. To my Mother, for encouraging me to dance, and to Jessica, for reminding me to keep dancing in the rain.

I am immensely grateful to all of my colleagues, collaborators, mentors, students, and friends at Memorial Sloan Kettering Cancer Center, across the United States, and around the world who have taken active roles in bringing the field of cancer caregiving forward and creating momentum that will not stop.

I am particularly grateful for my mentor, Dr. William Breitbart, who believed in a vision for a comprehensive program to support cancer caregivers, in the importance of family-centered care, and in me. I also re-main forever indebted to Dr. Jimmie Holland, who gave me no choice but to work on this incredible project—and to love this incredible field.

I am incredibly thankful for the contributions of Kelly Shaffer, PhD, Juliet Jenkelowitz, MS, Kara Buda, MA, and Micaela Raviv to this project. These women represent the next generation of clinician scientists who will surely continue to move this field forward.

Finally, my gratitude is extended to all of the cancer caregivers—my heroes—who walk the hospital hallways, who work overtime in isolation at home, who give their blood, sweat, and tears to this important role. You all are wearing invisible superhero capes, and you deserve to fly.

CONTRIBUTORS

Laurie Anderson, MD
Palliative Care Specialist
Florida Hospital Medical Group
Core Faculty for Florida Hospital
  Hospice and Palliative Care
  Program
Florida Hospital Orlando Campus
Orlando, FL

Allison J. Applebaum, PhD
Assistant Attending Psychologist
Memorial Sloan Kettering Cancer
  Center
Assistant Professor of Psychology
  in Psychiatry
Weill Cornell Medical College
New York, NY

Marie A. Bakitas, DNSc,
  APRN, FAAN
Professor, Marie L. O'Koren
  Endowed Chair
School of Nursing
University of Alabama at
  Birmingham
Birmingham, AL

Margaret Bevans, PhD, RN,
  AOCN, FAAN
Program Director
Scientific Resources, Clinical Nurse
  Scientist, Nursing Research and
  Translational Science
National Institutes of Health
  Clinical Center
Bethesda, MD

William S. Breitbart, MD
Chairman
Department of Psychiatry and
  Behavioral Sciences
The Jimmie C. Holland Chair in
  Psychiatry Oncology
Memorial Sloan Kettering
  Cancer Center
Professor of Clinical Psychiatry
Weill Medical College of Cornell
  University
New York, NY

Joanne S. Buzaglo, PhD
Executive Director, PRO Solutions
Vector Oncology
Memphis, TN

Rachel S. Cannady, BS
Strategic Director
Cancer Caregiver Support,
American Cancer Society
Atlanta, GA

Patricia Carter, PhD, RN, CNS
Associate Professor
School of Nursing
The University of Texas at Austin
Austin, TX

Wen-Ying Sylvia Chou, PhD, MPH
Program Director
Health Communication and
Informatics Research Branch,
Behavioral Research Program
National Cancer Institute
Bethesda, MD

**J. Nicholas Dionne-Odom, PhD,
RN, ACHPN**
Assistant Professor
School of Nursing
University of Alabama at
Birmingham
Birmingham, AL

Bonnie Dockham, LMSW
Program Facilitator, FOCUS
Program
Cancer Support Community
Ann Arbor, MI

**Betty Ferrell, PhD, MA, FAAN,
FPCN, CHPN**
Director and Professor
Division of Nursing Research and
Education
Department of Population Sciences
City of Hope National
Medical Center
Duarte, CA

David M. Fresco, PhD
Professor, Director of the
Psychopathology and Emotion
Regulation Laboratory (PERL)
CoDirector of the Kent
Electrophysiological
Neuroscience Laboratory
Department of Psychological
Sciences
Kent State University
Kent, OH

Sheila N. Garland, PhD
Assistant Professor
Department of Psychology
Memorial University of
Newfoundland
St. John's, Newfoundland, Canada

Login George, PhD
Postdoctoral Research Fellow
Department of Psychiatry and
Behavioral Sciences
Memorial Sloan Kettering
Cancer Center
New York, NY

**Barbara A. Given, PhD, RN,
FAAN, FAPOS**
University Distinguished Professor
Emerita
Interim Associate Dean for
Research, College of Nursing
Michigan State University
East Lansing, MI

Charles W. Given, PhD
Professor Emeritus
College of Nursing
Michigan State University
East Lansing, MI

William Goeren, LCSW-R, OSW-C, ACSW
Director of Clinical Programs
Cancer*Care*
New York, NY

Mitch Golant, PhD
Senior Consultant, Strategic
 Initiatives
Cancer Support Community
Los Angeles, CA

Cristina Pejoves Gorman, JD
Senior Staff Attorney
LegalHealth, New York Legal
 Assistance Group
New York, NY

Tamryn F. Gray, PhD, MSN, RN, BMTCN
Postdoctoral Research Fellow
Dana-Farber Cancer Institute
Harvard Medical School
Boston, MA

Joseph A. Greer, PhD
Assistant Professor
Department of Psychiatry, Harvard
 Medical School
Clinical Director, Center for
 Psychiatric Oncology and
 Behavioral Sciences
Massachusetts General Hospital
 Cancer Center
Boston, MA

Jamie M. Jacobs, PhD
Assistant Professor
Department of Psychiatry, Harvard
 Medical School
Psychologist, Massachusetts
 General Hospital Cancer Center
Boston, MA

Lauren B. Johnson, EdM
Doctoral Candidate
Department of Psychology
Drexel University
Philadelphia, PA

Sarah K. Kelly, MSW, LCSW
Clinical Supervisor
Cancer*Care*
New York, NY

Erin E. Kent, PhD, MS
Scientific Advisor
Outcomes Research Branch
Healthcare Delivery Research
 Program
National Cancer Institute
Bethesda, MD

Youngmee Kim, PhD
Professor
Department of Psychology
Director of the FAMILY Lab
University of Miami
Coral Gables, FL

David W. Kissane, MD
Professor of Psychiatry and Head
Department of Psychiatry
Monash University
Melbourne, Australia

Maria Kryzo-Lacombe, MA
Graduate Student Researcher
Department of Psychology
San Diego State University
San Diego, CA

Kristin Litzelman, PhD
Assistant Professor
Department of Human
 Development and Family Studies
University of Wisconsin-Madison
Madison, WI

Margaret L. Longacre, PhD
Assistant Professor
Department of Public Health
Arcadia University
Philadelphia, PA

Douglas S. Mennin, PhD
Professor
Department of Psychology
Teachers College
Columbia University
New York, NY

Hannah-Rose Mitchell, MPH
Graduate Research Assistant
Department of Psychology
FAMILY Lab
University of Miami
Coral Gables, FL

Michelle A. Mollica, PhD, MPH,
  RN, OCN
Program Director
Outcomes Research Branch,
  Healthcare Delivery Research
  Program
National Cancer Institute
Bethesda, MD

Arthur M. Nezu, PhD, DHL, ABPP
Distinguished University Professor
  of Psychology, Professor
  of Medicine, and Professor
  of Community Health and
  Prevention
Department of Psychology
Drexel University
Philadelphia, PA

Christine Maguth Nezu,
  PhD, ABPP
Professor of Psychology and
  Professor of Medicine
Department of Psychology
Drexel University
Philadelphia, PA

Laurel Northouse, PhD, RN, FAAN
Professor Emerita
University of Michigan School of
  Nursing
Ann Arbor, MI

Mia S. O'Toole, PhD
Associate Professor
Department of Psychology and
  Behavioral Sciences
Aarhus University
Aarhus, Denmark

Aliza A. Panjwani, MA
Doctoral Candidate
Health Psychology and Clinical
  Science Program at the
  Graduate Center
City University of New York
New York, NY

Patricia B. Pedreira, BS
Research Project Coordinator
Department of Psychology
FAMILY Lab
University of Miami
Coral Gables, FL

Laura C. Polacek, BA
Doctoral Student
Fordham University
New York, NY

Tammy A. Schuler, PhD
Director of Outreach and
  Partnerships
Association for Behavioral and
  Cognitive Therapies
New York, NY

Kelly M. Shaffer, PhD
Assistant Professor
Center for Behavioral Health and
  Technology
Department of Psychiatry and
  Neurobehavioral Sciences
University of Virginia
Charlottesville, VA

Katherine Sharpe, MTS
Senior Vice President
Patient and Caregiver Support,
  American Cancer Society
Atlanta, GA

Clayton Shuman, PhD, RN
Assistant Professor
Department of Systems,
  Populations and Leadership
University of Michigan School of
  Nursing
Ann Arbor, MI

Kimberson Tanco, MD
Assistant Professor
Department of Palliative,
  Rehabilitation and Integrative
  Medicine
Division of Cancer Medicine
The University of Texas MD
  Anderson Cancer Center
Houston, TX

Amanda Ting, BS
Graduate Research Assistant
Department of Psychology
FAMILY Lab
University of Miami
Coral Gables, FL

Marita Titler, PhD, RN, FAAN
Professor
Rhetaugh G. Dumas Endowed
  Professor
Department of Systems,
  Populations and Leadership
University of Michigan School of
  Nursing
Ann Arbor, MI

Lara Traeger, PhD
Assistant Professor
Department of Psychiatry
Harvard Medical School
Psychologist, Massachusetts
  General Hospital Cancer Center
Boston, MA

Moira Visovatti, PhD, RN
Assistant Professor
Department of Health Behavior
  and Biological Sciences
University of Michigan School of
  Nursing
Ann Arbor, MI

Emily A. Walsh, BA
Clinical Research Coordinator
Cancer Outcomes Research
  Program
Department of Psychiatry
Massachusetts General Hospital
Boston, MA

Debra Wolf, JD
Senior Supervising Attorney
LegalHealth, New York Legal
  Assistance Group
Adjunct Professor of Law, Fordham
  University
School of Law
New York, NY

Talia I. Zaider, PhD
Assistant Attending Psychologist
Memorial Sloan Kettering
  Counseling Center
New York, NY

Alexandra K. Zaleta, PhD
Senior Director of Research
Cancer Support Community
Philadelphia, PA

Describing the Population

CHAPTER 1

Who Are Informal Cancer Caregivers?

ERIN E. KENT, MARGARET L. LONGACRE,
WEN-YING SYLVIA CHOU, AND
MICHELLE A. MOLLICA

INTRODUCTION

Despite tremendous advances in treatment, cancer remains a pervasive and devastating disease for many individuals and families in the United States. In 2016, cancer was the second leading cause of death in the United States.[1] In 2018, more than 1.7 million Americans were projected to be diagnosed with cancer,[2] and through 2020 the overall number of Americans diagnosed with cancer is projected to increase.[3] Despite these concerning findings, an increasing number of Americans are surviving cancer. It is anticipated that by 2026, more than 20 million Americans will survive cancer, an increase of approximately 5.5 million individuals in 2016 who had a history of cancer and survived.[4]

The increasing number of individuals diagnosed with cancer in the United States is due largely to the aging population, coupled with greater use of early detection measures and advances in care.[3,4] Indeed, 62% of the 15.5 million US patients with cancer were 65 years of age or older in 2016, and by 2040, this demographic is anticipated to represent 73% of cancer patients.[5] Older adult cancer patients often present with comorbidities, and coordinating care among multiple providers and across treatment settings can be challenging.[5] Furthermore, because cancer as a health condition represents many unique diagnoses, broad differences in care and outcomes exist across sites, types, and stages of cancer. For example, between 2005 and 2011, the 5-year survival rate was 91% for breast cancer but 20% for esophageal cancer.[6] Cancer type also varies greatly by age at diagnosis, suggesting variability in disease management and life course needs.[7]

Cancer and its treatment can have a substantial impact on patient functioning and quality of life (QOL). Patients commonly suffer physical and emotional deficits that affect daily functioning and require assistance. These deficits vary depending on factors such as cancer type, disease progression or stage, and treatment.[8–10] For some patients, deterioration might be rapid; thus, assistance might be needed for only a short time, while for others, cancer requires long-term treatment and follow-up care. For example, despite advances in therapeutic management, pain remains a common and often persistent problem for cancer patients.[11] The need for assistance might extend into survivorship, as individuals are cancer free but continue to experience the lingering effects of cancer or treatment. Survivors are also susceptible to recurrence or secondary cancer in the future, and many survivors report fear of recurrence and need for psychosocial support into survivorship.[12]

A cancer diagnosis can have profound physical, financial, and psychosocial impacts on not only the patient, but also the patient's broader familial and community systems.[13] Though patients themselves individually experience the physical effects of cancer, the impact of cancer extends to relatives, friends, or community members, who contribute or assist in a variety of ways. Though definitions vary, *informal cancer caregivers* here are defined as those family members or friends who provide care to an individual with cancer; the care is typically uncompensated and at home, involving significant time and energy costs.[14]

The purpose of this chapter is to describe the prevalence of informal caregiving in cancer in the United States, characteristics of cancer caregivers, the roles these caregivers commonly fulfill at varied points and locations along the care trajectory, and the impact of caregiving on patient and caregiver outcomes. The chapter closes with implications for research, practice, and policy to improve understanding of this role and our addressing the needs of caregivers and patients alike.

US NATIONAL PREVALENCE ESTIMATES OF CANCER CAREGIVERS: HOW MANY CAREGIVERS ARE THERE?

Limited national data exist on the number of individuals who are providing care for a loved one with cancer. This gap in understanding of the prevalence of caregiving in cancer is due to many broad structural factors, such as (1) lacking an integrated (state-federal) surveillance system to collect data on caregiving and caregiver outcomes despite collecting patient diagnostic data in such a manner; (2) lacking an agreed-on descriptor or universal definition of a *caregiver* (e.g., primary vs. secondary or paid vs. unpaid) and the "caregiving" role (i.e., specified tasks/roles); (3) having a healthcare reimbursement system and processes that are centered on individual patients rather than on the delivery of patient- and family-centered care; and (4) having a fragmented national healthcare system that, despite improvement, still lacks integrated care and centralized data on patients (e.g., universal electronic health records). Recent prevalence estimates vary, and this variation is due largely to differences in assessment methods and measurement. For example, differences in prevalence estimates of caregivers vary depending on whether the data were collected from caregivers versus care recipients.[15] Additional discrepancies in prevalence arise depending on (1) whether those completing surveys about caregiving roles and tasks (i.e., care recipients or caregivers) were instructed or able to report multiple health conditions for which care is provided or only a single or primary health problem; (2) the time frame for providing care assessed by surveys; (3) whether primary caregivers or secondary carers were assessed; and (4) the intent of the research (raising awareness about caregiving or identifying health system needs).[16]

Table 1.1 provides available prevalence estimates of informal cancer caregivers in the United States and the sampling frame, descriptions of the data source, and sample size from which the estimates have been based. Some of the most recent US national estimates of cancer caregivers come from the National Alliance for Caregiving (NAC) data, which conducted a 2015 online probability-based survey of self-identified caregivers.[17] Respondents were asked to provide the main problem or illness that the recipient required care for, and approximately 2.8 million individuals, 7% of the 39.8 million caregivers included, were estimated to be actively providing care to an adult living with cancer. In contrast, according to the most recent cycle of the Health Information National Trends Survey (HINTS), fielded in 2017, as many as 6.1 million adult individuals were estimated to be providing care for an individual (adult or child) with cancer.[18] However, HINTS allowed respondents to endorse multiple health problems for which they were providing care, which likely explains the higher prevalence.

Another data source, the Medical Expenditure Panel Survey (MEPS), collects annual information from a nationally representative sample of households in the United States on utilization and costs of medical care and employment. In 2011, MEPS fielded a supplemental survey to individuals with a cancer history, and this survey assessed information

Table 1.1 US PREVALENCE ESTIMATES OF CANCER CAREGIVERS BY DATA SOURCE

Study	Description	Survey Participant	Time Period of Reference	Sampling Frame	Endorsement of Multiple Health Conditions Possible?	Sample Size	Prevalence Estimates
National Alliance for Caregiving, 2015[17,a]	Self-identified caregivers over the past 12 months, reporting on caregiving characteristics based on the main problem or illness of care recipient	Caregiver	Past 12 months	Online, probability-based sample of US adults	No	111 caregivers who indicated that cancer was the main problem of the adult for whom they were providing care	2.8 million caregivers of adults with cancer in the United States
Health Information National Trends Survey, 2017[18,b]	Self-identified caregivers, reporting on caregiving characteristics based on the main problem or illness of care recipient	Caregiver	Current (no specific time frame referenced)	Nationally representative survey of households, with one adult participant randomly selected from each residence	Yes	2,587 individuals who selected cancer as one of the conditions for which they were providing care	6.1 million caregivers of adults with cancer, and possibly other health conditions, in the United States

Survey	Description	Care recipient/caregiver	Time period	Survey design	Optional module	Sample	Estimate
Medical Expenditure Panel Survey, 2011[19,c]	Self-identified cancer survivors, reporting on the impact of employment and financial burden on caregivers from the perspective of care recipients	Care recipient/cancer survivor	Any time since cancer diagnosis	Nationally representative survey of households, sample drawn from the National Health Interview Survey	No	485 cancer survivors reporting an informal caregiver at some point since diagnosis	6.1 million survivors reporting have at least one caregiver at some point since diagnosis
Behavioral Risk Factor Surveillance System, 2015[21,d]	Self-identified caregivers, reporting on caregiving characteristics based on the main problem or illness of care recipient	Caregiver	Past month	Population-based survey of individuals randomly selected at the state level; 24 states fielded the optional Caregiving Module	Yes	1,574 who indicated that cancer was the main problem of the adult for whom they were providing care	1,131,461 cancer caregivers in 18 states (Alabama, Hawaii, Idaho, Illinois, Indiana, Iowa, Kentucky, Louisiana, Mississippi, New Jersey, Oregon, Pennsylvania, South Carolina, Tennessee, Virginia, West Virginia, Wisconsin, Wyoming)

Caregiver identification questions from the surveys cited:

a. At any time in the last 12 months, has anyone in your household provided unpaid care to a relative or friend 18 years or older to help them take care of themselves? This may include helping with personal needs or household chores. It might be managing a person's finances, arranging for outside services, or visiting regularly to see how they are doing. This adult need not live with you.

b. Are you currently caring for or making healthcare decisions for someone with a medical, behavioral, disability, or other condition?

c. Since the time you were first diagnosed with cancer, has any friend or family member provided care to you during or after your cancer treatment?

d. People may provide regular care or assistance to a friend or family member who has a health problem, long-term illness, or disability. During the past month, did you provide any such care or assistance to a friend or family member?

from survivors about the impact of the cancer experience on informal caregivers. Findings from this survey indicate that 37% (*n* = 458) of survivors reported having an informal cancer caregiver at any point since their diagnosis, which is estimated to represent approximately 6.1 million people in the United States.[19] Both MEPS and HINTS appear to have yielded similar prevalence estimates of current informal cancer caregivers in the United States, though their methods for assessing prevalence were quite different.

Other prevalence estimates are reported via the Behavioral Risk Factor Surveillance System (BRFSS), an annual survey that has included an optional caregiving module since 2006. In 2015, the module was fielded by 24 states; 24,034 (21.8% weighted) respondents endorsed the question of being a caregiver, and of those, 1,910 across 18 states (9.1% weighted) indicated cancer as the reason for providing care, with 1,831 (96.6% weighted) providing care for an adult with cancer.[20] In 2015, among these 18 states, an estimated 1.13 million were estimated to have served as a caregiver for an adult with cancer. Prevalence estimates of caregivers caring for an adult, with the main reason for care being cancer, can only be counted at the state level because not all states participated, but ranged between a high of about 5,700 in Wyoming to 177,000 in Pennsylvania (unpublished data).

CAREGIVER CHARACTERISTICS

Cancer incidence, prevalence, and mortality rates vary according to sociodemographic factors such as age, race/ethnicity, and socioeconomic status. These differences belie disparities in cancer outcomes suggestive of differential experiences of poverty, barriers in access to care, environmental exposures, behavioral risk factors, cultural differences, and clinical trial participation.[21] The varying distribution of patients with cancer relates in part to variation in the characteristics of caregivers, although caregiver characteristics are often documented in disparate data sources.

According to the 2015 NAC Caregiving in the US Study, most adult cancer caregivers were female (58%), with a mean age of 53.1, median of 52, and range of 18 to 88. Approximately 65% of caregivers reported non-Hispanic white ethnicity, followed by Hispanic (16%), non-Hispanic black (11%), and non-Hispanic Asian (8%). Cancer caregivers tended to have slightly higher educational attainment than noncancer caregivers and a median household income of $55,500. About half reported being employed in the past year while being a caregiver.[17]

CAREGIVING TASKS

There are several unique challenges of caring for an individual with cancer. The NAC report found that cancer caregiving is shorter and can be more intense than caring for noncancer patients,[17] which could be due in part to the acute nature of a cancer diagnosis and treatment trajectory. Cancer caregivers were found to provide an average of 1.9 years of care versus 4.1 years for noncancer caregivers. The number of hours of care and tasks provided each day are often greater, however, with estimates ranging from 1 to 8 hours per day[22,23] to an average of 32.9 hours per week.[24] Data from the 2015 BRFSS survey suggested that about 65% of cancer caregivers reported providing care up to 8 hours per week to an adult with cancer, 14% reported 9–19 hours per week, 8% reported 20–39 hours per week, and 13% reported 40 hours or more per week.[20]

Cancer caregivers assist with a range of tasks, including activities of daily living (ADLs) and medical/nursing tasks. Almost half of cancer caregivers indicate that they perform more than three ADLs,[24] including helping their care recipient to get dressed, transfer in and out of bed, go to the bathroom, and eat. In addition, cancer caregivers assist with instrumental ADLs, which include providing transportation, doing housework or grocery shopping, and preparing meals. Performing medical/nursing tasks requires specific knowledge and confidence to carry out and can thus be a challenge for caregivers. Between 52%[22] and 72%[24] of cancer caregivers participating in national surveys indicated that they perform some medical or nursing task. Data from the Share Thoughts on Care Caregiver Study conducted by the Cancer Care Outcomes Research and Surveillance (CanCORS) consortium, a cohort study of lung and colorectal cancer patients in the early 2000s, showed that almost two-thirds of caregivers managed care recipient symptoms (n = 504), more than half administered medications (n = 389), and some changed bandages (n = 173).[22] Notably, among the CanCORS caregivers surveyed who performed at least one medical or nursing task, most did not report receiving training for all of the care provided.

IMPACT OF CAREGIVING ON BOTH CAREGIVER AND PATIENT OUTCOMES

Caregiving has been shown via observational and intervention studies to have an impact on patient outcomes. The consequences of caregiving to caregivers themselves might manifest as several kinds of strain: physical,[24,25] psychosocial and emotional,[26,27] and financial/economic.[19,28]

The National Quality of Life Survey for Caregivers, initiated in 2002 and funded by the American Cancer Society, included over 1,200 caregivers at a 5-year follow-up after their care recipient's cancer diagnosis and assessed/ evaluated the experiences of former, bereaved, and current caregivers.[29] Older caregivers reported better psychosocial adjustment but worse physical health than younger caregivers. Caregivers who reported higher caregiving stress reported worse QOL years later, indicating a possible lasting impact of the caregiving burden. Spousal caregivers also reported experiencing worse QOL than other types of caregivers.

Several studies have demonstrated that efficacious interventions targeting caregivers tend to require large amounts of clinician time and involve symptom management components.[30] The number of intervention studies has increased dramatically in the past decade, with more studies targeting only caregivers and more studies delivered at a distance.[30] The impact that caregivers have on their care recipient's health outcomes and vice versa is thought to both vary and be reciprocal, especially in the context of intense caregiving. Studies that treat patient-caregiver pairs as dyads, particularly romantic couples, often find reciprocal effects of caregiving. Evidence of dyadic effects have been found for both illness stressors[31] and illness coping.[32,33] Various models of dyadic coping have been proposed, including the relationship-focused coping model, transactional model of stress and coping, systemic-transactional model of dyadic coping, collaborative coping, relationship intimacy model, communication models, and coping congruence. Each model emphasizes different components of coping, though one shared feature is the suggestion that impairments in the couple's communication generally lead to poor psychosocial outcomes in either partner.[33]

CAREGIVING ACROSS THE CANCER CARE CONTINUUM AND LIFE COURSE

Care recipient and caregiving needs fluctuate across the cancer care continuum, which can have an impact on both patients and caregivers alike.[34] Caregivers may play a role in the speed with which individuals access healthcare based on signs, symptoms, and testing results of cancer diagnosis. During the diagnostic period, they may play a role in treatment decision-making. As patient health needs and treatment experiences fluctuate, the demands placed on caregivers may vary. Caregivers may help care recipients transition through and beyond treatment and into survivorship or end-of-life care. Each phase of the continuum brings unique challenges for cancer patients, and this is also true for caregivers. Few studies have examined how caregiver needs change across the disease trajectory, in large part because there are few longitudinal studies that include caregivers. One review of end-of-life caregiving found that caregivers provided more extensive care and dealt with more care-related challenges than those caring for patients at earlier phases of the disease continuum.[35] Transitions in care are typically the most challenging times for caregivers, but given the need to change care plans at these points, transitions also present opportunities for caregiver engagement, skills training, and distress screening.[36]

In addition to considering the differences that arise across the course of the cancer care continuum, the needs and issues that arise for caregivers vary according to age and life course. For caregivers of individuals with serious illness, care recipients tend to be younger,[38] which can present unique and unexpected issues. One study found that over 40% of parents caring for a child with cancer reported anxiety, depression, or post-traumatic stress symptoms.[38] Standards of care that encourage a family-centered approach have been developed for treating children in cancer centers, and pediatric cancer centers are often very responsive to the needs of family members in the context of treating children with cancer.[38] Caregiving for adults at middle age is often done by partners, who might be in peak responsibility years in terms of childrearing, career, and other demands.[39] Older adults are more likely to experience cancer in concert with other chronic conditions, which also might exacerbate caregiving demands.[40] The variability in unmet needs among patients and caregivers across the life course suggests a need for a wide range of resources and services available to families as they navigate the cancer trajectory. The experience of caregivers based on their life stage and relationship to the patient are explored in detail in Chapter 3.

GEOGRAPHICAL DISTRIBUTION OF CAREGIVING IN CANCER

Informal cancer caregiving takes place in all regions of the United States. According to the 2015 NAC report, 71% of care recipients lived in urban or suburban areas, while 28% were in rural areas. In comparison, 84% of caregivers were estimated to live in urban/suburban areas, while just 16% lived in rural areas.[17] The differences in prevalence estimates between locations of care recipients and caregivers suggest that many caregivers do not live or work in close vicinity to their care recipients. Some travel a long distance or temporarily relocate in order to provide care, interrupting or altogether suspending normal routines. A recent review of distance caregiving showed that such caregivers tend to experience more anxiety related to their care recipient's health and more guilt about the extent of care they can provide.[41] Additional reported challenges for distance caregivers include limited firsthand information from the care team about the patient's condition and treatment options, being left out of family discussions, and anxiety and guilt, particularly when a parent has advanced cancer.

Technologically enabled interventions, through Internet and mobile devices, are poised to remedy some of these challenges, and research has recently begun to explore their efficacy and effectiveness. For example, web-based interventions, including online support groups and informational websites, can overcome geographic barriers and generally lower access barriers to support caregiver coping and reduce anxiety.[44] The growing prevalence of cancer-focused online networks (e.g., Facebook groups, illness blogs, caregivers' discussion boards on the American Cancer Society's Cancer Survivors Network) not only offer opportunities to remedy the challenges of distance caregiving, but also connect geographically dispersed cancer caregivers with one another. However, there may be risks associated with using online communities to share information about cancer caregiving, particularly in discussing treatment decisions. Individuals involved in online discussions over a long distance may not be adequately informed or experienced with a given situation (e.g., prognostic information, family dynamics, or exact symptoms) and as such may risk offering misinformation to other caregivers in need.[45] Professional monitoring of online forums can help mitigate misinformation risk, however. Another important technological solution to remedy the challenges in distance caregiving is the use of mobile devices (including smartphones, monitoring sensors, and telehealth applications) to connect patients and caregivers to providers over distance and increasing availability of remote sensors to offer informational, social, and instrumental support to caregivers.[44] These tools offer significant improvements in various patient and caregiver outcomes.[42, 44, 45]

Finally, only about an estimated 17% of cancer care recipients live in facilities (such as a nursing home, assisted living facility, or retirement community), while the majority (approximately 83%) are being cared for in their private homes by their caregivers.[17] As much of cancer care moves from inpatient to outpatient and home-based care, informal caregivers often are taking on tasks and responsibilities without training, supervision, or support.[30]

FINANCIAL IMPLICATIONS OF CANCER CAREGIVING

Cancer treatment can lead to financial problems and burden for families, due to both the increasingly high cost of cancer treatment[46] and the impact to both the cancer patient and caregiver's work productivity.[47] Lower income families are already at increased risk for high burden and negative impact to QOL.[48] After a cancer diagnosis, direct and indirect costs of treatment and loss of income can exacerbate pre-existing socioeconomic disparities.[49] Intensive and often debilitating cancer treatment, need to travel for treatment, high treatment costs, and change in work hours during cancer treatment have all been associated with decrements to productivity among cancer caregivers.[47] Time costs per year of informal caregiving were calculated using American Cancer Society national survey data (2003–2006) by cancer site for recently diagnosed (diagnosis to 2 years), with the highest sites being lung cancer (approximately $73,000) and ovarian cancer ($66,000).[50] A recent study of MEPS data indicated that approximately 25% of caregivers needed to make an extended employment change to accommodate their caregiving demands, with 8% making changes to work that lasted 2 months or longer.[17] Additional financial implications of informal caregiving can include loss of financial savings,[51] debt, and even bankruptcy.[52] Finally, in a review across health problems of the impact of caregiving for patients at end-of-life versus earlier stages of disease, cancer caregivers reported increased financial difficulties at end of life.[35,37]

FUTURE DIRECTIONS FOR RESEARCH, POLICY, AND PRACTICE
Research Implications

Gaps in existing literature point to the need for more longitudinal studies of cancer patients and their caregivers to understand the longer term impact of cancer caregiving. In addition, interventions to target underserved patient/caregiver populations, particularly in racial/ethnic minorities and low-income communities, are necessary. Despite burgeoning efforts to develop new interventions for cancer caregivers, the predominant focus continues to be white populations.[30] In addition, interventions that can be de novo developed or tailored to target caregiving for adolescent and young adult cancer populations, which have unique life course needs, are needed.

Other populations for which there are few interventions are several underserved populations, including racial/ethnic minorities, partners of sexual and gender minority cancer patients, and caregivers with limited English proficiency. One new cohort study of African American cancer survivors, the Detroit Research On Cancer Survivors (ROCS) Study, will include over 2,500 family members to help understand how cancer caregiving affects mental, physical, and financial health.[53] Work that extends beyond examining patient and caregiver effects in isolation, including dyadic data analysis and social network studies that treat the patient/caregiver dyad and family system as units of analysis, recognize and allow for measurement of the social context of illness and care.[32,54]

Finally, very little is understood about the costs and effects of informal caregiving in cancer, as economic evaluations are rarely included in the cancer context. Estimates of economic burden among caregivers of cancer patients are feasible, however, and have been calculated for caregivers of patients with localized prostate cancer.[55] Future studies should consider economic evaluations of informal caregiving to provide a comprehensive assessment and valuation of informal care.[56]

Practice Implications

Caregivers, though a fundamental presence in the care administered to cancer patients, are often not recognized or supported by the healthcare delivery centers they frequent alongside their care recipients. In addition, they are generally not formally recognized as a member of the care team. Privacy laws and regulations, including the Health Insurance Portability and Accountability Act (HIPAA), while designed to be protective of patients, often pose a challenge for caregivers who need access to health information or to communicate with providers to properly care and advocate for their care recipient. In addition, there is little competence assessment or distress screening taking place for family caregivers, regardless of family circumstances.[30] Fortunately, there has been a recent surge in the development of effective interventions to support family caregivers in cancer[30] and demonstrated potential to integrate many of these programs into practice through healthcare delivery systems and in the community.[57]

An overall paradigm shift from patient-centered to family-centered care is needed.[14] Recommendations at the practice and healthcare system level include the need to routinely assess and address the needs of caregivers, including those with language or literacy barriers; to educate them in the medical and nursing skills they need; to empower them to become engaged members of the healthcare team; and to provide ongoing support to them over the continuum of care.[58]

Policy Implications

The beginning of 2018 marked the bicameral passage of the RAISE (Recognize, Assist, Include, Support, and Engage) Family Caregivers Act (S. 1028/H.R. 3759), which requires the secretary of health and human services to develop a national strategy of multilevel actions to assist family caregivers. Some of the suggested actions include promoting patient- and family-centered care, service planning that involves family caregivers along with care recipients, respite options, and financial security and workplace issues. Several states (39 as of this writing) have already enacted the CARE (Caregiver Advise, Record, Enable) Act, which mandates that a family caregiver be identified on patient admission to a hospital, notified prior to patient discharge, and involved in discharge planning.[59] Neither piece of legislation is focused on cancer, but both have implications for cancer-specific caregiving, including being a first step to formally recognizing the vital role that thousands of individuals play in helping provide essential care to the seriously ill. These policies and their implications are discussed in detail in the final section of this textbook.

CONCLUSIONS

Caregivers are ubiquitous, and their tasks in caring for cancer patients are many, varied, and critical. Currently, it is estimated that between 2 and 6 million Americans are serving as cancer caregivers, caring for cancer patients across the care continuum. The majority of adult cancer caregivers have a median age of 52 and are female.[17] Caregivers have unique needs, including many that are unmet by the current healthcare delivery system. Future research efforts should consider interventions targeting not only patients and their families but also healthcare delivery systems and policies aimed at supporting caregivers through skills training, financial assistance, and psychosocial support. As cancer prevalence continues to rise, so will the burden placed on informal caregivers.

REFERENCES

1. National Center for Health Statistics. *Health, United States, 2016: With Chartbook on Long-Term Trends in Health.* Hyattsville, MD: National Center for Health Statistics; 2017.
2. Siegel RL, Miller KD, Jemal A. Cancer statistics, 2018. *CA Cancer J Clin.* 2018;68(1):7–30.
3. Weir HK, Thompson TD, Soman A, Moller B, Leadbetter S. The past, present, and future of cancer incidence in the United States: 1975 through 2020. *Cancer.* 2015;121(11):1827–1837.
4. Miller KD, Siegel RL, Lin CC, et al. Cancer treatment and survivorship statistics, 2016. *CA Cancer J Clin.* 2016;66(4):271–289.
5. Bluethmann SM, Mariotto AB, Rowland JH. Anticipating the "silver tsunami": Prevalence trajectories and co-morbidity burden among older cancer survivors in the United States. *Cancer Epidemiol Biomarkers Prev.* 2016;25(7):1029–1036.
6. Siegel RL, Miller KD, Jemal A. Cancer statistics, 2016. *CA Cancer J Clin.* 2016;66(1):7–30.
7. Howlader N, Noone AM, Krapcho M, et al. *SEER Cancer Statistics Review, 1975–2014, National Cancer Institute.* Bethesda, MD: National Cancer Institute; 2017.
8. Deshields TL, Potter P, Olsen S, Liu J, Dye L. Documenting the symptom experience of cancer patients. *J Support Oncol.* 2011;9(6):216–223.
9. Kent E, Mitchell SA, Oakley-Girvan I, Arora NK. The importance of symptom surveillance during follow-up care of leukemia, bladder, and colorectal cancer survivors. *Support Care Cancer.* 2014;22(1):163–172.
10. Burkett VS, Cleeland CS. Symptom burden in cancer survivorship. *J Cancer Surviv.* 2007;1(2):167–175.
11. Hackett J, Godfrey M, Bennett MI. Patient and caregiver perspectives on managing pain in advanced cancer: a qualitative longitudinal study. *Palliat Med.* 2016;30(8):711–719.
12. Mariotto AB, Rowland JH, Ries LA, Scopa S, Feuer EJ. Multiple cancer prevalence: a growing challenge in long-term survivorship. *Cancer Epidemiol Biomarkers Prev.* 2007;16(3):566–571.
13. Lund L, Ross L, Petersen MA, Groenvold M. Cancer caregiving tasks and consequences and their associations with caregiver status and the caregiver's relationship to the patient: a survey. *BMC Cancer.* 2014;14:541.
14. Biegel D, Sales E, Schulz R. *Family Caregiving in Chronic Illness: Alzheimer's Disease, Cancer, Heart Disease, Mental Illness, and Stroke.* Thousand Oaks, CA: Sage; 1991.
15. Giovannetti ER, Wolff JL. Cross-survey differences in national estimates of numbers of caregivers of disabled older adults. *Milbank Q.* 2010;88(3):310–349.
16. Kent EE, Rowland JH, Northouse L, et al. Caring for caregivers and patients: research and clinical priorities for informal cancer caregiving. *Cancer.* 2016;122(13):1987–1995.
17. Hunt GG, Longacre MLK, Kent EE, Weber-Raley L. *Cancer Caregiving in the US: An Intense, Episodic, and Challenging Experience.* Bethesda, MD: National Alliance for Caregiving; 2016.
18. National Cancer Institute. *Health Information National Trends Survey V, Cycle 1.* Rockville, MD: National Cancer Institute; 2017.
19. de Moor JS, Dowling EC, Ekwueme DU, et al. Employment implications of informal cancer caregiving. *J Cancer Surviv.* 2017;11(1):48–57.

20. Centers for Disease Control and Prevention (CDC). *Behavioral Risk Factor Surveillance System Survey Data.* Atlanta, GA: Department of Health and Human Services, Centers for Disease Control and Prevention; 2015.
21. Polite BN, Adams-Campbell LL, Brawley OW, et al. Charting the future of cancer health disparities research: a position statement from the American Association for Cancer Research, the American Cancer Society, the American Society of Clinical Oncology, and the National Cancer Institute. *J Clin Oncol.* 2017;35(26):3075–3082.
22. Mollica MA, Litzelman K, Rowland JH, Kent EE. The role of medical/nursing skills training in caregiver confidence and burden: a CanCORS study. *Cancer.* 2017;123(22):4481–4487.
23. van Ryn M, Sanders S, Kahn K, et al. Objective burden, resources, and other stressors among informal cancer caregivers: A hidden quality issue? *Psychooncology.* 2011;20(1):44–52.
24. Kim Y, Carver CS, Shaffer KM, Gansler T, Cannady RS. Cancer caregiving predicts physical impairments: roles of earlier caregiving stress and being a spousal caregiver. *Cancer.* 2015;121(2):302–310.
25. Kurtz ME, Kurtz JC, Given CW, Given BA. Depression and physical health among family caregivers of geriatric patients with cancer—a longitudinal view. *Med Sci Monit.* 2004;10(8):CR447–CR456.
26. Given CW, Given BA, Stommel M, Azzouz F. The impact of new demands for assistance on caregiver depression: tests using an inception cohort. *Gerontologist.* 1999;39(1):76–85.
27. Grosse J, Treml J, Kersting A. Impact of caregiver burden on mental health in bereaved caregivers of cancer patients: a systematic review. *Psychooncology.* 2018;27(3):757–767.
28. Van Houtven CH, Ramsey SD, Hornbrook MC, Atienza AA, van Ryn M. Economic burden for informal caregivers of lung and colorectal cancer patients. *Oncologist.* 2010;15(8):883–893.
29. Kim Y, Spillers RL, Hall DL. Quality of life of family caregivers 5 years after a relative's cancer diagnosis: follow-up of the national quality of life survey for caregivers. *Psychooncology.* 2012;21(3):273–281.
30. Ferrell B, Wittenberg E. A review of family caregiving intervention trials in oncology. *CA Cancer J Clin.* 2017;67(4):318–325.
31. Shaffer KM, Kim Y, Carver CS. Physical and mental health trajectories of cancer patients and caregivers across the year post-diagnosis: a dyadic investigation. *Psychol Health.* 2016;31(6):655–674.
32. Badr H, Acitelli LK. Re-thinking dyadic coping in the context of chronic illness. *Curr Opin Psychol.* 2017;13:44–48.
33. Regan TW, Lambert SD, Kelly B, Falconier M, Kissane D, Levesque JV. Couples coping with cancer: exploration of theoretical frameworks from dyadic studies. *Psychooncology.* 2015;24(12):1605–1617.
34. Given BA, Given CW, Sherwood PR. Family and caregiver needs over the course of the cancer trajectory. *J Support Oncol.* 2012;10(2):57–64.
35. Ornstein KA, Kelley AS, Bollens-Lund E, Wolff JL. A national profile of end-of-life caregiving in the United States. *Health Aff (Millwood).* 2017;36(7):1184–1192.
36. Blum K, Sherman DW. Understanding the experience of caregivers: a focus on transitions. *Semin Oncol Nurs.* 2010;26(4):243–258.
37. Girgis A, Abernethy AP, Currow DC. Caring at the end of life: do cancer caregivers differ from other caregivers? *BMJ Support Palliat Care.* 2015;5(5):513–517.

38. Kearney JA, Salley CG, Muriel AC. Standards of psychosocial care for parents of children with cancer. *Pediatr Blood Cancer*. 2015;62(suppl 5):S632–S683.
39. Lowenstein A, Gilbar O. The perception of caregiving burden on the part of elderly cancer patients, spouses and adult children. *Fam Syst Health*. 2000;18(3):1.
40. Jayani R, Hurria A. Caregivers of older adults with cancer. *Semin Oncol Nurs*. 2012;28(4):221–225.
41. Douglas SL, Mazanec P, Lipson A, Leuchtag M. Distance caregiving a family member with cancer: a review of the literature on distance caregiving and recommendations for future research. *World J Clin Oncol*. 2016;7(2):214–219.
42. Tang WP, Chan CW, So WK, Leung DY. Web-based interventions for caregivers of cancer patients: a review of literatures. *Asia Pac J Oncol Nurs*. 2014;1(1):9–15.
43. Vraga EK, Stefanidis A, Lamprianidis G, et al. Cancer and social media: a comparison of traffic about breast cancer, prostate cancer, and other reproductive cancers on Twitter and Instagram. *J Health Commun*. 2018;23(2):181–189.
44. Chi NC, Demiris G. A systematic review of telehealth tools and interventions to support family caregivers. *J Telemed Telecare*. 2015;21(1):37–44.
45. Kaltenbaugh DJ, Klem ML, Hu L, Turi E, Haines AJ, Hagerty Lingler J. Using web-based interventions to support caregivers of patients with cancer: a systematic review. *Oncol Nurs Forum*. 2015;42(2):156–164.
46. Institute of Medicine. *Delivering High-Quality Cancer Care: Charting a New Course for a System in Crisis*. Washington, DC: Institute of Medicine; 2013.
47. Kamal KM, Covvey JR, Dashputre A, et al. A systematic review of the effect of cancer treatment on work productivity of patients and caregivers. *J Manag Care Spec Pharm*. 2017;23(2):136–162.
48. Deniz H, Inci F. The burden of care and quality of life of caregivers of leukemia and lymphoma patients following peripheric stem cell transplantation. *J Psychosoc Oncol*. 2015;33(3):250–262.
49. Abbott DE, Voils CL, Fisher DA, Greenberg CC, Safdar N. Socioeconomic disparities, financial toxicity, and opportunities for enhanced system efficiencies for patients with cancer. *J Surg Oncol*. 2017;115(3):250–256.
50. Yabroff KR, Kim Y. Time costs associated with informal caregiving for cancer survivors. *Cancer*. 2009;115(18)(suppl):4362–4373.
51. Girgis A, Lambert S, Johnson C, Waller A, Currow D. Physical, psychosocial, relationship, and economic burden of caring for people with cancer: a review. *J Oncol Pract*. 2013;9(4):197–202.
52. Ramsey S, Blough D, Kirchhoff A, et al. Washington State cancer patients found to be at greater risk for bankruptcy than people without a cancer diagnosis. *Health Aff (Millwood)*. 2013;32(6):1143–1152.
53. National Cancer Institute. NCI launches study of African-American cancer survivors. https://www.cancer.gov/news-events/press-releases/2017/detroit-cancer-survivors-study. Published 2017. Accessed February 3, 2018.
54. Li Q, Loke AY. A systematic review of spousal couple-based intervention studies for couples coping with cancer: direction for the development of interventions. *Psychooncology*. 2014;23(7):731–739.
55. Li C, Zeliadt SB, Hall IJ, et al. Burden among partner caregivers of patients diagnosed with localized prostate cancer within 1 year after diagnosis: an economic perspective. *Support Care Cancer*. 2013;21(12):3461–3469.

56. Krol M, Papenburg J, van Exel J. Does including informal care in economic evaluations matter? A systematic review of inclusion and impact of informal care in cost-effectiveness studies. *Pharmacoeconomics*. 2015;33(2):123–135.
57. Longacre ML, Applebaum AJ, Buzaglo JS, et al. Reducing informal caregiver burden in cancer: evidence-based programs in practice. *Transl Behav Med*. 2018;8(2):145–155.
58. Berry LL, Dalwadi SM, Jacobson JO. Supporting the supporters: What family caregivers need to care for a loved one with cancer. *J Oncol Pract*. 2017;13(1):35–41.
59. The CARE Act: identifying and supporting family caregivers from hospitals to home. *Dimens Crit Care Nurs*. 2018;37(2):59–61.

CHAPTER 2

The Burden of Cancer Caregivers

BARBARA A. GIVEN AND CHARLES W. GIVEN

Each year, approximately 1.7 million new patients are diagnosed with cancer, and over 600,000 Americans die from this disease.[1] The National Alliance for Caregiving estimates 4 million individuals are caring for adult cancer patients. Caregivers of cancer patients represent about 8% of all caregivers. While demands exist across the entire cancer continuum, caregivers are more involved with providing care during three periods: during ongoing treatment (when they assist in managing side effects and frequent encounters with medical professionals); the first 2 years postdiagnosis; and during palliative care, as the patient's disease progresses toward death of the patient. Typically, caregivers of adult cancer patients are spouses or adult children[1] who have their own familial, employment, financial, and personal responsibilities, all of which have the potential to influence the degree of caregiver-related burden, the emotional and physical reactions to assisting a family member with cancer.[2,3]

The multidimensional components of caregiver burden need to be understood in order to extend research, guide practice, and formulate policy. Few researchers have examined changes in psychological distress and burden that accumulate among cancer caregivers across the care trajectory. The type and intensity of patient needs during each period described contribute to burden through the impact of caregiving demands on other normatively prescribed roles.[4] Indeed, persistent psychological distress and burden have been found in caregivers of cancer patients 1 year post-treatment completion. When left untreated, these concerns likely endure, though fewer studies have examined functioning 2 or 5 years post-treatment intervals.[5–7]

The purpose of this chapter is to present definitions of burden and discuss common conceptual models and frameworks used to study burden as experienced by caregivers of cancer patients. We also describe the roles and unmet needs of burdened caregivers and elaborate on the psychological and physiological sequelae of burden for caregivers of patients with cancer.

DEFINITIONS OF CAREGIVER BURDEN

There is no *International Classification of Diseases, Tenth Revision (ICD-10)* code for caregiver burden; therefore, it is not formally recognized as a health problem. However, there are several common definitions of burden used in the science of family caregiving, most of which originated outside of the oncology literature. Many reports use terms such as strain, stress, and burden (physical and emotional) interchangeably, but do not distinguish between the concepts. Indeed, much of the literature on family caregivers in general and cancer caregivers specifically does not include a clear definition of caregiver burden and how the demands and the settings of caregiving give rise to burden, but instead describe characteristics of burdened caregivers.

Zarit and collegues[8,9] and Gwyther and George[10] defined *caregiver burden* as a multidimensional response to the negative appraisal and perceived stress resulting from taking care of an ill individual. Caregiver burden was also further defined by Given and collegues[2,11] as the negative reaction to the impact of providing care on caregivers' social, occupational, and personal roles, as well as on their physical, psychological, and emotional health. Montgomery and collegues[12] introduced the concept of "objective" and "subjective" burden. *Objective* dimensions of caregiver burden consider the time spent providing care and support and are assessed through examining physical or instrumental components of care. *Subjective* burden includes psychological and emotional dimensions of burden (depression, anxiety, and quality of life [QOL]).[12] It is evident that caregiving is an individualized experience with risk factors for burden emanating from circumstances surrounding the care or from patient and caregiver characteristics. As such, interventions implemented to alleviate caregiver burden should be tailored to the type (objective, subjective, or both) of burden experienced.

In summary, caregiver burden is the "stress" perceived by family caregivers who care for patients, and the stress results from the imbalance between demands (objective and subjective) and their coping resources. This chapter focuses on caregiver burden stemming from family caregivers' negative appraisals (burden) of the care they provide to patients with cancer. This resulting burden may threaten the patient-caregiver dyadic relationship and result in negative physical, psychological, and social outcomes for the caregiver. The balance between demands and resources determines the level of burden and the consequences on the care situation. Note *family* is defined broadly for this chapter.

FRAMEWORKS

A number of theoretical frameworks have been used to examine the concept of caregiver burden. By far the most common is the stress process model, which was used and validated originally in the setting of Alzheimer's disease and subsequently in the setting of cancer caregiving.[7,13,14] Considering stress and coping models, caring for a family member with cancer is a complex and challenging role to which the caregiver must adapt. Patients' disease stage, prognosis, treatment trajectory, and associated care coordination all represent primary stressors that require different modes of coping responses, ranging from new physical tasks and emotional reactions to negotiations with the healthcare system and other family members. Secondary stressors related to other dimensions of the caregiver's life, such as role changes, family and employment demands, and daily schedule disruption, also contribute to the experience of burden, as do caregivers' personality, coping strategies, social support, and distress appraisal. As the intensity of role demands increase and stressors mount, they begin to overwhelm caregivers' resources and in turn contribute to burden, which negatively impacts their emotional and physical health. Notably, the quality of the patient-caregiver relationship prior to the onset of care will impact the stress-coping balance, as will factors that give rise to unmet needs where coping is no longer adequate.

In the stress processes model, the stressor and resource balance interact to influence caregiver well-being, which includes mental and physical health, mental adjustment mastery, and overall QOL.[13] The stress appraisal model[14,15] guided Northouse and colleagues in their conceptualization of burden,[7,16,17] which considers personal and illness-related factors and determines how they influence an individual's appraisals of the demands of caring and their coping with cancer. Both the inequity of demands in relation to available resources and the way in which the caregiver's role is appraised affect the QOL of both the patient and family member.[17]

Barbara Swore developed an updated model of Lazarus and Folkman's stress appraisal model[14,15] that focuses on cancer caregivers, and Fletcher and collegues[18] used more recent literature (2000–2010) to examine the concepts used specifically in family caregiving of cancer patients. The Fletcher model includes the stress process, contextual factors, and the cancer trajectory and highlights five broad constructs that are associated with burden: primary stressors, secondary stressors, appraisal, cognitive behavioral responses, and health and well-being outcomes. By incorporating external stressors (e.g., the appraisal, cognitive, and behavioral processes produced by the stressors), this model represents a valuable approach to clarifying the interplay among possible contributors to caregiver burden.

The self-determination theory of Ryan and Deci[19] focuses on types of motivation (i.e., autonomous motivation, controlled motivation, and amotivation) as predictors of performance and well-being outcomes. Actions are driven by autonomy and compliance, as well as intrinsic and extrinsic motivations. Self-determination theory addresses self-regulation: Individuals explore experiences and events and, based on that reflection, make adaptive changes in their goals, behaviors, and relationships. Autonomous motivation predicts persistence and is related to psychological health. Cognitive behavioral therapy approaches are consistent with self-determination theory and can be used to achieve change by promoting caregiver self-endorsed transformation through choice of value directions and goals. Through this process, caregivers can develop a greater sense of autonomy.

Early in the descriptions of caregiving and the study of caregiver burden, role theory was also used as a guiding framework. Role theory focused on role stress and strain that accumulate when a family member adds caregiving to other ongoing roles, such as those of spouse, parent, or employee.[20] Role theory describes both role overload and role conflict evolving from expectations and expanding time constraints that challenge the limited resources of the caregiver. In this model, as new demands in one or possibly several roles overwhelm coping resources, caregivers experience increased burden and distress.[21] Role theory also facilitates our understanding of how burden may differ depending on the relationship to the patient (e.g., family and nonfamily) and requires a review of various roles concurrently inhabited by a caregiver and limitations in conflict resolution. Few researchers have used this framework to explain how role conflict arises and produces burden and how coping strategies may account for variations in the resulting burden. More recently, Bastawrous[3] recommended combining the stress process model with role theory to derive a more comprehensive model for determining the mechanisms driving caregiver burden.

Another more recent model from family research is the actor-partner interdependence model (APIM).[22] The APIM specifies that the influence of one's own casual variable on his or her own outcome variable (actor effect) affects the outcome variable of the dyadic partner (called the *partner effect*). This allows for the examination of relationship patterns within dyadic partners as a means of determining the impact of patient factors on caregiver burden.[23] The APIM posits that the caregiver-patient dyad reacts to caregiving distress as an emotional system, thereby highlighting the interdependent nature of the unit. Using this model, Kim and colleagues[24] found that each person's psychological distress is the strongest predictor of life and partner distress, and that discordant levels of distress between patients and caregivers negatively affect caregiver QOL.

Van Houtven and colleagues[25] developed an organizing framework for describing and categorizing caregiver skill sets and activities and caregiver and patient outcomes to guide intervention development for informal caregivers. They reviewed 121 studies of cancer caregivers to determine variables and activities to include in the framework. These patient and caregiver baseline characteristics and four domains of caregiver activities (clinical knowledge [problem-solving, decision-making], psychological [self-efficacy, coping], support seeking, and quantity of caregiving [time spent]). Outcomes are the psychological, physical, and economic status of the caregiver and their utilization of services, which may indicate the psychophysiologic toll (burden) the caregiver experiences. This model introduces aspects of the care recipient and care activities and skills needed by both the patient and the caregiver to cope with the demands of facing cancer.

ROLE OF CAREGIVERS IN CANCER CARE THAT LEADS TO BURDEN

At this point, we have summarized the frameworks and key concepts that may give rise to caregiver burden. In this section, we explore the cancer and care trajectory context to determine their contributions to the rise of caregiver burden. Such an understanding of the context of burden will help to clarify how the models mentioned may be most optimally applied.

Today, with short hospital stays and more outpatient-based cancer care, family caregivers are involved with and provide much of the care for patients. The care roles and demands of care depend on the patient's disease status, physical and mental states, and treatment plan, as well as caregivers' competing roles. The demands of caregiving vary across the care trajectory, from the point of diagnosis, through treatment, survivorship, and recurrence and into palliative and end-of-life care. Tasks are multifaceted and often specific to treatment type, length, and the patient's response (physical and emotional) to that treatment. Caregiver burden results from the added demands placed on caregivers, shifts in the dyadic patient-caregiver relationship and the unpredictability and uncontrollability of the care situation.[26] The uncertainty of treatment response, disease progression, and recurrence may lead to an increased temporal demand of care that further challenges caregivers' capacity to cope and gives rise to burden.

Van Houtven and colleagues[25] highlighted that caregiving requires knowledge and confidence to manage patient care and self-efficacy for task mastery. Additionally, they described the role as encompassing care manager, gatekeeper, and provider, all of which require knowledge and organizational, tactical, and recruiting skills (e.g., to obtain resources, needed information, and direction and to know when to seek assistance). Frequently, this means coordinating multiple providers and community agencies that are needed to sustain patient care.

Caregiving includes assistance with numerous basic and instru-mental care tasks and often the provision of ongoing emotional support. Instrumental tasks of caregiving may include decision-making; helping patients to adhere to care guidelines; medication administration; assistance with drains, ports, and wound care; and care of intravenous sites. During active treatment, caregivers often assist patients with management of symptoms and side effects that occur from chemotherapy, radiation, immu-notherapy, or biologics. As patients receiving palliative or end-of-life care lose the ability to engage in self-care, caregivers provide more direct care with assistance with eating, dressing, and mobility. Additionally, the emo-tional, psychological, and cognitive tasks of care include supporting and managing patients' anxiety or depression, engaging in problem-solving and decision-making, providing encouragement, assisting with scheduling the multiple components of care, and accompanying patients to clinical visits. Those (often spousal) caregivers who live with the patient report needing more assistance, perhaps because their accessibility makes them suscep-tible to assuming increased role demands compared to those who live apart.

CAREGIVER UNMET NEEDS

Given the complexity of cancer care and the shifts in the types of care needed, caregivers often experience a number of unmet needs or areas where they feel inadequate, insecure, unprepared, or unsupported to provide patient care. An overview of categories of unmet needs is presented in Table 2.1.

Table 2.1 CATEGORIES OF UNMET NEEDS AMONG CAREGIVERS

Needs Category	Needs Include Assistance With . . .
Patient's healthcare	Navigating the healthcare system and care coordination Obtaining information to understand the patient's medical condition, treatment, and prognosis Communicating effectively with healthcare providers
Caregiving responsibilities	Problem-solving around expanding the caregiver support network Managing and limiting uncertainty about care expectations Obtaining advice and information to manage the patient's side effects and symptoms (especially pain management) Skills training Providing emotional support to the patient (especially addressing anxiety and depression)
Emotional needs	General support to manage caregiver stress and feelings of being overwhelmed by the role Addressing emotional and psychological needs (fears) about the patient's condition/potential decline
Practical needs	Accessing financial support Accessing community resources for care for the patient and themselves

Kim and colleagues[27] examined five domains of caregiving needs and concern (psychosocial, cognitive, financial, medical, and physical function [activities of daily living]) and found that younger caregivers had more unmet needs than older caregivers, and women had more unmet needs than men. They also found that individuals with unmet social needs reported deficient emotional, but ample financial, support. Without sufficient information, caregivers often feel that they are unprepared for their role and cannot adequately provide care,[28-30] especially when they are required to carry out complex medical tasks and engage in critical decision-making. Indeed, difficulty with care coordination is often identified as an area contributing to unmet needs,[28] and caregivers report cognitive unmet needs, including educational support and decision-making support.[31]

Sklenarova and colleagues[32] reported that 44% of caregivers had at least 10 unmet needs related to health services and information, followed by emotional, psychological, and spiritual needs. At more advanced phases of patient illness, caregivers were found to report more unmet needs.[32] Kim and colleagues found that caregivers, after 2 years of providing care, indicated that their needs included managing their own emotions, improving communication with providers, and obtaining information about patient care.[33] At 5 years, caregivers reported that their own distress remained, as did the need for assistance with medical and insurance coverage.[30,33] Taken together, the shift in caregiving demands over the cancer care trajectory often result in unmet needs that, if left unaddressed, are likely to contribute to increased burden.

Caregivers who are depressed, are socially isolated, or have additional family obligations, lower education, and greater financial stress are at higher risk for reporting unmet needs.[34] Increased needs have been associated with increased amount of time spent providing care.[32,34] Importantly, unmet needs are often reported by caregivers in the context of expressing fears about patients' deterioration when engaging in care coordination, when discussing patients' prognosis and treatment options, and when making decisions in the setting of uncertainty. As unmet needs tend to be heightened during care transitions, interventions to support caregivers should target these particularly vulnerable moments in the care trajectory. Though literature examining the association between unmet needs and burden is limited, researchers[28,32,35] have recently reported an association between unmet needs and burden, such that greater unmet needs were associated with greater burden.[35]

CONSEQUENCES OF CAREGIVER BURDEN

The consequences of caregiver burden are substantial. These include poor self-care and a decline in caregivers' own physical and mental health.[36–38] Indeed, the prevalence of clinically significant psychological distress (i.e., anxiety and depression) in caregivers is between 20% and 30%.[37–39] For physical health, studies have documented consequences for caregivers' sleep, fatigue, immune response, and health-related behaviors (e.g., increased substance use), as well as hypertension, heart disease, endocrine dysregulation, and arthritis (all common midlife comorbidities likely exacerbated in the setting of cancer caregiving).[40] A general decline in healthcare service utilization has also been documented, suggesting that caregivers forgo preventive services, delay screening, and delay general healthcare follow-ups for themselves. Kim and colleagues[41] looked at physical impairments among cancer caregivers over a 6-year period and found increased heart disease, arthritis, and chronic back pain several years after caregiving. These effects were independent of age, sex, education, or income. Their results suggest adverse long-term effects of early caregiver distress when left untreated. Although few have examined these effects, Ji and colleagues[42] demonstrated that spouses of patients with cancer had more cardiovascular disease (i.e., heart disease and stroke) that persisted over time, and such medical morbidity was more pronounced among those caring for patients with high mortality rates (i.e., those with pancreatic and lung cancers).

Unintentional injuries, such as muscle injuries, falls, cuts, scrapes, and bruises, resulting from care tasks (i.e., transferring patients from bed to wheelchair) have not been systematically studied in cancer caregivers but are likely more common among overburdened and older caregivers, as has been found in studies of non–cancer caregiver populations.[43]

The impact of caregiving on employment and career trajectories is also not well documented.[44] Similarly, changes in social activities and relationships are seldom examined in investigations of caregiver burden. Studies have focused on marital distress but seldom look at leisure activities or general lifestyle disruption. As such, assessments need to more comprehensively examine disruptions in lifestyle and roles due to caregiving.[45]

Although numerous authors suggested that caregiver burden will have a negative consequence on the quality of care provided to the patient, few studies have systematically examined this relationship. Litzelman and colleagues[46] evaluated the association of caregiver well-being and perceived quality of care (QOC) among patients with cancer and found that high levels of caregiver depressive symptoms were associated with patient report of fair-to-poor QOC provided. More research is needed to determine if some aspects of care are ignored while others endure or to what extent the care provided by caregivers benefits patient outcomes. Similarly, structural and environmental factors and community resources have the potential to improve caregivers' ability to function in their role, though few studies documented any effect.

To help prevent these potential negative effects of caregiver burden, screening processes need to be implemented early in the caregiving trajectory.[37] Such screening should evaluate risk factors (level and type) and unmet needs, as described previously and presented in Box 2.1. Risk assessment should also include sex, age, financial stress, depression, anxiety, hours of care, complexity of care, changes in patient status, role conflict, perceived communication challenges, and competence and sense of self-efficacy.[47] The tools outlined in Chapter 6 may be used for more detailed assessment of risk factors for burden in caregivers. Together, these screening processes can help identify caregivers who can most benefit from psychosocial interventions (see Sections 2 and 3 of this textbook).

In addition to these risk factors for—and correlates of—caregiver burden, research is needed to understand what allows some caregivers

---

Box 2.1
CAREGIVER ASSESSMENT FACTORS

Sex

Age

Symptoms of depression and anxiety

Physical care needs of patient

Hours of care

Roles (work, family, social)

Relationship to the care recipient

Communication adequacy with patient and providers

Feeling of competency to provide care (knowledge and skills)

Living with the care recipient

Care environment

Financial adequacy

---

to experience benefits of the role. Positive aspects of caregiving, such as feelings of gratification and satisfaction derived from the caregiving experience, have been documented.[48] Such positive responses have the potential to enhance caregiver well-being through a reduction in distress and heightened sense of resilience, competence, and appreciation for the positive aspects of caregiving.[49] Future research is needed to clearly delineate the association between such positive responses to caregiving and caregiver burden.

STRATEGIES TO PREVENT AND LOWER CAREGIVER BURDEN

So, what does this all mean? We need more systematic, rigorous studies with consistent measurement strategies. There is little work that shows how burden is experienced differently across cultural, racial, and ethnic groups. More understanding of these differences is required for the purposes of designing appropriate interventions. Until then, programs should educate caregivers in how to prevent and ameliorate caregiver burden and guide them to maintain their own health. Providers in cancer care settings not only need to concern themselves with the patients' health, but also must attend to caregivers' physical and mental health to recognize and address early signs of burden. Caregivers need preparation, including skills training, for their responsibilities and demands of caregiving. Therefore, interventions are needed to assist with such education.[50] Importantly, as the risk for burden may shift across the caregiving trajectory, professionals must continually assess fluctuating needs and risks for developing burden.

A more comprehensive picture of contributing factors to burden is also needed. This should include the unique types of care provided and the existence of informal and professional (i.e., home health aides) care networks, as well as personality factors that predispose caregivers to burden. As family caregivers take on more dimensions of care, the adverse effects of caregiver burden and duration of that burden need to be acknowledged and strategies introduced to prevent and assist caregivers to manage the care required of them.

More broadly, policies need to acknowledge caregiver burden as a national healthcare issue. This perspective will assist with the implementation and legitimization of strategies to support caregivers. To that end, caregivers must be considered a part of the patient care unit by cancer care professionals. The reciprocal relationships of responses to the care situation that continue to be identified make this an imperative.[7,24,51] Family caregivers need our continued support, as they are a crucial—but often hidden—part of the cancer support system.

REFERENCES

1. American Cancer Society. *Cancer facts & figures 2017*. Atlanta, GA: American Cancer Society;2017.
2. Given B, Given CW, Kozachik S. Family support in advanced cancer. *CA Cancer J Clin*. 2001;51(4):213–231.
3. Bastawrous M. Caregiver burden—a critical discussion. Int J Nurs Stud. 2013;50(3):431–441.
4. Kim Y, Spillers RL. Quality of life of family caregivers at 2 years after a relative's cancer diagnosis. *Psychooncology*. 2010;19(4):431–440.
5. Hagedoorn M, Buunk BP, Kuijer RG, Wobbes T, Sanderman R. Couples dealing with cancer: role and gender differences regarding psychological distress and quality of life. *Psychooncology*. 2000;9(3):232–242.
6. Mellon S, Northouse LL, Weiss LK. A population-based study of the quality of life of cancer survivors and their family caregivers. *Cancer Nurs*. 2006;29(2):120–131.
7. Northouse LL, Mood D, Templin T, Mellon S, George T. Couple's patterns of adjustment to colon cancer. *Soc Sci Med*. 2000;50(2):271–284.
8. Zarit SH, Reever KE, Bach-Peterson J. Relatives of the impaired elderly: correlates of feelings of burden. *Gerontologist*. 1980;20(6): 649–655.
9. Zarit SH, Todd PA, Zarit JM. Subjective burden of husbands and wives as caregivers: a longitudinal study. *Gerontologist*. 1986;26(3):260–266.

10. Gwyther LP, George LK. Caregivers for dementia patients: complex determinants of well-being and burden. *Gerontologist*. 1986;26(3):245–247.
11. Given CW, Given B, Stommel M, Collins C, King S, Franklin S. The Caregiver Reaction Assessment (CRA) for caregivers to persons with chronic physical and mental impairments. *Res Nurs Health*. 1992;15(4):271–283.
12. Montgomery RJ, Gonyea JG, Hooyman NR. Caregiving and the experience of subjective and objective burden. *Family Relations*. 1985;34(1):19–26.
13. Weitzner MA, Haley WE, Chen H. The family caregiver of the older cancer patient. *Hematol Oncol Clin North Am*. 2000;14(1):269–281.
14. Lazarus RS, Folkman S. *Stress Appraisal and Coping*. New York, NY: Springer; 1984.
15. Lazarus R. *Psychological Stress and the Coping Process*. New York, NY: McGraw-Hill; 1966.
16. Northouse L, Templin T, Mood D. Couples' adjustment to breast disease during the first year following diagnosis. *J Behav Med*. 2001;24(2):115–136.
17. Northouse L, Kershaw T, Mood D, Schafenacker A. Effects of a family intervention on the quality of life of women with recurrent breast cancer and their family caregivers. *Psychooncology*. 2005;14:478–491.
18. Fletcher BS, Miaskowski C, Given B, Schumacher K. The cancer family caregiving experience: an updated and expanded conceptual model. *Eur J Oncol Nurs*. 2012;16(4):387–398.
19. Ryan RM, Deci EL. A self-determination theory approach to psychotherapy: the motivational basis for effective change. *Can Psychol*. 2008;49(3):186–193.
20. Biddle BJ. Recent developments in role theory. *Annu Rev Sociol*. 1986;12(1):67–92.
21. Rozario PA, Morrow-Howell N, Proctor E. Comparing the congruency of self-report and provider records of depressed elders' service use by provider type. *Med Care*. 2004;42(10):952–959.
22. Kashy DA, Kenny DA. The analysis of data from dyads and groups. In Reiss HT, Judd CM, eds. *Handbook of Research Methods in Social and Personality Psychology*. New York, NY: Cambridge University Press; 2000:451–477.
23. Kenny DA, Ledermann T. Detecting, measuring, and testing dyadic patterns in the actor-partner interdependence model. *J Fam Psychol*. 2010;24(3):359–366.
24. Kim Y, Kashy DA, Wellisch DK, Spillers RL, Kaw CK, Smith TG. Quality of life of couples dealing with cancer: dyadic and individual adjustment among breast and prostate cancer survivors and their spousal caregivers. *Ann Behav Med*. 2008;35(2):230–238.
25. Van Houtven CH, Volis CI, Weinberger M. An organizing framework for informal caregiver interventions: detailing caregiving activities and caregiver and care recipient outcomes to optimize evaluation efforts. *BMC Geriatr*. 2011;11:77.
26. Schulz R, Sherwood PR. Physical and mental health effects of family caregiving. *Am J Nurs*. 2008;108(9)(Suppl):23–27; quiz 27.
27. Kim Y, Baker F, Spillers RL. Cancer caregivers' quality of life: effects of gender, relationship, and appraisal. *J Pain Symptom Manage*. 2007;34(3):294–304.
28. Campbell HS, Sanson-Fisher R, Taylor-Brown J, Hayward L, Wang XS, Turner D. The cancer support person's unmet needs survey: psychometric properties. *Cancer*. 2009;115(14):3351–3359.
29. Girgis A, Lambert S, Lecathelinais C. The supportive care needs survey for partners and caregivers of cancer survivors: Development and psychometric evaluation. *Psychooncology*. 2011;20(4):387–393.

30. Lambert SD, Girgis A. Unmet supportive care needs among informal caregivers of patients with cancer: opportunities and challenges in informing the development of interventions. *Asia Pac J Oncol Nurs*. 2017;4(2):136–139.

31. Hashemi M, Irajpour A, Taleghani F. Caregivers needing care: the unmet needs of the family caregivers of end-of-life cancer patients. *Support Care Cancer*. 2018;26(3):759–766.

32. Sklenarova H, Krümpelmann A, Haun MW, et al. (2015). When do we need to care about the caregiver? Supportive care needs, anxiety, and depression among informal caregivers of patients with cancer and cancer survivors. *Cancer*. 2015;121(9):1513–1519.

33. Kim Y, Kashy DA, Spillers RL, Evans TV. Needs assessment of family caregivers of cancer survivors: three cohort's comparison. *Psychooncology*. 2010;19(6):573–582.

34. McCarthy B. Family members of patients with cancer: what they know, how they know and what they want to know. *Eur J Oncol Nurs*. 2011;15(5):428–441.

35. Saxton C, Buzaglo J, Rochman S, Zaleta A. Helping cancer patients and caregivers navigate immunotherapy treatment. *Am J Manag Care*. 2017;23(2)(Spec No.):SP78–SP80.

36. Shaffer KM, Kim Y, Carver CS. Physical and mental health trajectories of cancer patients and caregivers across the year post-diagnosis: a dyadic investigation. *Psychol Health*. 2016;31(6):655–674.

37. Shaffer KM, Kim Y, Carver CS, Cannady RS. Depressive symptoms predict cancer caregivers' physical health decline. *Cancer*. 2017;123(21):4277–4285.

38. Shaffer KM, Kim Y, Carver CS, Cannady RS. Effects of caregiving status and changes in depressive symptoms on development of physical morbidity among long-term cancer caregivers. *Healthy Psychol*. 2017;36(8):770–778.

39. Pitceathly C, Maguire P. The psychological impact of cancer on patients' partners and other key relatives: a review. *Eur J Cancer*. 2003;39(11):1517–1524.

40. Mellon S. Comparison between cancer survivors and family members on meaning of the illness and family quality of life. *Oncol Nurs Forum*. 2002;29(7):1117–1125.

41. Kim Y, Carver CS, Shaffer KM, Gansler T, Cannady RS. Cancer caregiving predicts physical impairments: roles of earlier caregiving stress and being a spousal caregiver. *Cancer*. 2015;121(2):302–310.

42. Ji J, Zöller B, Sundquist K, Sundquist J. Increased risks of coronary heart disease and stroke among spousal caregivers of cancer patients. *Circulation*. 2012;125(14):1742–1747.

43. Hayes J, Chapman P, Young LJ, Rittman M. The prevalence of injury for stroke caregivers and associated risk factors. *Top Stroke Rehabil*. 2009;16(4):300–307.

44. Stenberg U, Ruland CM, Miaskowski C. Review of the literature on the effects of caring for a patient with cancer. *Psychooncology*. 2010;19(10):1013–1025.

45. Carlsen K, Dalton SO, Frederiksen K, Diderichsen F, Johansen C. Are cancer survivors at an increased risk for divorce? A Danish cohort study. *Eur J Cancer*. 2007;43(14):2093–2099.

46. Litzelman K, Kent EE, Mollica M, Rowland JH. How does caregiver well-being relate to perceived quality of care in patients with cancer? Exploring associations and pathways. *J Clin Oncol*. 2016;34(29):3554–3560.

47. Romito F, Goldzweig G, Cormio C, Hagedoorn M, Anderson BL. Informal caregiving for cancer patients. *Cancer*. 2013;119(S11):2160–2169.

48. Tarlow BJ, Wisniewski SR, Belle SH, Rubert M, Ory MG, Gallagher-Thompson D. Positive aspects of caregiving: contributions of the REACH project to

the development of new measures for Alzheimer's caregiving. *Res Aging.* 2004;26(4):429–453.

49. Palacio C, Krikorian A, Limonero JT. The influence of psychological factors on the burden of caregivers of patients with advanced cancer: resiliency and caregiver burden. *Palliat Support Care.* 2017;3:1–9.

50. Mollica M, Litzelman K, Rowland JH, Kent EE. The role of medical/nursing skills training in caregiver confidence and burden: a CanCORS study. *Cancer.* 2017;15;123(22):4481–4487.

51. Kim Y, Carver CS, Deci EL, Kasser T. Adult attachment and psychological well-being in cancer caregivers: the mediational role of spouses' motives for caregiving. *Health Psychol.* 2008;27(S2):S144–S154.

CHAPTER 3

The Unique Experience of Caregivers Based on Their Life Stage and Relationship to the Patient

KRISTIN LITZELMAN

Although we often think of caregivers as middle-aged or older adults, cancer caregiving spans the life course. Regardless of when cancer occurs, it has a considerable impact on the family. While cancer caregivers across the life course share many experiences, they also face differences that contribute to unique challenges and opportunities at each life stage.

In this chapter, I examine cancer caregiving across the life course. For convenience, the population is divided into three life stages—early adulthood, encompassing 18–44 years of age; middle age (45–64 years of age); and older age (65 years of age and older). For each life stage, I describe the population (including the distribution of relationship types, the typical caregiving load, and relevant sociodemographic characteristics) and draw on existing literature to comment on the unique considerations at each time period. Special attention is paid to the caregiver's relationship to the patient at each life stage.

A methodological note: Key points in this chapter are supported with nationally representative data from the 2015 Behavioral Risk Factor Surveillance System (BRFSS).[1] The 2015 BRFSS included caregiving questions in the core survey (used by all states). These questions asked all adults in the sample to report on whether they had been a caregiver in the past 30 days. Caregivers then reported their relationship to the person they cared for; how long they had been providing care; how many hours of care they provided in an average week; the main health problem, illness, or disability of their care recipient; and whether they helped manage personal care tasks (e.g., giving medications, feeding, dressing, bathing) or household care tasks (e.g., cleaning, managing finances, preparing meals). In total, there were 1,910 cancer caregivers in the sample. For this chapter, data are described using frequency distributions and cross-tabulations. Where appropriate, chi-squared analyses were employed to test whether differences between age groups were statistically significant. All analyses employed survey weights to account for the complex sampling structure of the BRFSS.

EARLY ADULTHOOD (18–44 YEARS OF AGE)

Early adulthood caregivers made up 43% of adult cancer caregivers in the United States. They most often provided care to a parent or in-law (42%), and a considerable proportion provided care to a grandparent (23%), friend (15%), or other relative (13%). Figure 3.1 shows the relationship of the care recipient to the caregiver (e.g., the care recipient was the caregiver's parent/in-law) by the caregiver's life stage. Figure 3.2 depicts the distribution of caregiving responsibility by life stage. Nearly half of early adulthood caregivers had been providing care for less than 6 months (48%); only 13% had been providing care for 5 or more years. The majority provided fewer than 8 hours of care per week (58%), while 1 in 10 provided more than 40 hours of care per week (11%). Nearly all reported helping with household

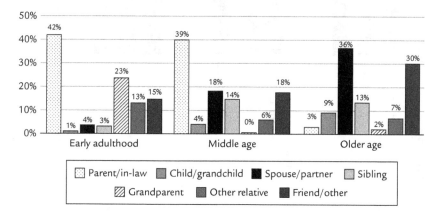

Figure 3.1: Care recipient relationship, by caregiver life stage.

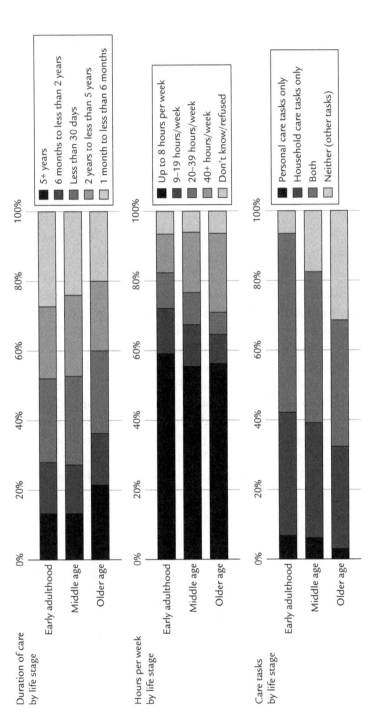

Figure 3.2: Distribution of caregiving responsibility by life stage.

care tasks such as cleaning, managing finances, or preparing meals (87%), and the majority reported helping with personal care tasks, such as giving medications, feeding, dressing, or bathing (58%).

Early adulthood is a time of self-discovery and developing independence. Individuals in this age group are exploring their identity and making choices related to marriage, family, education, and career. This puts cancer caregivers in this age group in a unique situation. First, caregiving in early adulthood is particularly nonnormative,[2] adversely impacting these individuals' experiences with caregiving. Caregivers in this age group may not know anyone else providing care and may struggle to find formal or informal support from similarly aged peers. Indeed, early adulthood caregivers have reported the need for emotional support from other caregivers of the same age.[3] The relationship to the care recipient also brings challenges. As noted, nearly two-thirds of caregivers in this age group are caring for a parent, in-law, or grandparent with cancer. Dealing with the potential death of a parent at a young age is a struggle for many young adults[4] and may be particularly poignant among those who have assumed a caregiving role. Moreover, taking on a caregiving role for a parent or grandparent can result in role reversal,[4-6] which may be uncomfortable for both the caregiver and the care recipient. In one qualitative study, 36% of early adulthood caregivers reported role reversal as a strain, particularly when the care recipient had high personal care needs (e.g., bathing, toileting).[6] This may result in feelings of grief for younger caregivers (who normatively expect to continue to receive emotional and substantive support from their parents or grandparents throughout early adulthood) and may inhibit younger caregivers' ability to develop their autonomy and independence. As a result, both the caregiver and care recipient may need to learn how to navigate new relationship dynamics.

Second, cancer caregivers in this age group may be particularly vulnerable to life disruption. Nearly half of caregivers in this age group were married (47%; Table 3.1), and more than two-thirds were employed outside the home (69%). More than half (58%) had children living in their home (by contrast, only a quarter of middle-aged caregivers [27%] and very few older age caregivers [3%] had children in the home). This has implications for role functioning and adult development. Across the life course, many cancer caregivers report making employment changes to accommodate the demands of caregiving, including working a flexible schedule, cutting back on work hours, changing jobs, or declining a promotion, among others.[7,8] Many early adulthood caregivers report having to quit a job, missing job promotion opportunities, and negative impacts to long-term career goals due to caregiving demands.[3,6]

Table 3.1 CHARACTERISTICS BY LIFE STAGE

	Early Adulthood (%)	Middle Age (%)	Older Age (%)	p Value
Gender				.3675
Male	41.22	35.63	40.43	
Female	58.78	64.37	59.57	
Children in the household				<.0001
No	42.49	72.23	96.83	
Yes	57.51	27.77	3.17	
Income				.3192
<$25,000	22.93	25.44	30.48	
≥$25,000	61.78	62.04	54.09	
Unknown/refused	15.29	12.52	15.43	
Employment				<.0001
Employed for pay	68.68	63.07	14.19	
Not employed for pay	31.32	36.93	85.81	
Marital status				<.0001
Never married	39.46	6.54	5.47	
Married/partnered	46.72	64.63	59.59	
Divorced/widowed/separated	13.82	28.83	34.94	
Education				.9539
High school or less	46.80	47.91	48.37	
Some college or more	53.20	52.09	51.63	

Data are from the 2015 Behavioral Risk Factor Surveillance System; frequencies are weighted to account for the complex sampling frame.

These career and employment choices in early adulthood have a ripple effect on adult opportunities. At a time when their peers are establishing and advancing their careers, such employment changes may have a dramatic cumulative impact on career advancement potential, lifetime earning potential, or retirement savings.[9–11] On the other hand, the caregiving role confers new skill sets and may help some caregivers in their career.[12] Qualitative work in young adults caring for their grandparents suggests that the caregiving role may help guide future career and educational interests.[5]

Caregiving may also be a strain on romantic relationships and family functioning or act as a barrier to development in this area. Caregivers often face time constraints and struggle with self-care; for early adults, this—in addition to emotional burden and facing a nonnormative life situation—may pose a particular barrier for dating. A majority of young adult caregivers report difficulty establishing or maintaining dating relationships.[3] They struggle with less time for dating and may give up on dating entirely.[6] Among those in committed relationships, a majority report that caregiving negatively impacted their relationship,[3] specifically indicating strains related to having less time for their significant other or their partner being unsupportive of their caregiving role.[6]

Finally, 58% of early adulthood caregivers had children in the home. Balancing cancer caregiving and childrearing presents a unique challenge for these families,[13] including role and identity conflicts that may cause stress and burden for the caregiver and impact family functioning. Early adulthood caregivers frequently report that caregiving negatively impacts the amount of time they are able to dedicate to parenting.[3] At the same time, parents may consider it a priority to maintain a normative lifestyle for the children in the family (e.g., keeping up with school and extracurricular activities), but this effort can come with costs in the form of increased burden and time constraints.[14-16] Juggling multiple role obligations contributes to distress and burden, and these caregivers may not recognize when they need help or accept available help.[17]

Young spousal caregivers, in particular, may face significant and unique challenges, especially if they have young children in the home. Although accounting for only a small percentage of cancer caregivers, they are likely to have few (if any) peer spousal caregivers. The emotional impact of caregiving may be exacerbated by the nonnormative circumstances of cancer and their caregiving role: These caregivers may be facing widowhood at a young age or years of treatment and uncertainty (including ongoing fear of recurrence), which can impact their well-being, family functioning, and identity.

Nearly a quarter of these caregivers were in emerging adulthood (18–24 years of age), a time when most individuals are establishing their independence, beginning careers, pursuing higher education, or starting families. Caregivers in this age group may feel that developmental milestones, like work or school, can wait while they are in the caregiving role[5] or may choose to pursue career or educational opportunities that are close to home (even if that comes at the expense of potential prospects at a geographical distance). They frequently report having less time for family and friends and giving up hobbies or social/extracurricular activities.[18-20]

As noted, many of these caregivers were providing care to a grandparent. In the BRFSS sample explored here, across age groups, grandparental care was associated with longer duration of care. Specifically, 28% of those caring for a grandparent had been providing care for 5 or more years, compared to 21% of those caring for their child/grandchild and 21% of those caring for their spouse/partner, with lower proportions across other relationship types ($p<.0001$). This potentially puts emerging adult caregivers on developmental life trajectories that differ considerably from their peers. It is not surprising, therefore, that emerging adult caregivers experience greater symptoms of depression and anxiety than their peers.[19] These caregivers are also at risk of being unaware of the services and supports available to them or their care recipient and family.[20]

MIDDLE AGE (45–64 YEARS OF AGE)

Middle-aged caregivers made up 40% of adult cancer caregivers in the United States. These caregivers were most likely to be taking care of a parent or in-law (40%), followed by their spouse/partner (18%), friend (18%), or sibling (14%) (Figure 3.1). Nearly half had been providing care for less than 6 months (47%), while 13% had been providing care for 5 or more years. The majority provided less than 8 hours of care per week (56%), while nearly one in five provided 40 or more hours of care per week (18%). Three-quarters helped with household care tasks, such as cleaning, managing finances, or preparing meals (76%), and nearly half reported helping with personal care tasks such as giving medications, feeding, dressing, or bathing (49%) (Figure 3.2).

At middle age, many working adults are reaching the apex of their career. In the general population, more than 90% of men and 80% of women in this age group are employed.[21] Among caregivers, the employment rate was lower: In the BRFSS data, approximately 60% of US caregivers reported being employed for pay (63%) (Table 3.1). Caregivers in this age group often face complicated and challenging decisions regarding their working lives. They are not yet eligible for many retirement benefits, and the family may rely on their job for income or health insurance; at the same time, caregiving demands may make it extremely challenging for caregivers to continue their employment. Indeed, more than a quarter of cancer survivors report that their caregiver made extended employment changes because of the cancer.[8] These employment changes took a wide array of forms, including taking extended paid or unpaid leave (8%), changing from full- to part-time work (2.5%), changing to a less demanding job (2.4%,) retiring early (2.1%), delaying retirement (3.6%), and other changes (21%), including adjustments to workload, schedule, or job responsibilities; changing jobs; turning down a promotion; and delaying looking for work.[8] This is reflective of the complex considerations these family members must undertake in balancing work and caregiving and assessing the long- and short-term consequences of such changes. As with caregivers in early adulthood, the career decisions undertaken by middle-aged caregivers have long-term consequences for their families' financial well-being due to impacts on career potential, cumulative retirement savings, and lifetime earnings. Employment changes may also impact caregivers' psychological well-being or self-image by changing or removing a source of social status, self-esteem, or social support. Indeed, while managing multiple roles can be a strain for caregivers, employment also brings some psychosocial benefits.[13]

In addition to financial and employment challenges, caregivers in middle age may experience the onset of their own health problems. Chronic diseases become more common in middle age,[22] with potential implications for caregiving duties. The increased prevalence of health problems in middle age may have a direct impact on caregivers' ability to provide care. For example, caregivers with arthritis may be less able to help with the physical needs of their care recipients due to pain or weakness or may be less able to complete household tasks. In addition, caregivers with their own chronic health problems may face increased burden of condition management— managing their own medications, appointments, and symptoms in addition to their care recipient's. This burden is likely greatest for those who are caring for someone who is unable to fully participate in their own care management, including care recipients with the greatest mental or physical impact of the cancer or treatment, or those with comorbid conditions such as dementia or frailty. As noted, 40% of caregivers in this age group were caring for a parent, who might be more likely to need extra help as they age.

Many adults at middle age find themselves situated between the older and the younger generations.[23] For some adults, middle age may bring about the lessening of responsibilities around the house as children mature and move away or take on more household responsibilities. This may mean less role conflict for some caregivers in this age group. For spousal caregivers in particular, however, household burdens may increase as the caregiver attempts to compensate for their spouse's activity restrictions in order to maintain their family life and household.[24]

Access to formal supports and resources may continue to be a challenge for cancer caregivers at middle age. For example, to be eligible for the National Family Caregiver Support Program, caregivers must be generally be 55 years of age or older themselves or caring for someone 60 years of age or older (or any individual with dementia).[25] Middle-aged caregivers who are caring for an age peer or younger friend or relative may therefore not have access to the services and supports this program provides. Although other resources exist at the national, state, and local levels, caregivers may struggle to find the time and focus to access these services. Therefore, early and middle adulthood caregivers, particularly those who are also juggling work, parenting, and other responsibilities, may benefit from additional support in accessing and navigating the services available to them.

OLDER AGE (65+ YEARS OF AGE)

Older caregivers made up 17% of the total cancer caregiving population in the United States. Cancer caregivers in the older age bracket were most likely to be caring for their spouse/partner (36%) or a friend (30%), significantly more than caregivers in the other age groups ($p < .0001$ and $p = .003$, respectively; Figure 3.1). A considerable proportion were caring for their sibling (13%) or their child or grandchild (9%). More than one in five older age caregivers had been providing care for more than 5 years (21%) and provided more than 40 hours per week of care (22%; Figure 3.2).

In older adulthood, many responsibilities and goals change. Adults in this age group turn their attention to new life goals, making sense of the past and preparing for the future.[26,27] Those who work are making decisions about retirement or other changes to paid employment, and most adult children have moved out and have reached a stage of relative independence. In the BRFSS sample, more than 85% of late life cancer caregivers were not employed for pay, a much larger proportion than at other life stages (31% and 37% for early adulthood and midlife caregivers, respectively, $p < .0001$; Table 3.1). Furthermore, only 3% had children in the home, compared to 58% of young adult caregivers and 28% of middle-aged caregivers ($p < .0001$). As such, these caregivers may have more time to dedicate to caregiving and care coordination. This supposition is supported by the distribution of caregiving load: In the BRFSS sample, older adult caregivers were the most likely to report providing more than 40 hours of care per week (22% vs. 11% for younger and 18% for middle-aged adults; Figure 3.2) and having been a caregiver for 5 or more years (21% vs. 13% for younger and middle-aged adults), although these differences did not reach statistical significance. Older age also brings an increase in the prevalence of chronic conditions and health problems.[22]

These normative changes may have both positive and negative consequences in the caregiving context, possibly simultaneously. Caregiving itself is far more normative in older age than other life stages; with this comes a greater supply of both formal and informal support, from caregiver support groups with greater age peer validation to support from common experiences among friends and acquaintances. Reductions in work and childcare responsibilities leave later life caregivers with fewer competing demands and more time for caregiving responsibilities.[28,29] This may lead to fewer role conflicts and less burden or strain. Indeed, some evidence suggests that older age caregivers may be more satisfied with their role than younger caregivers,[30] possibly due to fewer time commitments or demands that facilitate reduced role strain and greater satisfaction with care. Older cancer caregivers are also less likely to report disruption to their daily routine, compared to their younger counterparts.[31] However, such advantages may come with concomitant challenges. Taking on greater care responsibilities or more hours of care may contribute to stress, burden, and burnout if not balanced with support and resources. Caregivers without outside responsibilities or activities may conceivably be at greater risk of social isolation, which has serious implications for older adult health and well-being.[32] Furthermore, older adults are more likely to be on a fixed income, which may have implications for their ability to pay for out-of-pocket or unexpected caregiving expenses. However, some evidence suggests that financial distress may be lower among older adult cancer patients and their families compared to their younger counterparts.[31,33]

Later life caregivers may experience distinct aging-related stress during caregiving,[34] in part related to the unique challenges of dealing with their own health problems while simultaneously supporting the cancer patient. In one qualitative study, older spousal cancer caregivers indicated that meeting their spouses' care needs was confounded by their own aging process, which they felt was accelerated by caregiving.[34] These caregivers listed their own health conditions as obstacles to caregiving.[34] Not only may health problems make it physically more difficult or time consuming to provide cancer care, but also may increase the cognitive load of coordinating care, monitoring symptoms, and managing appointments and prescriptions for both themselves and their care recipient. Qualitative case studies indicate that health problems also lead caregivers to question their ability to provide care and play a role in decision-making around the use of assisted living or other supportive services.[34]

The availability of time and reduction in competing demands may explain the high prevalence of friend caregiving at this life stage. Previous research has indicated that among friend or nonkin caregivers, work and family responsibilities predicted amount of care provided.[35,36] Spousal caregiving was also particularly prevalent at this life stage. Spouses are particularly likely to act as primary caregivers,[28,29] and older spousal caregivers provide more hours of care than their middle-aged counterparts.[15,16] This is consistent with the BRFSS data on cancer caregivers examined here, which showed that 57% of spousal caregivers provided more than 20 hours of care per week, compared to 39% of those caring for a child or grandchild,

25% of those caring for a parent, and 24% of those caring for a grandparent ($p < .0001$; Table 3.1).

Caregivers over age 75 may be a particularly vulnerable population. Although individual health and functional capacity vary dramatically as individuals age, this time period is characterized by increasing vulnerability to illness and physical decline (including both chronic diseases and sensory limitations) and concomitant decreases in independence and autonomy.[26] In a general study of caregivers,[37] nearly half of those age 75 or older reported a high burden of care (compared to 40% across age groups). These caregivers provided care for more hours per week (34 hours, on average, compared to an average of 21.7 hours for caregivers age 18–49) and had been providing care for longer (5.6 years on average) than younger caregivers (2.8 years for millennials[38]). They were also more likely to report having no other unpaid help. Some research suggests that caregivers in this age group may be at particular risk for adverse physical or psychological health outcomes related to their caregiving role (summarized by Harden et al.[26]), although this may vary based on competing time demands.[31] However, in a recent report, caregivers over age 75 reported less strain than younger caregivers.[37,39] There may be a normative coming to terms with mortality or fewer concerns about cancer recurrence in this age group,[26] potentially contributing to different perceptions and impacts of the caregiving role.

OTHER LIFE STAGES: CAREGIVING IN CHILDHOOD

It should be noted that cancer caregiving is not limited to adults. While only a small body of literature has examined caregiving during childhood and adolescence, adolescents and even younger children sometimes provide care for their parents, grandparents, or other relatives. Although many children help out in the home, a child caregiver is distinguished as "assuming a level of responsibility that would usually be associated with an adult."[40] These young caregivers most often engage in household care tasks (e.g., cooking, cleaning),[18,41] though they also take on personal care (e.g., bathing) and even medical care tasks for their loved one.[41,42]

Estimates from a 2005 survey[18] suggest that there were more than 50,000 children under the age of 18 providing informal cancer care in the United States. While they typically were not doing this work alone,[18] caregiving has impacts on these children. They report dualities around these responsibilities: Caregiving is both hard and gratifying,[42] and children may feel ambivalent about the role.[43] While families often seek to keep the home life as normal as possible, including maintaining school participation, child caregivers report having less time for themselves.[18,42] They also report that the caregiving role negatively impacted their academic performance and learning.[44,45] Caregiving may be particularly isolating for child caregivers: Teachers, peers, even family members may not recognize that these children have taken on a caregiving role, resulting in their feeling invisible or unsupported.[43] These children may struggle to obtain both emotional and functional support for their underrecognized role in the care of a loved one with cancer. Caregiving at a young age may also affect children's development and identity formation.[43]

POSITIVE ASPECTS OF CAREGIVING

Although this chapter deals primarily with the unique challenges that cancer caregivers may face across the life course, it is important to note that many caregivers also experience positive outcomes and personal growth as a result of their role. Although little work has assessed how life stage and caregiver–care recipient relationship impacts these positive outcomes, some research suggests that spousal caregivers are less likely to report that caregiving is a positive experience, compared to other types of caregivers.[46] It is not yet clear whether age or life stage predict caregivers' perceptions of positive aspects of caregiving.

CONCLUSIONS: IMPLICATIONS AND OPPORTUNITIES FOR FUTURE RESEARCH

Just as cancer spans the life course, so does cancer caregiving. Caregivers at each life stage experience unique challenges. Understanding caregivers' unique and individual situations is critical to assessing their needs and providing adequate guidance and support.

There are several implications and opportunities for future research that build on our existing knowledge about the role of life stage and relationship in cancer caregiving. From a clinical perspective, understanding the prevalence of caregiving across the life course and the challenges these individuals face can facilitate clinicians' abilities to support caregivers. This may be especially important for "off-time" caregivers, who may not fit the caregiver archetype. Clinicians can support caregivers through a variety of formal and informal means, ranging from informal emotional support and nonmedical referrals (e.g., referrals to a medical social worker, respite care support, support groups, etc.), to the systematic integration of caregivers into formal healthcare settings[47] (e.g., deployment of needs assessment tools and follow-up,[48] training caregivers on medical tasks,[49] among other strategies). Recognizing that caregivers may struggle more than other individuals or be at particularly high risk for isolation or adverse outcomes—especially at some life stages or with certain relationships to the cancer survivor—may help clinicians to normalize the caregiving experience and provide support.

From a policy perspective, the recognition of caregiving as a life course issue is important to maximize the impact of caregiving resources. Eligibility for formal caregiving resources (e.g., financial support) is often tied to age of the caregiver or care recipient or the care recipient's health condition(s). For example, the National Family Caregiver Support Program provides services primarily to caregivers who are 55 year of age or older themselves or caring for someone 60 years of age or older (or someone with dementia, regardless of age).[25] This program therefore may not cover some off-time caregivers (e.g., a cancer patient and their spouse in middle age). The proportion of caregivers who fall outside those eligibility criteria has not been systematically examined. Better understanding of how caregivers across life stages access (or fail to access) support services will provide an opportunity to improve policy, service availability, and utilization for caregivers.

Finally, there are opportunities to better understand how caregiver needs and impacts differ across the life course and across relationship types. For example, theory suggests that caregiver and cancer survivor well-being are intertwined.[50] However, the nature of that interrelationship may differ by the relationship type or relationship quality of the caregiver and care recipient. Given the proliferation of interventions intended to help family caregivers, dissemination and implementation studies might be particularly helpful in determining how well existing interventions work for caregivers at different life stages and other life circumstances and how further tailoring can enhance outcomes.

As we continue to understand and appreciate cancer caregiving as a life course phenomenon, we will continue to improve our ability to support families and improve outcomes for both cancer survivors and their loved ones.

REFERENCES

1. Centers for Disease Control and Prevention. Behavioral Risk Factor Surveillance System (BRFSS). https://www.cdc.gov/brfss/annual_data/annual_2015.html). Published 2015. Accessed November 15, 2017

2. Marks NF. Caregiving across the lifespan: National prevalence and predictors. *Fam Relat.* 1996;45(1):27–36.
3. Dellmann-Jenkins M, Blankemeyer M, Pinkard O. Young adult children and grandchildren in primary caregiver roles to older relatives and their service needs. *Fam Relat.* 2000;49(2):177–186.
4. Puterman J, Cadell S. Timing is everything. *J Psychosoc Oncol.* 2008;26(2):103–121.
5. Fruhauf CA, Jarrott SE, Allen KR. Grandchildren's perceptions of caring for grandparents. *J Fam Issues.* 2006;27(7):887–911.
6. Dellmann-Jenkins M, Blankemeyer M, Pinkard O. Incorporating the elder caregiving role into the developmental tasks of young adulthood. *Int J Aging Hum Dev.* 2001;52(1):1–18.
7. Hunt GG, Longacr ML, Kent EE, Weber-Raley L. *Cancer Caregiving in the US: An Intense, Episodic, and Challenging Care Experience.* Washington, DC: NAC/AARP; 2016.
8. de Moor JS, Dowling EC, Ekwueme DU, et al. Employment implications of informal cancer caregiving. *J Cancer Surviv.* 2017;11(1):48–57.
9. Women's Institute for a Secure Retirement. *The Effects of Caregiving.* Washington, DC: Women's Institute for a Secure Retirement; 2012.
10. National Alliance for Caregiving and AARP. *Caregiving in the US 2009.* Bethesda, MD: AARP and National Alliance for Caregiving; 2009.
11. Keating NC, Fast JE, Lero DS, Lucas SJ, Eales J. A taxonomy of the economic costs of family care to adults. *J Econ Ageing.* 2014;3:11–20.
12. Phillips SS, Ragas DM, Hajjar N, Tom LS, Dong X, Simon MA. Leveraging the experiences of informal caregivers to create future healthcare workforce options. *J Am Geriatr Soc.* 2016;64(1):174–180.
13. Kim Y, Baker F, Spillers RL, Wellisch DK. Psychological adjustment of cancer caregivers with multiple roles. *Psychooncology.* 2006;15(9):795–804.
14. Rashi C, Wittman T, Tsimicalis A, Loiselle CG. Balancing illness and parental demands: coping with cancer while raising minor children. *Oncol Nurs Forum.* 2015;42(4):337–344.
15. Moore CW, Rauch PK, Baer L, Pirl WF, Muriel AC. Parenting changes in adults with cancer. *Cancer.* 2015;121(19):3551–3557.
16. Aamotsmo T, Bugge KE. Balance artistry: the healthy parent's role in the family when the other parent is in the palliative phase of cancer—challenges and coping in parenting young children. *Palliat Support Care.* 2014;12(4):317–329.
17. Given CW, Given BA, Sherwood P, DeVoss D. Early adult caregivers: characteristics, challenges, and intervention approaches. In: Talley RC, Montgomery RJV, eds. *Caregiving Across the Lifespan.* New York, NY: Springer; 2013:81–103.
18. Hunt GG, Levine C, Naiditch L. *Young Caregivers in the US: Findings From a National Survey.* Bethesda, MD: National Alliance for Caregiving, in collaboration with United Hospital Fund; 2005.
19. Greene J, Cohen D, Siskowski C, Toyinbo P. The relationship between family caregiving and the mental health of emerging young adult caregivers. *J Behav Health Serv Res.* 2017;44(4):551–563.
20. Becker F, Becker S. *Young Adult Carers in the UK: Experiences, Needs and Services for Carers aged 16–24.* London, UK: Princess Royal Trust for Carers; 2008.
21. Eggebeen DJ, Sturgeon S. Demography of the baby boomers. In: Whitbourne S, Willis S, eds. *The Baby Boomers Grow Up: Contemporary Perspectives on Midlife.* London, UK: Routledge; 2006:3–22.
22. Saad L. *Chronic Illness Rates Swell in Middle Age, Taper Off After 75.* Princeton, NJ: Gallup News; 2011.

23. Lachman ME, Teshale S, Agrigoroaei S. Midlife as a pivotal period in the life course: balancing growth and decline at the crossroads of youth and old age. *Int J Behav Dev*. 2015;39(1):20–31.

24. Jakobsson L, Hallberg IR, Loven L. Experiences of daily life and life quality in men with prostate cancer. An explorative study. Part I. *Eur J Cancer Care (Engl)*. 1997;6(2):108–116.

25. Administration for Community Living. National Family Caregiver Support Program. https://www.acl.gov/programs/support-caregivers/national-family-caregiver-support-program. Published 2017. Accessed March 7, 2018.

26. Harden J. Developmental life stage and couples' experiences with prostate cancer: a review of the literature. *Cancer Nurs*. 2005;28(2):85–98.

27. Baltrusch HJ, Seidel J, Stangel W, Waltz ME. Psychosocial stress, aging and cancer. *Ann N Y Acad Sci*. 1988;521(1):1–15.

28. Lima JC, Allen SM, Goldscheider F, Intrator O. Spousal caregiving in late midlife versus older ages: implications of work and family obligations. *J Gerontol B Psychol Sci Soc Sci*. 2008;63(4):S229–S238.

29. Wolff JL, Kasper JD. Caregivers of frail elders: updating a national profile. *Gerontologist*. 2006;46(3):344–356.

30. Given BA, Given CW. Family caregiving for the elderly. *Annu Rev Nurs Res*. 1991;9:77–101.

31. Mor V, Allen S, Malin M. The psychosocial impact of cancer on older versus younger patients and their families. *Cancer*. 1994;74(7)(Suppl):2118–2127.

32. Luo Y, Hawkley LC, Waite LJ, Cacioppo JT. Loneliness, health, and mortality in old age: a national longitudinal study. *Soc Sci Med*. 2012;74(6):907–914.

33. Meeker CR, Wong YN, Egleston BL, et al. Distress and financial distress in adults with cancer: an age-based analysis. *J Natl Compr Canc Netw*. 2017;15(10):1224–1233.

34. Wittenberg-Lyles E, Demiris G, Oliver DP, Burchett M. Exploring aging-related stress among older spousal caregivers. *J Gerontol Nurs*. 2014;40(8):13–16.

35. LaPierre TA, Keating N. Characteristics and contributions of non-kin carers of older people: a closer look at friends and neighbours. *Ageing Soc*. 2013;33(8):1442–1468.

36. Himes CL, Reidy EB. The role of friends in caregiving. *Res Aging*. 2000;22(4):315–336.

37. National Alliance for Caregiving and AARP Public Policy Institute. *Caregiver Profile: The Caregiver Age 75 and Older*. Washington, DC: National Alliance for Caregiving and AARP Public Policy Institute; 2015.

38. National Alliance for Caregiving and AARP Public Policy Institute. *Caregiver Profile: The Millennial Caregiver*. Washington, DC: National Alliance for Caregiving and AARP Public Policy Institute; 2015.

39. National Alliance for Caregiving and AARP. *Caregiving in the US*. Bethesda, MD: AARP and National Alliance for Caregiving; 2015.

40. Becker S. Young Carers. In: Davies M, ed. *The Blackwell Encyclopedia of Social Work*. Oxford: Blackwell; 2000:378.

41. Lackey NR, Gates MF. Adults' recollections of their experiences as young caregivers of family members with chronic physical illnesses. *J Adv Nurs*. 2001;34(3):320–328.

42. Gates MF, Lackey NR. Youngsters caring for adults with cancer. *J Nurs Scholarsh*. 1998;30(1):11–15.

43. Rose HD, Cohen K. The experiences of young carers: a meta-synthesis of qualitative findings. *J Youth Stud*. 2010;13(4):473–487.

44. Pakenham KI. Children who care for their parents: the impact of parental disability on young lives. In: Marshall CA, Kendall E, Banks ME, Gover RMS, eds.

Disabilities: Insights From Across Fields and Around the World. Westport, CT: Praeger; 2009:39–60.
45. Siskowski C. Young caregivers: effect of family health situations on school performance. *J Sch Nurs.* 2006;22(3):163–169.
46. Associated Press-NORC Center for Public Affairs Research. *Long-Term Care in America: Expectations and Reality.* Chicago, IL: Associated Press-NORC Center for Public Affairs Research; 2014.
47. Kent EE, Rowland JH, Northouse L, et al. Caring for caregivers and patients: research and clinical priorities for informal cancer caregiving. *Cancer.* 2016;122(13):1987–1995.
48. Aoun SM, Grande G, Howting D, et al. The impact of the Carer Support Needs Assessment Tool (CSNAT) in community palliative care using a stepped wedge cluster trial. *PLoS One.* 2015;10(4):e0123012.
49. Mollica MA, Litzelman K, Rowland JH, Kent EE. The role of medical/nursing skills training in caregiver confidence and burden: a CanCORS study. *Cancer.* 2017;123(22):4481–4487.
50. Northouse LL, Katapodi MC, Schafenacker AM, Weiss D. The impact of caregiving on the psychological well-being of family caregivers and cancer patients. *Semin Oncol Nurs.* 2012;28(4):236–245.

CHAPTER 4

Burden Among Caregivers of Patients With Unique Sites of Cancer or Treatment and Comorbid Psychopathology

MARIA KRYZO-LACOMBE, TAMRYN F. GRAY,
MARGARET BEVANS, LOGIN GEORGE,
AND WILLIAM S. BREITBART

The burden experienced by cancer caregivers is well documented, as evidenced by the previous chapters. While all caregivers are at risk for a host of negative psychosocial and medical outcomes, specific groups may be at unique risk for burden because of their loved one's cancer or treatment or comorbid conditions. In this chapter, we provide an overview of three such groups of caregivers who may be at particular risk for burden and in need of psychosocial support.

CAREGIVERS OF PATIENTS WITH BRAIN TUMORS OR NEUROCOGNITIVE SEQUELAE OF CANCER/ TREATMENT
Maria Kryza-Lacombe

In 2017 in the United States alone, approximately 23,800 individuals received a diagnosis of brain or other nervous system cancer,[1] and it is estimated that between 200,000 and 300,000 people develop brain metastases each year.[2] Caregivers of these patients must navigate a complex symptom profile that includes cognitive, neuropsychiatric, and functional decline.[3] As such, the associated support needs of these patients place a unique burden on caregivers.

Understanding the Patient's Brain Tumor and Neurocognitive Changes

The idiosyncratic behavioral and functional deficits of the patient with a brain tumor may include language deficits, facial recognition difficulties, difficulty making decisions, impaired judgment, decreased reasoning ability, changes in emotional control and personality, motor deficits such as the coordination of motor movements or weakness affecting motor activities, or a combination of any of these.[4–6] Additionally, treatment of the tumor may lead to fatigue and further impact existing cognitive and functional deficits.[6] Disease progression is met with an increase in responsibilities for caregivers who are tasked with eventually assisting patients with many (to all) activities of daily living (ADLs), navigating treatment decision-making, and end-of-life planning.[7]

Even early in the disease trajectory, cognitive difficulties such as memory and attention problems may require caregivers to give repeated reminders and directions for routine activities when the patient's physical status may still allow them to complete ADLs independently. In addition to cognitive changes, the patient may experience neuropsychiatric changes, such as hallucinations and delusions, as well as anxiety, depression, irritability, anger, apathy, and mania.[6] The combination of cognitive and neuropsychiatric changes can lead to unpredictable and problematic behaviors, such as forgetting to turn off the stove, violent disinhibited behaviors, and confusion. The severity of these symptoms is distressing and difficult to gauge and may lead to safety concerns.[6,8] Cognitive and behavioral changes are usually accompanied by deficits in functional status, which can range from having to discontinue employment and traveling alone, to being unable to perform ADLs such as bathing and dressing. When the patient is no longer able to independently engage in self-care and treatment-related activities, it creates a demand for caregivers to assist with, or assume the, functional tasks completely.[6]

Caregivers often reframe the experience associated with the patients' physical, cognitive, and psychological changes as "the new normal."[9] As caregivers get settled into this new normal, they report that it is often difficult for others to understand the physical, cognitive, and personality

changes in the patient with a brain tumor and that members of their social network withdraw from social interactions with the patient and their
family[10] during a time social support is especially needed.[11] This specific
concern regarding the perception of their loved one's disease by others
tends to be unique among caregivers of patients with brain tumors and
exacerbates their overall risk for burden.[10]

The Unique Burden of Providing Care for Patients With Brain Tumors and Neurocognitive Sequelae of Cancer and Its Treatment

The devastating neurologic changes and sequelae of cancer treatment for
patients with brain malignancies puts caregivers at particular risk for
burden. On average, caregivers of brain tumor patients spend approximately 12 (though up to 24) hours per day caring for their loved one, mostly
consisting of supervision time, which is likely related to deteriorating cognitive autonomy, risk of falls, seizures, and incontinence.[12] Indeed, functional, cognitive, and neuropsychiatric status of the patient has been
linked to global caregiver burden.[13] Poorer functional status, in particular,
is linked to sleep disturbances,[14] poorer psychological well-being,[15,16] and
higher self-reported burden among caregivers, as well as increased hours
per day spent providing care.[12] The burden associated with caring for a
loved one with brain malignancy may result in a strong stress response,
which may be linked to decreased overall health and social functioning and
increased mortality risk.[6,15] Physical[6,14] and emotional well-being of these
caregivers may be compromised,[5,12,13] and existential questions frequently
emerge.[7] Compared to the general population, caregivers of brain tumor
patients have higher levels of anxiety and depression, with one study reporting clinically relevant levels of anxiety and depression in 50% and 20%
of caregivers, respectively.[15] These symptoms may have broad impact on
caregiver well-being as anxiety has been linked to sleep disturbances[14] and
both anxiety and depression to low social support[11] in this population.

Caregivers' mental health is affected by the patient's status. Anxiety is particularly prevalent among brain tumor patient caregivers who have been providing care for less than 10 months and those who provide care for patients
with a low functional status (Karnofsky Performance Scale [KPS] < 80).[15]
Neuropsychiatric symptoms in the patient, which may include hallucinations,
delusions, irritability, anger, and mania, have been linked to both caregiver anxiety[6] and depression, as well as other manifestations of caregiver
burden, including health, financial difficulties, self-esteem, and feelings of

abandonment.[13] Higher levels of depressive symptoms among caregivers are especially prevalent when the number of the patient's neuropsychiatric symptoms is very high.[13] Additionally, neurocognitive and associated personality changes add to the burden and have been predictive of a negative caregiving experience overall.[17]

Such cognitive changes in patients may ignite an early grieving process in caregivers[6,7] and leave them feeling like they are caring for someone different from who they knew before.[8] The patient's cognitive and personality changes may also alter the patient-caregiver relationship and lead to feelings of isolation and a changing sense of identity.[7] Thus, the psychological burden caregivers of brain tumor patients experience extends beyond anxiety and depression and includes impactful existential struggles. The immense new responsibility that comes with providing care, feelings of powerlessness over the situation, as well as emerging feelings of guilt that arise whenever there are conflicting priorities in the caregiver's life likewise contribute to burden.[7]

Caregiver burden may be moderated by access to external and internal resources. Financial resources can ameliorate burden with hired care,[6] but when such assets are not available, financial strain can contribute to burden, especially when caregivers discontinue paid employment to care for their loved one. However, even when working, caregiver wages and careers may be affected.[12] Social support has been widely documented as a critical resource that can alleviate burden in caregivers of brain tumor patients[9] and has been shown to make a notable difference in their well-being.[7,11,13] Alternatively, sparse or absent social support contributes to burden.[11,12] Caregivers report that support from family and friends is vital, especially as caregiving demands increase and the time to seek out support decreases.[9] Internal resources, such as feeling mastery in the ability to provide care, the ability to engage in problem-focused coping strategies,[6] as well as the ability to derive meaning from the caregiving experience[7] may also alleviate burden. Additionally, spiritual well-being among caregivers has been found to be positively associated with caregiver quality of life (QOL).[18]

Caring for a Child With a Brain Tumor or Its Neurocognitive Sequelae

Parenting a child with a brain tumor brings unique challenges. Parents may fear that they are responsible for their child's illness[19] and are conflicted between having to meet both their medical and their emotional needs.[20]

Survival rates of childhood brain malignancies are high,[21] but the current and long-term effects of treatment are challenging. Therefore, many concerns about potential obstacles, such as navigating school accommodations, as well as developmental, cognitive, and psychosocial treatment sequelae, are prevalent.[22] Discussions with children and adolescents about death are especially distressing to these parent caregivers, but their absence has been associated with notable guilt.[20] Findings regarding well-being among such parents is consistent with nonparent caregivers of brain tumor patients: Physical and psychosocial health-related QOL is associated with caregiving demand, caregiving competence, as well as supportive factors.[23]

Supporting the Informal Caregivers of Patients With Brain Tumors

Caregivers of patients with brain tumors need targeted support to protect their well-being and that of their loved one. Indeed, mastery in the caregiving role has been associated with patient survival, above and beyond known covariates such as patient age, functional status, and postsurgical treatment.[24] Interventions for caregivers are therefore needed to minimize burden and help them maintain physical and mental well-being. Efforts to minimize initial burden may be an especially impactful way to address long-term sequelae, as lower burden at diagnosis is associated with positive caregiver outcomes along the illness trajectory.[11] Caregivers of brain tumor patients are unique in several ways, but perhaps most notably because of their significant and immediate need for information.[10] Thus, empowering caregivers by providing greatly desired early high-quality information about their loved one's diagnosis, the disease trajectory (including functional, cognitive, and neuropsychiatric deficits), as well as practical hands-on information and training in how to support the patient, is a critical first step.[10] For example, not understanding neurocognitive changes makes it more challenging for caregivers to manage their sequelae, but understanding that the patient is unable to control their own behavior helps caregivers be more resilient and find ways to cope.[5] Providing educational resources may thus decrease caregivers' negative stress responses.

Accurate understanding of prognosis has been associated with favorable medical outcomes for the patient at the end of life[25] and psychosocial outcomes for caregivers through bereavement.[26] Because of the functional and cognitive decline of patients with brain malignancy, caregivers often become the main person to communicate with the healthcare team about treatment. In this context, they may advocate for the patient and act as a healthcare proxy. Interventions are therefore needed to help caregivers develop skills to navigate prognostic communication with their loved ones and with healthcare providers, which will help caregivers advocate for their loved one's wishes.[26]

Interventions are also needed for physicians and other members of the healthcare team who communicate prognostic information to the family. Most caregivers feel that prognostic information is extremely important and actively seek information. This may be the reason why many caregivers have full awareness of the incurability of malignant glioma and have accurate estimates of their loved one's life expectancy. Despite this, caregivers desire more prognostic information[26] but report that physicians are frequently unable to address their questions[5] and that the timing and content of the information provided by their oncologists is problematic.[26,27] Additionally, caregivers desire prognostic information but concurrently strive to maintain hope for their loved one. Therefore, it is important for prognostic information to be delivered in a sensitive and flexible manner that is attuned to the family's values and preferences.[26] Healthcare providers should also understand the importance of acknowledging the challenges of providing informal care for a patient with a brain tumor and validate the caregiver's effort.[8]

It is likewise critical that families of patients with brain tumors receive information and access to resources that will support the caregiving experience. Sleep interventions, assistance in accessing and navigating financial supports, as well as education on maintaining self-care and social support throughout the caregiving experience are important as each has been shown to have a meaningful impact on caregiver and patient well-being.[11,12,14,16] Access to psychosocial support is likewise critical considering the high prevalence of clinically relevant levels of anxiety and depression among caregivers of brain tumor patients.[15] Such formal support should include targeted intervention to address existential distress and ameliorate feelings of identity loss, isolation, guilt, and death anxiety.

Providing care to a loved one with a brain tumor or neurocognitive sequelae of cancer and its treatment is uniquely challenging. Targeted interventions are needed to empower these caregivers to provide skilled care to the patient while maintaining their own health and well-being.

CAREGIVERS OF PATIENTS UNDERGOING HEMATOPOIETIC STEM CELL TRANSPLANTATION
Tamryn F. Gray and Margaret Bevans

Cancer and its treatment not only affect the individuals with the illness but also have a broader impact on family members.[28] In addition to coping with the diagnosis and uncertainty of the disease, family members often have added caregiving responsibilities when loved ones undergo care and treatment.[28,29] One such intense treatment, hematopoietic stem cell transplantation (HSCT), is available for a growing number of patients with high-risk hematologic malignancies, such as leukemia, and nonmalignant diseases sensitive to immune modulation.[30]

Many factors influence the approach to an HSCT. Depending on the underlying diseases, age of the patient, availability and human leukocyte antigen compatibility of a donor, the HSCT intensity varies, thus creating a more unique experience for the patient and family. Each patient receives a conditioning regimen (myeloablative, reduced-intensity, nonmyeloablative) that often includes chemotherapy and radiation therapy followed by an infusion of the stem cells: peripheral blood, bone marrow, or cord blood. When the stem cells are harvested from the patient, the procedure is considered an autologous HSCT compared to an allogeneic HSCT, where the stem cells are harvested from a related or unrelated donor.

Here, we focus on the care of allogeneic HSCT patients. Although an allogeneic HSCT can be life-saving, the treatment course is often complicated by multiple toxicities[31,32] that require close monitoring and specialized care, often leading to a prolonged inpatient hospital stay and frequent readmissions and outpatient visits.[33] Allogeneic HSCT recipients may spend multiple weeks as inpatients, and 50% are readmitted to receive treatment for transplant-related complications.[34] When the patient is an inpatient, caregiving often includes psychological and social support, advocacy, and building skills related to medication administration, symptom management, and problem identification.[29,35] Additionally, the caregiver often has home care duties to manage, including those at a secondary/temporary residence close to the transplantation center—along with providing care for other family members.[33,36]

Because the risk of morbidity and mortality remains high after the HSCT procedure, patients and a caregiver are required to remain close to the transplant center for approximately 100 days.[37,38] After discharge, the caregiver assumes responsibility 24 hours a day for symptom management in addition to monitoring for problems and coordination of care.[39] This includes monitoring the patient for infection, tracking complex medication regimens, providing specialized dietary restrictions, and providing transportation to and from the center.[40] Advances in HSCT conditioning regimens (e.g., nonmyeloablative) and supportive care approaches have allowed some centers to move patients into the outpatient setting more quickly. However, we have little knowledge about the impact of these changes on caregiver burden.[41]

Approximately 3 months following allogeneic HSCT, patients experience a turning point toward the chronic phase of transplant recovery and prepare to transition from the transplant center to their home community.[36] Almost 25% of long-term survivors, however, present with chronic consequences of the transplant requiring continued care from family members.[42,43] This extended need for support continues to affect caregiver health and QOL.[44,45]

Caregiver Experiences During HSCT

Allogeneic HSCT is a physically and psychologically exhausting treatment.[43] The challenges of this intense procedure and its recovery mandate the presence of a caregiver who can provide, at minimum, instrumental support to the patient.[46] Caregivers may also face intensive responsibilities involving the provision of emotional support for transplant patients.[38] Although caregivers frequently put the needs of the patient above their own, they often report challenges in many dimensions of their life and seldom seeking help.[37] These caregivers are tasked with quickly learning how to provide care to patients during HSCT and in preparation for their return home.[29] Furthermore, the long transplant recovery period creates a long-term commitment for the caregiver to patient care.[32] The uncertainty and complexity associated with the transplantation process increases the level of distress for the patient and the caregiver.[39] Table 4.1 highlights the common problems that caregivers experience during HSCT.

Implications for Practice

It is essential to provide care and support for caregivers in their new role. The types of support for caregivers are fluid and may occur at various times throughout the treatment trajectory by different members of the care team. An initial assessment of the HSCT patient is standard of care and includes determination that a caregiver has been identified. Screening the caregiver for their needs or baseline distress is not routine in HSCT care. Approaches to assessing the caregiver are outlined in Chapter 6.

Although few evidence-based interventions specific to caregivers of HSCT patients are available, extensive evidence exists in the cancer caregiver literature at large and is summarized in Sections 2 and 3 of this textbook, as well as in the Oncology Nursing Society's discussion of caregiver strain and burden (https://www.ons.org/practice-resources/pep/caregiver-strain-and-burden).

Table 4.1 CAREGIVER OUTCOMES AND TARGETED INTERVENTIONS

Literature Highlights	Targeted Interventions
Psychological Health	
• High psychological morbidity related to the caregiving experience.[32] Some psychological issues include concealing their fears and worries about the cancer and the transplant,[28] post-traumatic stress disorder after HSCT,[47] intensive medical treatments for the patient, isolation in hospitals, and living with unknown prognosis.[31]	• Access to telepsychiatry. • Refer to mental health services and facilitate continuity of care. • Provide education to prepare for the severity and duration of emotional and physical changes in patients.[48]
Physical Health	
—**Sleep Disturbances**	
• Related to increased stress, fatigue, and decreased quality of life,[34,36] more frequent night-time interruptions in the hospital setting than at home,[34] and daytime dysfunction.[49]	• Promote healthy eating and physical activity. • Promote stress reduction activities such as mindfulness and meditation, yoga, progressive relaxation, massage, and biofeedback. • Refer to provider for pharmacology treatment. • Suggest noise-cancelling options (e.g., sound machines). • In hospital—clustering care during the overnight hours. • Encourage caregivers to identify family or friends for support and respite.
— **Fatigue**	
• Major concern for caregivers. • Fatigue is often positively correlated with depression.[37]	• Promote healthy eating and physical activity. • Recommend that the caregiver cluster care. • Incorporate spiritual care. • Join a caregiving support group. • Encourage the caregiver to enlist support and assistance from friends and family. • Provide respite care for the caregiver.
Social Health	
— **Social Isolation**	
• Social isolation is commonly reported and perceived among caregivers.	• Encourage supportive interpersonal relationships with family and friends. • Provide respite care for caregivers. • Encourage caregivers to take part in new hobbies and activities to help cope with caregiving stress. • Provide education about handwashing and other infection precautions when in public places.

Table 4.1 CONTINUED

Literature Highlights	Targeted Interventions
	• Inform caregivers about caregiver support groups.
	• Recommend web-based sharing systems such as blogging, emailing, and other social networking sites.[48]
— **Relationship quality**	
• Disruption to family structure, family interaction, and family relationships.[48]	• Enlist family and friends to help with chores at home.
• New roles and responsibilities.[28]	• Promote open communication, dialogue, and problem-solving between caregivers, patients, and family members and friends.
	• Recommend caregivers and patients schedule time together as a dyad.
	• Discuss discharge strategies with the nurse coordinator or hospital social worker to reduce burden for caregivers as patients transition home.
	• Provide anticipatory guidance about sexual issues with caregivers.
— **Employment and Financial Concerns**	
• Disruptions to family and work routines.[32]	• Alternate hospital duties between caregivers.
• Financial burden is a major barrier to transplantation.[50]	• Promote open communication, dialogue, and problem-solving.
• Financial toxicity associated with long-term recovery and complications post-HSCT.	• Encourage caregivers to ask for support from employers, family members, friends, and the care team.
	• Schedule consultation with the hospital social worker or nurse coordinator related to financial concerns.
	• Cluster and coordinate hospital visits and medical rounds, keeping in mind the caregiver's other responsibilities and daily work schedule.
	• Assist caregivers in receiving medical leave from employer.
	• Inform patients about the option of creating a fundraising group to help support the costs of HSCT.
— **Housing Barriers and Relocation**	
• Need to relocate for temporary housing to be closer to a transplant center.[51]	• Schedule consultation with the hospital social worker or nurse coordinator related to financial or housing concerns.
	• Assist in relocation during the transplant and post-transplant periods.

Overall, the supportive resources for caregivers can be individually focused or provided as a component of dyadic or family care, and many resources are a component of the interdisciplinary team-based approach. These interventions can include skills building, psychoeducational approaches, problem-solving strategies, and self-care, including stress reduction strategies. Other resources can be in the HSCT center or in the community, such as cancer or HSCT support groups. At times, caregivers may require more advanced support, such as cognitive behavioral therapy, to manage psychological distress (e.g., anxiety, depression) and should be referred to experienced providers for care.

Summary

Caregivers of HSCT patients need support in adjusting and adapting to a new role in caring for a loved one undergoing this intense and uncertain medical therapy. HSCT yields much psychological distress and financial, physical, and social concerns for caregivers. It is important to utilize a multidisciplinary team approach and assess and address caregiver burden during the pre-HSCT phase. Moreover, as recovery at home is a family experience and, hence, the success of recovery is contingent in large part on functioning of caregivers, evaluating family function pre-HSCT will highlight potential challenges at discharge.[41] Research showed that without a caregiver's support, the transplant experience and patient outcomes may be negatively affected.[52] Therefore, interventions should be tailored to the unique needs of caregivers and promote self-care, health, and resilience. Healthcare systems should facilitate the implementation of early supportive care services and referrals as well as closely monitor the impact that HSCT has on the caregiver over time.

CAREGIVERS OF PATIENTS WITH CANCER AND COMORBID PSYCHIATRIC DISORDERS
Login George and William S. Breitbart

Psychiatric comorbidity may add a layer of complexity to the challenges that caregivers face, exacerbating burden and negative outcomes.[53] While there is a paucity of research examining how psychiatric comorbidity impacts caregivers, existing research suggests that such comorbidity likely poses additional challenges to a significant portion of caregivers, exacerbating the negative impact of the caregiving role.

Psychiatric comorbidity is not uncommon among cancer patients.[54] Due to the stressful nature of cancer, patients are at increased risk of developing psychopathology, most commonly depression, adjustment disorder, and anxiety. Prevalence estimates vary based on the assessment methods used and the specific sample characteristics (e.g., early vs. advanced cancer). A recent meta-analysis of 70 interview-based studies in oncological and hematological settings showed prevalence rates of depression at 16.3%, adjustment disorder at 19.4%, and anxiety at 10.3%[55] and the prevalence of any mood disorder at 38.2%. Another recent study examined the 4-week prevalence of psychiatric disorders in German cancer patients and found that 31.8% had any one psychiatric disorder.[56] Another study from Germany compared cancer patients to the general population and found that the odds of being depressed (defined as Patient Health Questionnaire [PHQ]-9 score of 10 or greater) were more than five times higher in cancer patients.[57]

As psychiatric comorbidity is a challenge faced by a significant portion of cancer patients, it is important to understand the impact of such comorbidity on the experience of caregivers. Only a few studies have examined the impact of patient psychopathology on caregiving and suggest, not surprisingly, the impact is a negative one. For example, higher patient depression was associated with higher caregiver depression,[58] as well as higher caregiver burden and impact on schedule and lower social functioning.[59,60] Patient anxiety was similarly found to be positively associated with caregiver burden and depression.[59] More broadly, in one study, when patients met criteria for any psychiatric diagnosis, caregivers were 7.9 times more likely to meet criteria for a psychiatric diagnosis themselves.[53] These studies suggest the possibility that patients' comorbid psychiatric difficulties may bleed into caregivers' functioning and well-being.

Psychiatric comorbidity may also take the form of more chronic and severe mental illnesses, such as schizophrenia and bipolar disorder.[61] Schizophrenia is characterized by distortions in thinking and perception and may include delusions, hallucinations, disorganized speech, and disorganized behavior (the positive symptoms) or avolition and diminished emotions (the negative symptoms). Bipolar disorder involves two or more episodes of markedly disturbed mood, energy, and activity levels wherein patients feel manic or hypomanic (mood and energy levels are increased) or depressed (mood and energy levels are decreased). Prevalence estimates in the general population are 0.5% to 1.5% for schizophrenia and 0.4% to 1.6% for bipolar disorder, and the prevalence among patients with cancer is likely the same.[54] Although relatively more uncommon, the severity of these disorders means that they are likely posing significant additional hardship on caregivers.

A significant body of literature suggests that cancer patients with severe mental illnesses, such as schizophrenia or bipolar disorder, may have a more complicated course of cancer treatment and more negative outcomes.[61,62] For example, studies have documented that patients with severe mental illness may be more likely to experience diagnostic delays, be diagnosed at a more advanced stage of cancer, and not receive treatment.[63,64] Treatment is more likely to be disrupted or delayed,[65] and in one study, this was associated with recurrence of breast cancer at 5 years.[66] Postsurgery complications and mortality have also been found to be higher among those with schizophrenia.[67] Such disparities may be due to the cognitive, emotional, and behavioral deficits associated with severe mental illness, which lead to poor health behaviors and poor compliance and adherence to treatment recommendations.[68] Further, the higher incidence of medical comorbidities among the severely mentally ill, and provider and systemic factors (e.g., stigma, fragmented physical and mental health treatment), negatively contribute to care and outcomes.[62,69] These difficulties with treatment are exacerbated in the context of other psychosocial issues affecting the severely mentally ill and their families, including poverty, stigma, victimization, behavioral problems, social isolation, and lower family functioning.[70,71] Thus, caregivers of cancer patients with persistent or severe mental illness likely face multiple significant challenges.

Broadly, the demands faced by caregivers of patients with cancer and comorbid psychiatric illness may take several forms. Patients may be more reliant on caregivers to understand their illness and remain motivated to engage in their treatment.[61] Cognitive deficits are often present in individuals with severe mental illness[72] and can negatively impact patients' capacity to engage in clear and ongoing communication with healthcare providers. Such patients may also lack insight into their cancer diagnosis and prognosis and may even refuse treatment that is potentially curative. Indeed, case examples from the literature of patients with serious mental illness highlight inadequate illness understanding and refusal of treatment as salient issues.[68,73] In such cases, caregivers are often responsible to ensure that patients understand their illness and engage in appropriate treatment in line with patients' values. Indeed, this literature emphasizes the importance of caregivers taking these responsibilities to address challenges with patient engagement in care.[68,74]

Ensuring adequate adherence to treatment recommendations, such as properly taking medications and regularly attending appointments, may also fall on caregivers. Individuals with depression, for example, have three times greater odds of being noncompliant to medical treatment recommendations according to a quantitative review of the literature.[75]

Similarly, patients with psychosis have higher frequencies of nonadherence than those who are not psychotic.[76,77] Although little research has examined the exact role that caregivers may play in addressing such adherence issues in the face of cancer and mental illness, research on other populations suggests that caregivers may be working to foster adherence. For example, qualitative interviews with caregivers of HIV-infected adults suggest that caregivers may enhance adherence by helping patients with access to and knowledge of medications, fostering motivation, and providing cues to action (e.g., reminders[78]). In another study of patients with chronic obstructive pulmonary disease (COPD), those with informal caregivers were more likely to be adherent to their medications and less likely to engage in poor health-related behaviors (e.g., smoking) than those without caregivers.[79]

Helping patients coordinate adequate treatment of psychiatric illness alongside their cancer treatments is another task faced by caregivers. For example, some oncologic medications may interact with psychotropic drugs and result in adverse side effects.[61,68] As such, caregivers may often be relied on to recognize the signs and symptoms of drug interactions and communicate these events to healthcare professionals so that timely changes in medication regimens may be made. Finally, caregivers' provision of instrumental support, such as assisting patients with transportation to and from appointments, may be more challenging due to the disproportionately high rates of poverty and other social issues affecting this patient population.[70,71] Similarly, providing patients with emotional support may be particularly challenging as depression, anxiety, and other psychiatric difficulties may impair patients' coping abilities and exacerbate their baseline needs.

Psychiatric comorbidity is therefore likely an added challenge faced by a significant portion of caregivers. The few relevant studies that documented the unique experience of such caregivers highlighted associations between comorbid psychiatric illness and worse caregiver well-being, functioning, and burden.[59,60] Further research is needed on the full breadth of impact that psychiatric comorbidity may have on caregivers. Are these caregivers in fact experiencing greater challenges and feeling more distress, and consequently, are they in need of additional support? Research is also needed on caregivers of patients with severe and chronic mental illness, as the negative impact on this group may be much greater. It will also be important to examine aspects of resilience and strength among these caregivers, who may have a long history of providing care for someone with a chronic mental illness, which may translate into strengths in providing cancer-related care.

Research is also needed to determine if existing approaches for supporting caregivers are sufficient to address the unique needs of caregivers of patients with comorbid psychiatric illness. The unique contexts of severe mental illness (stigma, poverty, and discrimination) may contribute to disparities in this population's interest and skepticism of caregiver interventions and accessibility to them.[70,71] As such, interventions may further need to be tailored to their unique contexts and needs. For example, psychoeducation and skills on how psychiatric difficulties may manifest in the context of cancer care (e.g., adherence problems, poor health behaviors, poor understanding of treatment, communication difficulties, or conflict with oncology care providers) may be helpful. Communication skills training to assist caregivers to convey to healthcare providers the unique needs of patients due to their psychiatric status, as well as education on the importance of coordinating psychiatric and oncologic care, may also be helpful.[61] Caregivers have a vital role to play as members of treatment teams, as they assist with many of the challenges involved in treating patients with psychiatric illness. Interventions are therefore needed to help them to successfully carry out this responsibility.

REFERENCES

1. Siegel, R. L., Miller, K. D., & Jemal, A. (2017). Cancer statistics, 2017. *CA Cancer J Clin, 67*(1), 7–30. doi:10.3322/caac.21387
2. American Brain Tumor Association. (2017). Metastatic brain tumor. http://www.abta.org/brain-tumor-information/types-of-tumors/metastatic-brain-tumor.html. Published 2017.
3. Ostgathe, C., Gaertner, J., Kotterba, M., et al.; for the Hospice and Palliative Care Evaluation (HOPE) Working Group in Germany. (2010). Differential palliative care issues in patients with primary and secondary brain tumours. *Support Care Cancer, 18*(9), 1157–1163. doi:10.1007/s00520-009-0735-y
4. Packer, R. J., & Mehta, M. (2002). Neurocognitive sequelae of cancer treatment. *Neurology, 59*(1), 8–10.
5. Schubart, J. R., Kinzie, M. B., & Farace, E. (2008). Caring for the brain tumor patient: family caregiver burden and unmet needs. *Neuro Oncol, 10*(1), 61–72. doi:10.1215/15228517-2007-040
6. Sherwood, P., Given, B., Given, C., Schiffman, R., Murman, D., & Lovely, M. (2004). Caregivers of persons with a brain tumor: a conceptual model. *Nurs Inq, 11*(1), 43–53.
7. Applebaum, A., Kryza-Lacombe, M., Buthorn, J., DeRosa, A., Corner, G., & Diamond, E. (2016). Existential distress among caregivers of patients with brain tumors: a review of the literature. *Neuro-Oncology Practice, 3*(4), 232–244.
8. Whisenant, M. (2011). Informal caregiving in patients with brain tumors. *Oncol Nurs Forum, 38*(5), E373–E381. doi:10.1188/11.ONF.E373-E381
9. Hricik, A., Donovan, H., Bradley, S. E., et al. (2011). Changes in caregiver perceptions over time in response to providing care for a loved one with a primary malignant brain tumor. *Oncol Nurs Forum, 38*(2), 149–155. doi:10.1188/11.ONF.149-155

10. Heckel, M., Hoser, B., & Stiel, S. (2018)Caring for patients with brain tumors compared to patients with non-brain tumors: experiences and needs of informal caregivers in home care settings. *J Psychosoc Oncol*, 36(2), 189–202. doi:10.1080/07347332.2017.1379046

11. Reblin, M., Small, B., Jim, H., Weimer, J., & Sherwood, P. (2018). Mediating burden and stress over time: caregivers of patients with primary brain tumor. *Psychooncology*, 27(2), 607–612. doi:10.1002/pon.4527

12. Bayen, E., Laigle-Donadey, F., Proute, M., Hoang-Xuan, K., Joel, M. E., & Delattre, J. Y. (2017). The multidimensional burden of informal caregivers in primary malignant brain tumor. *Support Care Cancer*, 25(1), 245–253. doi:10.1007/s00520-016-3397-6

13. Sherwood, P. R., Given, B. A., Given, C. W., et al. (2006). Predictors of distress in caregivers of persons with a primary malignant brain tumor. *Res Nurs Health*, 29(2), 105–120. doi:10.1002/nur.20116

14. Pawl, J. D., Lee, S. Y., Clark, P. C., & Sherwood, P. R. (2013). Sleep characteristics of family caregivers of individuals with a primary malignant brain tumor. *Oncol Nurs Forum*, 40(2), 171–179. doi:10.1188/13.ONF.171-179

15. Finocchiaro, C. Y., Petruzzi, A., Lamperti, E., et al. (2012). The burden of brain tumor: a single-institution study on psychological patterns in caregivers. *J Neurooncol*, 107(1), 175–181. doi:10.1007/s11060-011-0726-y

16. Ownsworth, T., Henderson, L., & Chambers, S. K. (2010). Social support buffers the impact of functional impairments on caregiver psychological well-being in the context of brain tumor and other cancers. *Psychooncology*, 19(10), 1116–1122. doi:10.1002/pon.1663

17. Pinquart, M., & Sorensen, S. (2003). Associations of stressors and uplifts of caregiving with caregiver burden and depressive mood: a meta-analysis. *J Gerontol B Psychol Sci Soc Sci*, 58(2), P112–P128.

18. Pawl, J. D., Lee, S. Y., Clark, P. C., & Sherwood, P. R. (2013b). Sleep loss and its effects on health of family caregivers of individuals with primary malignant brain tumors. *Res Nurs Health*, 36(4), 386–399. doi:10.1002/nur.21545

19. Nicholas, D. B., Chahauver, A., Brownstone, D., Hetherington, R., McNeill, T., & Bouffet, E. (2012). Evaluation of an online peer support network for fathers of a child with a brain tumor. *Soc Work Health Care*, 51(3), 232–245. doi:10.1080/00981389.2011.631696

20. Zelcer, S., Cataudella, D., Cairney, A. E., & Bannister, S. L. (2010). Palliative care of children with brain tumors: a parental perspective. *Arch Pediatr Adolesc Med*, 164(3), 225–230. doi:10.1001/archpediatrics.2009.284

21. Deatrick, J. A., Hobbie, W., Ogle, S., et al. (2014). Competence in caregivers of adolescent and young adult childhood brain tumor survivors. *Health Psychol*, 33(10), 1103–1112. doi:10.1037/a0033756

22. Forinder, U., & Lindahl Norberg, A. (2010). "Now we have to cope with the rest of our lives." Existential issues related to parenting a child surviving a brain tumour. *Support Care Cancer*, 18(5), 543–551. doi:10.1007/s00520-009-0678-3

23. Quast, L. F., Turner, E. M., McCurdy, M. D., & Hocking, M. C. (2016). Health-related quality of life in parents of pediatric brain tumor survivors at the end of tumor-directed therapy. *J Psychosoc Oncol*, 34(4), 274–290. doi:10.1080/07347332.2016.1175535

24. Boele, F. W., Given, C. W., Given, B. A., et al. (2017). Family caregivers' level of mastery predicts survival of patients with glioblastoma: a preliminary report. *Cancer*, 123(5), 832–840. doi:10.1002/cncr.30428

25. Wright, A. A., Zhang, B., Ray, A., et al. (2008). Associations between end-of-life discussions, patient mental health, medical care near death, and caregiver bereavement adjustment. *JAMA, 300*(14), 1665–1673. doi:10.1001/jama.300.14.1665

26. Applebaum, A., Buda, K., Kryza-Lacombe, M., et al. (2018). Prognostic awareness and communication preferences among caregivers of patients with malignant glioma. *Psychooncology, 27*(3), 817–823. doi:10.1002/pon.4581

27. Wasner, M., Paal, P., & Borasio, G. D. (2013). Psychosocial care for the caregivers of primary malignant brain tumor patients. *J Soc Work End Life Palliat Care, 9*(1), 74–95. doi:10.1080/15524256.2012.758605

28. Beattie, S., Lebel, S., Petricone-Westwood, D., et al. (2017). Balancing give and take between patients and their spousal caregivers in hematopoietic stem cell transplantation. *Psychooncology, 26*(12), 2224–2231.

29. Beattie, S., & Lebel, S. (2011). The experience of caregivers of hematological cancer patients undergoing a hematopoietic stem cell transplant: a comprehensive literature review. *Psychooncology, 20*(11), 1137–1150.

30. D'Souza, A., & Fretham, C. (2017). Current uses and outcomes of hematopoietic cell transplantation (HCT): CIBMTR summary slides, 2017. https://www.cibmtr. org/ReferenceCenter/SlidesReports/SummarySlides/pages/index.aspx. Accessed 22 October 2018.

31. Arnaout, K., Patel, N., Jain, M., El-Amm, J., Amro, F., & Tabbara, I.A. (2014). Complications of allogeneic hematopoietic stem cell transplantation. *Cancer Investig, 32*, 349–362. doi:10.3109/07357907.2014.919301

32. Gemmill, R., Cooke, L., Williams, A. C., & Grant, M. (2011). Informal caregivers of hematopoietic cell transplant patients: a review and recommendations for interventions and research. *Cancer Nurs, 34*(6), E13.

33. Sabo, B., McLeod, D., & Couban, S. (2013). The experience of caring for a spouse undergoing hematopoietic stem cell transplantation: opening Pandora's box. *Cancer Nurs, 36*(1), 29–40.

34. Coleman, K., Flesch, L., Petiniot, L., et al. (2018). Sleep disruption in caregivers of pediatric stem cell recipients. *Pediatr Blood Cancer, 65*(5), e26965.

35. Beattie, S., Lebel, S., & Tay, J. (2013). The influence of social support on hematopoietic stem cell transplantation survival: a systematic review of literature. *PloS One, 8*(4), e61586

36. Bevans, M. F., Mitchell, S. A., & Marden, S. (2008). The symptom experience in the first 100 days following allogeneic hematopoietic stem cell transplantation (HSCT). *Support Care Cancer, 16*(11), 1243–1254.

37. Ross, A., Yang, L., Klagholz, S. D., Wehrlen, L., & Bevans, M. F. (2016). The relationship of health behaviors with sleep and fatigue in transplant caregivers. *Psychooncology, 25*(5), 506–512.

38. Langer, S. L., Yi, J. C., Storer, B. E., & Syrjala, K. L. (2010). Marital adjustment, satisfaction and dissolution among hematopoietic stem cell transplant patients and spouses: a prospective, five-year longitudinal investigation. *Psychooncology, 19*(2), 190–200.

39. Sundaramurthi, T., Wehrlen, L., Friedman, E., Thomas, S., & Bevans, M. (2017). Hematopoietic stem cell transplantation recipient and caregiver factors affecting length of stay and readmission. *Oncol Nurs Forum, 44*(5), 571–579. doi:10.1188/ 17.ONF.571-579.

40. Sannes, T. S., Mikulich-Gilbertson, S. K., Natvig, C. L., Brewer, B. W., Simoneau, T. L., & Laudenslager, M. L. (2018). Caregiver sleep and patient neutrophil engraftment in allogeneic hematopoietic stem cell transplant: a secondary analysis. *Cancer Nurs, 41*(1), 77–85. doi:10.1097/NCC.0000000000000447.

41. Applebaum, A. J., Bevans, M., Son, T., et al. (2016). A scoping review of caregiver burden during allogeneic HSCT: lessons learned and future directions. *Bone Marrow Transplant, 51*(11), 1416.
42. Socié, G., Salooja, N., Cohen, A., et al. (2003). Nonmalignant late effects after allogeneic stem cell transplantation. *Blood, 101*(9), 3373–3385.
43. Poloméni, A., Lapusan, S., Bompoint, C., Rubio, M. T., & Mohty, M. (2016). The impact of allogeneic-hematopoietic stem cell transplantation on patients' and close relatives' quality of life and relationships. *Eur J Oncol Nurs, 21*, 248–256.
44. Bishop, M. M., Curbow, B. A., Springer, S. H., Lee, J. A., & Wingard, J. R. (2011). Comparison of lasting life changes after cancer and BMT: perspectives of long-term survivors and spouses. *Psychooncology, 20*(9), 926–934. doi:10.1002/pon.1812. Epub 2010 Aug 4.
45. Wulff-Burchfield, E. M., Jagasia, M., & Savani, B. N. (2013). Long-term follow-up of informal caregivers after allo-SCT: a systematic review. *Bone Marrow Transplant, 48*(4), 469.
46. Bevans, M., Wehrlen, L., Castro, K., et al. (2014). A problem-solving education intervention in caregivers and patients during allogeneic hematopoietic stem cell transplantation. *J Health Psychol, 19*(5), 602–617. doi:10.1177/1359105313475902. Epub 2013 Mar 7.
47. Armoogum, J., Richardson, A., & Armes, J. (2013). A survey of the supportive care needs of informal caregivers of adult bone marrow transplant patients. *Support Care Cancer, 21*(4), 977–986. doi:10.1007/s00520-012-1615-4. Epub 2012 Oct 20.
48. Jim, H. S., Quinn, G. P., Barata, A., et al. (2014). Caregivers' quality of life after blood and marrow transplantation: a qualitative study. *Bone Marrow Transplant, 49*(9), 1234.
49. Kotronoulas, G., Wengstrom, Y., & Kearney, N. (2013). Sleep patterns and sleep-impairing factors of persons providing informal care for people with cancer: a critical review of the literature. *Cancer Nurs, 36*(1), E1–E15.
50. Majhail, N. S., Rizzo, J. D., Hahn, T., et al. (2013). Pilot study of patient and caregiver out-of-pocket costs of allogeneic hematopoietic cell transplantation. *Bone Marrow Transplant, 48*(6), 865.
51. Preussler, J. M., Mau, L. W., Majhail, N. S., et al. (2016). Patient housing barriers to hematopoietic cell transplantation: results from a mixed-methods study of transplant center social workers. *Support Care Cancer, 24*(3), 1167–1174. doi:10.1007/s00520-015-2872-9. Epub 2015 Aug 15.
52. Bevans, M., Wehrlen, L., Castro, K., et al. (2014). A problem-solving education intervention in caregivers and patients during allogeneic hematopoietic stem cell transplantation. *J Health Psychol, 19*(5), 602–617.
53. Bambauer, K. Z., Zhang, B., Maciejewski, P. K., et al. (2006). Mutuality and specificity of mental disorders in advanced cancer patients and caregivers. *Soc Psychiatry Psychiatr Epidemiol, 41*, 819–824.
54. Miovic, M., & Block, S. (2007). Psychiatric disorders in advanced cancer. *Cancer, 110*, 1665–1676.
55. Mitchell, A. J., Chan, M., Bhatti, H., et al. (2011). Prevalence of depression, anxiety, and adjustment disorder in oncological, haematological, and palliative-care settings: a meta-analysis of 94 interview-based studies. *Lancet Oncol, 12*, 160–174.
56. Mehnert, A., Brähler, E., Faller, H., et al. (2014). Four-week prevalence of mental disorders in patients with cancer across major tumor entities. *J Clin Oncol, 32*, 3540–3546.

57. Hartung, T. J., Brähler, E., Faller, H., et al. (2017). The risk of being depressed is significantly higher in cancer patients than in the general population: prevalence and severity of depressive symptoms across major cancer types. *Eur J Cancer*, 72, 46–53.

58. Kurtz, M. E., Kurtz, J. C., Given, C. W., & Given, B. (1995). Relationship of caregiver reactions and depression to cancer patients' symptoms, functional states and depression—a longitudinal view. *Soc Sci Med*, 40, 837–846.

59. Cotrim, H., & Pereira, G. (2008). Impact of colorectal cancer on patient and family: implications for care. *Eur J Oncol Nurs*, 12, 217–226.

60. Kurtz, M. E., Kurtz, J. C., Given, C. W., & Given, B. A. (2005). Depression and physical health among family caregivers of geriatric patients with cancer—a longitudinal view. *Med Sci Monit*, 10, CR447–CR456.

61. Howard, L. M., Barley, E. A., Davies, E., et al. (2010). Cancer diagnosis in people with severe mental illness: practical and ethical issues. *Lancet Oncol*, 11, 797–804.

62. Seeman, M. V. (2017). Schizophrenia and cancer: low incidence, high mortality. *Res J Oncol*, 1, 1–6.

63. Baillargeon, J., Kuo, Y. F., Lin, Y. L., Raji, M. A., Singh, A., & Goodwin, J. S. (2011). Effect of mental disorders on diagnosis, treatment, and survival of older adults with colon cancer. *J Am Geriatr Soc*, 59, 1268–1273.

64. Iglay, K., Santorelli, M. L., Hirshfield, K. M., et al. (2017). Impact of preexisting mental illness on all-cause and breast cancer–specific mortality in elderly patients with breast cancer. *J Clin Oncol*, 35, 4012–4018.

65. Iglay, K., Santorelli, M. L., Hirshfield, K. M., et al. (2017). Diagnosis and treatment delays among elderly breast cancer patients with pre-existing mental illness. *Breast Cancer Res Treat*, 166, 267–275.

66. Irwin, K. E., Park, E. R., Shin, J. A., et al. (2017). Predictors of disruptions in breast cancer care for individuals with schizophrenia. *Oncologist*, 22, 1–9.

67. Liao, C. C., Shen, W. W., Chang, C. C., Chang, H., & Chen, T. L. (2013). Surgical adverse outcomes in patients with schizophrenia: a population-based study. *Ann Surg*, 257, 433–438.

68. Cole, M., & Padmanabhan, A. (2012). Breast cancer treatment of women with schizophrenia and bipolar disorder from Philadelphia, PA: lessons learned and suggestions for improvement. *J Cancer Educ*, 27, 774–779.

69. Irwin, K. E., Henderson, D. C., Knight, H. P., & Pirl, W. F. (2014). Cancer care for individuals with schizophrenia. *Cancer*, 120, 323–334.

70. Perese, E. F. (2007). Stigma, poverty, and victimization: roadblocks to recovery for individuals with severe mental illness. *J Am Psychiatr Nurses Assoc*, 13, 285–295.

71. Saunders, J. C. (2003). Families living with severe mental illness: a literature review. *Issues Mental Health Nurs*, 24, 175–198.

72. Trivedi, J. K. (2006). Cognitive deficits in psychiatric disorders: current status. *Indian J Psychiatry*, 48, 10–20.

73. Akaho, R., Sasaki, T., Yoshino, M., Hagiya, K., Akiyama, H., & Sakamaki, H. (2003). Bone marrow transplantation in subjects with mental disorders. *Psychiatry Clin Neurosci*, 57, 311–315.

74. Danzer, G., & Rieger, S. M. (2016). Improving medication adherence for severely mentally ill adults by decreasing coercion and increasing cooperation. *Bull Menninger Clin*, 80, 30–48.

75. DiMatteo, M. R., Lepper, H. S., & Croghan, T. W. (2000). Depression is a risk factor for noncompliance with medical treatment: meta-analysis of the effects of anxiety and depression on patient adherence. *Arch Intern Med*, 160, 2101–2107.

76. Kane, J. M., Kishimoto, T., & Correll, C. U. (2013). Non-adherence to medication in patients with psychotic disorders: epidemiology, contributing factors and management strategies. *World Psychiatry, 12*, 216–226.
77. Lacro, J. P., Dunn, L. B., Dolder, C. R., Leckband, S. G., & Jeste, D. V. (2002). Prevalence of and risk factors for medication nonadherence in patients with schizophrenia: a comprehensive review of recent literature. *J Clin Psychiatry, 63*, 892–909.
78. Fredriksen-Goldsen, K. I., Shiu, C. S., Starks, H., et al. (2011). "You must take the medications for you and for me": family caregivers promoting HIV medication adherence in China. *AIDS Patient Care STDs, 25*, 735–741.
79. Trivedi, R. B., Bryson, C. L., Udris, E., & Au, D. H. (2012). The influence of informal caregivers on adherence in COPD patients. *Ann Behav Med, 44*, 66–72.

CHAPTER 5

Sociocultural Investigation of Cancer Caregiving

PATRICIA B. PEDREIRA,
HANNAH-ROSE MITCHELL, AMANDA TING,
AND YOUNGMEE KIM

Family members and close friends play an integral role in providing care and support to cancer patients and survivors along the disease trajectory, making an invaluable contribution to the medical system and to society. Yet, substantial variation exists regarding who is likely to engage in caregiving and, when engaged, how stressful the experience is.[1,2] This is probably because the complexity and scope of care provided by family caregivers depend not only on patients' disease characteristics, but also on the sociocultural factors embedded in caregivers. This chapter provides theoretical perspectives and empirical findings to develop a comprehensive understanding of the role of sociocultural factors in caregiving involvement, caregiving stress, caregivers' unmet needs, and caregivers' quality-of-life (QOL) outcomes (Figure 5.1). Due to a paucity of studies investigating the role of sociocultural factors in cancer caregiving, we broadened our review to caregiving research in general.

ROLE OF SOCIOCULTURAL FACTORS IN CAREGIVING INVOLVEMENT

Who cares for relatives with cancer? When a circumstance arises in which a relative or member of society is in need of care, those who have been

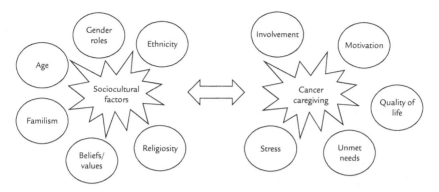

Figure 5.1: Sociocultural correlates of cancer caregiving.

reinforced for their nurturing behaviors are often expected to engage in caregiving and are more likely to do so. This is according to the gender role socialization perspective,[3,4] which assumes gender differences in caregiving: Women and highly feminine individuals engage in caregiving behaviors largely as a byproduct of social, developmental, and learning processes.[5] On the other hand, a "doing gender" approach emphasizes that gender is a social construct that emerges by enacting the internalized ideals of behaviors formed by interactions with others.[6] This approach suggests that a behavior (e.g., caregiving) is not determined by an individual's gender identity, but by the relational and institutional context in which the individual enacts his or her gendered self and sexual identity.[7] From this perspective, those who have culturally embedded characteristics related to communalism and nurturing the family, regardless of gender per se, are likely to assume the caregiving role.

Family caregiving is more prevalent among African Americans,[8,9] Asians,[10,11] and Hispanics/Latinos[12-14] than European Americans, as ethnic minority populations are growing at a faster rate in the United States and are less likely to use formal support services.[15] One key construct related to communal cultural values is *familism*, which refers to a "strong identification and attachment of individuals with their families (nuclear and extended) and strong feelings of loyalty, reciprocity and solidarity among members of the same family" (p. 398).[14] Familism is a motivating factor for providing informal care.[16] It conveys the expectation that the extended family will assist with the care of older relatives.[17,18] It is widely demonstrated that minorities in the United States have high levels of familism, which is not the case for the majority group. For many African Americans, Asian Americans, and Hispanic/Latino Americans, providing care for one's family is culturally ingrained, and assuming the caregiver role is done without question. In contrast, caregiving does not appear to be culturally prescribed for European Americans.[19]

ROLE OF SOCIOCULTURAL FACTORS
IN CAREGIVING STRESS

The model of caregiving stress and health[20,21] posits that the likelihood that a stressor (e.g., illness in the family) will create psychological distress and trigger poor health habits depends on the caregiver's characteristics, both hardwired (e.g., gender and disposition) and mutable (e.g., coping and social support). Supporting this model, a plethora of studies has shown several *nonmodifiable, demographic factors* as significant predictors of caregiving stress, including younger age, female gender, low socioeconomic status, and lack of health insurance.[2] In contrast, the role of *mutable, sociocultural factors* in determining caregiving stress has been studied far less, despite the fact that stress appraisal of the caregiving situation may be particularly relevant to understand individual and group differences in health disparities among minorities. In this section, we review the sociocultural factors that are relevant to caregiving stress and propose future studies that will fill the current gap in our knowledge on the role of sociocultural factors in caregiving stress.

Familism has generally been viewed as a protective factor against caregiving stress among minority caregivers.[22] In Asian culture, family caregiving is considered a key virtue and an integral element, as it is seen as a way to repay parents and other family members.[23] For example, family caregivers in Thailand report lower levels of caregiving burden, as taking care of ill relatives is considered an ordinary responsibility in Thai culture, in which it is believed one should repay the goodness received from one's relatives.[24] From this perspective, the caregiver role is more welcomed, a perspective that may be protective against stress. Yet, there are also ways in which familism appears to aggravate caregiving stress, such as predicting less use of formal support services,[25-27] thus keeping more burden on the family.[28,29] Caregiving responsibilities often create demands that make family caregivers vulnerable to psychological distress and hinder their social engagement outside the family.[30-33] Therefore, those high in familism may face these additional burdens as they take on the caregiver role out of obligation.

Ethnic/racial minority caregivers in the United States are likely to be part of the "sandwich generation" with multiple social roles, including being caregivers for both the younger and older generations.[34-37]

Compared with white caregivers, African American caregivers have reported more hours spent caregiving throughout the illness phases. Although they also reported receiving greater instrumental social support 1 year after diagnosis, independent of cancer stage and comorbidities,[38] African American and Hispanic caregivers reported significantly more difficulty with taking time off from work, compared with white counterparts.[39] The commitment to caregiving for ill family members in the absence of adequate social support may create problems in other social roles (e.g., employment), thereby exacerbating stress. Thus, a strong sense of familism, *familial obligation* in particular, may be related to greater caregiving stress.

Support networks are shown to be wider and stronger among ethnic/racial minority caregivers than among white caregivers. This is reflective of the cultural values of collectivism, interdependence, and strong family ties.[40–45] Other studies regarding social support network size, however, were inconsistent, suggesting that informal support may not always be so available for ethnic/racial minority caregivers. One study found that Mexican American caregivers had smaller social support networks and received less support than white caregivers.[13] It may be that the disruption of social ties associated with *immigration* might remove culturally expected sources of assistance and diminish available support.[46] Thus, examining the effects of social support in conjunction with length of residence in the United States is required.

Gender is another social factor consistently shown to be pertinent to caregiving stress, beyond caregiving involvement. Women are expected to be family caregivers in many cultures[4,47] and represent 75% of caregivers in the United States.[34] Thus, they often perceive providing care as doing simply what they are supposed to do. With this expectation, and often being the sole caregivers of sick husbands, female caregivers have reported more burden and less self-esteem from providing care than do male caregivers.[48,49] In contrast, when men fulfill a caregiver role that is typically not expected of them, they often report feeling good about themselves as a result.[50–53] These studies suggest that female *gender-stereotypic* individuals would report greater caregiving stress.

Religiosity has also been implicated in caregiver adjustment, especially among ethnic/racial minority caregivers.[22,54] The use of religious coping to find personal and spiritual meaning in the caregiving experience appears to buffer caregiving stress.[55,56] Similarly, higher religious commitment and greater availability of informal support from one's religious community or fellow church members appear to contribute to lessening caregiving stress among African Americans and Hispanics/Latinos.[56]

Preexisting stressors include various types of chronic stress, such as minority status, lower socioeconomic status, and perceived discrimination. The burden from preexisting stressors may reduce the ability to manage a new stressor, such as caregiving.[57] Ethnic minorities (African Americans and Hispanic/Latino Americans), compared to non-Hispanic whites, have displayed dysregulated patterns of neuroendocrine functioning that are a manifestation of greater stress, regardless of caregiver status.[58,59] Supporting the common assumption of the chronic stress literature, caregivers of lower socioeconomic status—particularly when managing more advanced illness—reported greater caregiving stress, which is consistent across different ethnic groups and countries.[60] Individuals who perceive discrimination, such as being mistreated or disrespected by other people, are also vulnerable to experiencing elevated caregiving stress, as perceived discrimination has been a significant predictor of various aspects of QOL, independent of the effects of ethnicity/race.[61,62]

Perceived discrimination has been associated with poor mental and physical health of patients with chronic illnesses,[63] poor neuroendocrine functioning,[64,65] and dysregulated sympathetic nervous system activity, marked by shorter telomere length.[66,67] Among caregivers of patients with traumatic brain injury, perceived discrimination was significantly associated with caregiving stress.[68] However, the role of perceived discrimination in stress among cancer caregivers is unknown to date. Findings suggest the need for investigating chronic preexisting stressors, such as low socioeconomic status and perceived discrimination, in conjunction with the other sociocultural factors reviewed previously to better understand cancer caregiving stress.

ROLE OF SOCIOCULTURAL FACTORS IN CAREGIVERS' UNMET NEEDS

Caregiver needs related to caring for oneself, the patient, and other family members span the psychosocial, medical, financial, and daily activity domains.[69] Results from a nationwide study in the United States that surveyed caregivers 2 months, 2 years, and 5 years after the patients' diagnoses showed that caregivers had a variety of unmet needs. Among those, psychosocial unmet needs were consistently the most prevalent (36.0%–67.9%) across the three survivorship phases studied. Although unmet needs in all domains declined, with fewer reported in longer term survivorship than around the time of diagnosis and treatment, a substantial proportion of caregivers continued to report their needs not being met at longer term survivorship phases.[69,70] These findings underscore the urgent call to develop comprehensive programs that address the diverse needs of family caregivers throughout the illness trajectory.

Studies have reported inconsistent findings regarding the associations of caregivers' demographic characteristics (age, gender, education, employment, and spousal relationship) and unmet needs.[71] On the other hand, psychosocial characteristics, such as greater levels of anxiety and depression and low social support and relationship satisfaction, have been consistently associated with increased caregivers' unmet needs.[71,72] Findings suggest that healthcare providers should screen and consider caregivers' existing psychosocial conditions to provide them with quality care. Future studies should investigate the sociocultural and biobehavioral mechanisms influencing the relationship between caregivers' psychosocial characteristics and their unmet needs. Additionally, studies should cross-culturally examine changing patterns of cancer caregivers' unmet needs throughout the survivorship trajectory and identify their common and unique sociocultural factors.

ROLE OF SOCIOCULTURAL FACTORS
IN CAREGIVERS' QUALITY-OF-LIFE OUTCOMES

Quality of life is a multidimensional construct with mental/social, physical, psychological, and spiritual components.[1,54,73,74] The levels of caregivers' QOL vary depending on the patient's illness trajectory. For example, around 2 years after the initial diagnosis, caregivers from a nationwide survey study in the United States reported comparable levels of QOL to US norms in various domains, except the spiritual, in which caregivers reported heightened awareness of spirituality compared to population norms. Caregivers' age and income and their patients' mental and physical functioning were significantly associated with caregivers' QOL.[75] However, around 8 years postdiagnosis, caregivers reported comparable levels of QOL with US norms across various domains. Caregivers' demographic (i.e., age) and early caregiving characteristics (i.e., caregiving stress and caregiver esteem) were significantly associated with QOL at the 8-year mark. In addition, being bereaved at that point predicted poorer mental health and greater psychological distress, independent of contributions of demographic and early caregiving characteristics.[76]

Importantly, cultural values, beliefs, and family systems appear to account for substantial variations in psychosocial correlates of caregivers' QOL.[77] For instance, patients' emotional QOL was not significantly related to their caregivers' QOL in Taiwan[78]; in contrast, it was related in the United States and the Netherlands.[79,80] This cross-cultural difference might be due in part to Taiwanese people's greater emphasis on values of modesty and harmony, which lead them to minimize or even avoid expressing emotions (particularly distress), thus experiencing less awareness of each other's emotional state. Other sociocultural factors, such as social support and family hardiness, have also been shown to buffer caregiving stress effects on QOL.[24]

IMPLICATIONS OF SOCIOCULTURAL FACTORS' IMPACT ON CANCER CAREGIVING

Elevated caregiving stress is a concern not only because stressed caregivers may be inefficient at providing quality care to ill relatives,[81] but also because it impairs caregivers' own mental and physical health.[21,33,82] Caregivers' perceptions of their role, which are influenced by sociocultural norms, may contribute to their appraisal of stress.[83] Thus, identifying demographic and sociocultural factors associated with caregiving stress would be the first step in addressing subsequent health disparities in cancer caregivers. The studies reviewed in this chapter have begun to provide valuable evidence that sociocultural factors play a significant role in caregiving involvement and subsequent experiences.

Generalizability of the existing broad caregiving literature that is mainly from non–cancer caregivers to cancer caregivers, however, needs to be carefully evaluated for two primary reasons. First, cancer caregiving has a trajectory and associated burdens that differ from those of other chronic diseases.[84] Family members of cancer patients often face a sudden diagnosis of cancer, which brings immediate turmoil, as cancer is typically perceived as a life-threatening disease. In addition, family caregivers are "on call" throughout different phases of cancer survivorship; the patients' need for care tends to be sporadic, although it peaks around the time of diagnosis and treatment, again if there is cancer recurrence, and at end of life. Therefore, caregiver involvement may depend heavily on who is immediately available and present, especially among individualistic societies.

In individualistic societies, the caregiver is most likely an adult who lives with the patient in the same household or nearby to help manage practical concerns. To help manage emotional and psychosocial concerns, however, the caregiver is likely to be any family member or close friend. In contrast, in collectivistic societies, whoever is defined as a "family-like" member would be involved in caregiving, making themselves available and present. Caregiving tasks may be more evenly distributed among a larger number of family members and close friends, although friends are more likely to be in and out of the caregiver role throughout the illness trajectory. Investigating caregiver networks across various sociocultural groups and their differences in caregiving stress and QOL is highly warranted. Such information will set the cornerstone of research on health disparities and precision medicine in caregivers.

Multigenerational involvement in caregiving is another area of research and clinical practice that is unique to cancer caregiving but requires further study. Grandparents involved in caregiving for grandchildren with cancer and grandchildren involved in cancer caregiving for their grandparents are two of the most understudied yet fastest growing groups of caregivers.[34] Multigenerational involvement is also common in ethnic minorities.[34] Whether and how the involvement in cancer caregiving at an early age would exert a long-term impact on the caregivers' life and whether grandparental caregiving may be associated with different caregiver and patient outcomes need to be investigated. Furthermore, the role of sociocultural factors reviewed previously and its interplay with age, cohort/generation, and life span are currently unknown. Whether the patterns and consequences of caregiving may be influenced by the sociocultural factors reviewed in this chapter, as well as the extent to which the bidirectional relationship holds true, as depicted in Figure 5.1, should also be further investigated.

A fatalistic or deterministic view of cancer may result in avoiding getting screened, diagnosed, or treated, which is likely related to being diagnosed at a later cancer stage and having a poor prognosis.[85] Investigations of fatalistic or deterministic views and behaviors may have major implications for cancer prevention and control. Findings may help uncover the key factors related to cancer preventive behaviors, such as cancer screening, healthy diet, and exercise, as well as identify crucial sociocultural factors protecting against or aggravating the adverse effects of cancer on informal caregivers, cancer patients, and survivors.

Investigating the role of sociocultural factors in caregiving has begun to gain momentum, even though it is still in its infancy in the field of cancer caregiving research and clinical practice. Taking socioculturally tailored and targeted approaches is necessary to identify subgroups of caregivers who are vulnerable to the adverse effects of cancer in the family and to develop evidence-based interventions. Integration of issues related to caregiver sociocultural resources and risk factors, life span stage, and the medical trajectory of the patients to the emerging area of cancer caregiver research and practice is warranted for improving the QOL of those touched by cancer and minimizing their premature mortality and morbidity. Transdisciplinary and cross-cultural collaborations are necessary to achieve this ultimate mission globally.

REFERENCES

1. Kim Y, Given BA. Quality of life of family caregivers of cancer survivors. *Cancer*. 2008;112(S11):2556–2568.
2. Pinquart M, Sörensen S. Gender differences in caregiver stressors, social resources, and health: an updated meta-analysis. *J Gerontol B Psychol Sci Soc Sci*. 2006;61(1):P33–P45.
3. Barusch AS, Spaid WM. Gender differences in caregiving: why do wives report greater burden? *Gerontologist*. 1989;29(5):667–676.
4. Gilligan C. *In a Different Voice: Psychological Theory and Women's Development*. Cambridge, MA: Harvard University Press; 1982.
5. Friedemann ML, Buckwalter KC. Family caregiver role and burden related to gender and family relationships. *J Fam Nurs*. 2014;20(3):313–336.
6. West C, Zimmerman DH. Doing gender. *Gend Soc*. 1987;1(2):125–151.
7. Schofield T, Connell RW, Walker L, Wood JF, Butland DL. Understanding men's health and illness: a gender-relations approach to policy, research, and practice. *J ACH*. 2000;48(6):247–256.
8. Dilworth-Anderson P, Brummett BH, Goodwin P, Williams SW, Williams RB, Siegler IC. Effect of race on cultural justifications for caregiving. *J Gerontol B Psychol Sci Soc Sci*. 2005;60(5):S257–S262.
9. Franklin DL, James AD. *Ensuring inequality: The structural transformation of the African-American family*. New York, NY: Oxford University Press; 2015.
10. Chan SWC. Family caregiving in dementia: the Asian perspective of a global problem. *Dement Geriatr Cogn Disord*. 2010;30(6):469–478.
11. Tang ST, Li C-Y, Liao Y-C. Factors associated with depressive distress among Taiwanese family caregivers of cancer patients at the end of life. *Palliat Med*. 2007;21(3):249–257.
12. Gallagher-Thompson D, Aréan P, Coon D, et al. Development and implementation of intervention strategies for culturally diverse caregiving populations. In: Schulz R, ed. *Handbook on Dementia Caregiving: Evidence-Based Interventions for Family Caregivers*. New York, NY: Springer; 2000:151–185.
13. Phillips LR, Ardon ETd, Komnenich P, Killeen M, Rusinak R. The Mexican American caregiving experience. *Hisp J Behav Sci*. 2000;22(3):296–313.
14. Sabogal F, Marín G, Otero-Sabogal R, Marín BV, Perez-Stable EJ. Hispanic familism and acculturation: what changes and what doesn't? *Hisp J Behav Sci*. 1987;9(4):397–412.
15. Napoles AM, Chadiha L, Eversley R, Moreno-John G. Reviews: Developing culturally sensitive dementia caregiver interventions: are we there yet? *Am J Alzheimers Dis Other Demen*. 2010;25(5):389–406.
16. Becker G, Beyene Y, Newsom E, Mayen N. Creating continuity through mutual assistance: intergenerational reciprocity in four ethnic groups. *J Gerontol B Psychol Sci Soc Sci*. 2003;58(3):S151–S159.
17. Clark M, Huttlinger K. Elder care among Mexican American families. *Clin Nurs Res*. 1998;7(1):64–81.

18. Cox C, Monk A. Hispanic culture and family care of Alzheimer's patients. *Health Soc Work*. 1993;18(2):92–100.
19. Pharr JR, Dodge Francis C, Terry C, Clark MC. Culture, caregiving, and health: exploring the influence of culture on family caregiver experiences. *ISRN Public Health*. 2014;2014:8.
20. Pearlin LI, Mullan JT, Semple SJ, Skaff MM. Caregiving and the stress process: an overview of concepts and their measures. *Gerontologist*. 1990;30(5):583–594.
21. Vitaliano PP, Zhang J, Scanlan JM. Is caregiving hazardous to one's physical health? A meta-analysis. *Psychol Bull*. 2003;129(6):946–972.
22. Coon DW, Rubert M, Solano N, et al. Well-being, appraisal, and coping in Latina and Caucasian female dementia caregivers: findings from the REACH study. *Aging Ment Health*. 2004;8(4):330–345.
23. Cui J, Song LJ, Zhou LJ, Meng H, Zhao JJ. Needs of family caregivers of advanced cancer patients: a survey in Shanghai of China. *Eur J Cancer Care*. 2014;23(4):562–569.
24. Meecharoen W, Sirapo-ngam Y, Monkong S, Oratai P, Northouse LL. Factors influencing quality of life among family caregivers of patients with advanced cancer: a causal model. *Pac Rim Int J Nurs Res Thail*. 2013;17(4):304–316.
25. Horowitz CR. The role of the family and the community in the clinical setting. In: Loue S, ed. *Handbook of Immigrant Health*. Boston, MA: Springer; 1998: 163–182.
26. Kosloski K, Montgomery RJV, Youngbauer JG. Utilization of respite services: a comparison of users, seekers, and nonseekers. *J Appl Gerontol*. 2001;20(1): 111–132.
27. Strain LA, Blandford AA. Community-based services for the taking but few takers: reasons for nonuse. *J Appl Gerontol*. 2002;21(2):220–235.
28. Gaugler JE, Kane RL, Kane RA, Clay T, Newcomer R. Caregiving and institutionalization of cognitively impaired older people: utilizing dynamic predictors of change. *Gerontologist*. 2003;43(2):219–229.
29. Yaffe K, Fox P, Newcomer R, et al. Patient and caregiver characteristics and nursing home placement in patients with dementia. *JAMA*. 2002;287(16):2090–2097.
30. Covinsky KE, Goldman L, Cook EF, et al. The impact of serious illness on patients' families. SUPPORT Investigators. Study to understand prognoses and preferences for outcomes and risks of treatment. *JAMA*. 1994;272(23):1839–1844.
31. Donelan K, Hill CA, Hoffman C, et al. Challenged to care: informal caregivers in a changing health system. *Health Aff (Millwood)*. 2002;21(4):222–231.
32. Pinquart M, Sörensen S. Differences between caregivers and noncaregivers in psychological health and physical health: a meta-analysis. *Psychol Aging*. 2003;18(2):250–267.
33. Schulz R, Beach SR. Caregiving as a risk factor for mortality: the Caregiver Health Effects Study. *JAMA*. 1999;282(23):2215–2219.
34. National Alliance for Caregiving and AARP Public Policy. *Caregiving in the US. 2015*. Bethesda, MD, & Washington, DC: AARP Public Policy Institute; 2015.
35. Toseland RW, McCallion P, Gerber T, Banks S. Predictors of health and human services use by persons with dementia and their family caregivers. *Soc Sci Med*. 2002;55(7):1255–1266.
36. Ho CJ, Weitzman PF, Cui X, Levkoff SE. Stress and service use among minority caregivers to elders with dementia. *J Gerontol Soc Work*. 2000;33(1):67–88.
37. Wallace SP, Lew-Ting CY. Getting by at home. Community-based long-term care of Latino elders. *West J Med*. 1992;157(3):337–344.

38. Martin MY, Sanders S, Griffin JM, et al. Racial variation in the cancer caregiving experience: a multisite study of colorectal and lung cancer caregivers. *Cancer Nurs.* 2012;35(4):249–256.

39. Siefert ML, Williams A-L, Dowd MF, Chappel-Aiken L, McCorkle R. The caregiving experience in a racially diverse sample of cancer family caregivers. *Cancer Nurs.* 2008;31(5):399–407.

40. Connell CM, Gibson GD. Racial, ethnic, and cultural differences in dementia caregiving: review and analysis. *Gerontologist.* 1997;37(3):355–364.

41. Giunta N, Chow J, Scharlach AE, Dal Santo TS. Racial and ethnic differences in family caregiving in California. *J Hum Behav Soc Environ.* 2004;9(4):85–109.

42. Dilworth-Anderson P, Williams IC, Gibson BE. Issues of race, ethnicity, and culture in caregiving research: a 20-year review (1980–2000). *Gerontologist.* 2002;42(2):237–272.

43. Aranda MP, Knight BG. The influence of ethnicity and culture on the caregiver stress and coping process: a socio-cultural review and analysis. *Gerontologist.* 1997;37(3):342–354.

44. Smerglia VL, Deimling GT, Barresi CM. Black/white family comparisons in helping and decision-making networks of impaired elderly. *Fam Relat.* 1988;37(3):305–309.

45. Tennstedt SL, Chang B-H, Delgado M. Patterns of long-term care: a comparison of Puerto Rican, African-American, and non-Latino white elders. *J Gerontol Soc Work.* 1998;30(1–2):179–199.

46. Neufeld A, Harrison MJ, Stewart MJ, Hughes KD, Spitzer D. Immigrant women: making connections to community resources for support in family caregiving. *Qual Health Res.* 2002;12(6):751–768.

47. Chodorow N. *The Reproduction of Mothering.* Berkeley, CA: University of California Press; 1978.

48. Collins C, Jones R. Emotional distress and morbidity in dementia carers: a matched comparison of husbands and wives. *Int J Geriatr Psychiatry.* 1997;12(12):1168–1173.

49. Rose-Rego SK, Strauss ME, Smyth KA. Differences in the perceived well-being of wives and husbands caring for persons with Alzheimer's disease. *Gerontologist.* 1998;38(2):224–230.

50. Allen SM, Goldscheider F, Ciambrone DA. Gender roles, marital intimacy, and nomination of spouse as primary caregiver. *Gerontologist.* 1999;39(2):150–158.

51. Majerovitz SD, Revenson TA. Sexuality and rheumatic disease: the significance of gender. *Arthritis Care Res.* 1994;7(1):29–34.

52. Kaye LW, Applegate JS. Men as elder caregivers: a response to changing families. *Am J Orthopsychiatry.* 1990;60(1):86–95.

53. Kim Y, Loscalzo MJ, Wellisch DK, Spillers RL. Gender differences in caregiving stress among caregivers of cancer survivors. *Psychooncology.* 2006;15(12):1086–1092.

54. Haley WE, LaMonde LA, Han B, Burton AM, Schonwetter R. Predictors of depression and life satisfaction among spousal caregivers in hospice: application of a stress process model. *J Palliat Med.* 2003;6(2):215–224.

55. Colgrove LA, Kim Y, Thompson N. The effect of spirituality and gender on the quality of life of spousal caregivers of cancer survivors. *Ann Behav Med.* 2007;33(1):90–98.

56. Pinquart M, Sorensen S. Ethnic differences in stressors, resources, and psychological outcomes of family caregiving: a meta-analysis. *Gerontologist.* 2005;45(1):90–106.

57. Cohen S, Janicki-Deverts D, Miller GE. Psychological stress and disease. *JAMA*. 2007;298(14):1685–1687.

58. Gallagher-Thompson D, Shurgot GR, Rider K, et al. Ethnicity, stress, and cortisol function in Hispanic and non-Hispanic white women: a preliminary study of family dementia caregivers and noncaregivers. *Am J Geriatr Psychiatry*. 2006;14(4):334–342.

59. McCallum TJ, Sorocco KH, Fritsch T. Mental health and diurnal salivary cortisol patterns among African American and European American female dementia family caregivers. *Am J Geriatr Psychiatry*. 2006;14(8):684–693.

60. Pinquart M, Sörensen S. Correlates of physical health of informal caregivers: a meta-analysis. *J Gerontol B*. 2007;62(2):P126–P137.

61. Lewis TT, Barnes LL, Bienias JL, Lackland DT, Evans DA, Mendes de Leon CF. Perceived discrimination and blood pressure in older African American and white adults. *J Gerontol A Biol Sci Med Sci*. 2009;64(9):1002–1008.

62. Williams DR, Yu Y, Jackson JS, Anderson NB. Racial differences in physical and mental health: socio-economic status, stress and discrimination. *J Health Psychol*. 1997;2(3):335–351.

63. Major B, Mendes WB, Dovidio JF. Intergroup relations and health disparities: a social psychological perspective. *Health Psychol*. 2013;32(5):514–524.

64. Adam EK, Heissel JA, Zeiders KH, et al. Developmental histories of perceived racial discrimination and diurnal cortisol profiles in adulthood: a 20-year prospective study. *Psychoneuroendocrinology*. 2015;62:279–291.

65. Zeiders KH, Hoyt LT, Adam EK. Associations between self-reported discrimination and diurnal cortisol rhythms among young adults: the moderating role of racial-ethnic minority status. *Psychoneuroendocrinology*. 2014;50:280–288.

66. Chae DH, Nuru-Jeter AM, Adler NE, et al. Discrimination, racial bias, and telomere length in African-American men. *Am J Prev Med*. 2014;46(2):103–111.

67. Lee DB, Kim ES, Neblett EW. The link between discrimination and telomere length in African American adults. *Health Psychol*. 2017;36(5):458–467.

68. Phelan SM, Griffin JM, Hellerstedt WL, et al. Perceived stigma, strain, and mental health among caregivers of veterans with traumatic brain injury. *Disabil Health J*. 2011;4(3):177–184.

69. Kim Y, Kashy DA, Spillers RL, Evans TV. Needs assessment of family caregivers of cancer survivors: three cohorts comparison. *Psychooncology*. 2010;19(6):573–582.

70. Girgis A, Lambert SD, McElduff P, et al. Some things change, some things stay the same: a longitudinal analysis of cancer caregivers' unmet supportive care needs. *Psychooncology*. 2013;22(7):1557–1564.

71. Lambert SD, Harrison JD, Smith E, et al. The unmet needs of partners and caregivers of adults diagnosed with cancer: a systematic review. *BMJ Support Palliat Care*. 2012;2(3):224–230.

72. Balfe M, O'Brien K, Timmons A, et al. The unmet supportive care needs of long-term head and neck cancer caregivers in the extended survivorship period. *J Clin Nurs*. 2016;25(11–12):1576–1586.

73. Ferrell BR, Dow KH, Grant M. Measurement of the quality of life in cancer survivors. *Qual Life Research*. 1995;4(6):523–531.

74. Ferrell B, Grant M, Padilla G, Vemuri S, Rhiner M. The experience of pain and perceptions of quality of life: validation of a conceptual model. *Hospice J*. 1991;7(3):9–24.

75. Kim Y, Spillers RL. Quality of life of family caregivers at 2 years after a relative's cancer diagnosis. *Psychooncology*. 2010;19(4):431–440.

76. Kim Y, Shaffer KM, Carver CS, Cannady RS. Quality of life of family caregivers 8 years after a relative's cancer diagnosis: follow-up of the National Quality of Life Survey for Caregivers. *Psychooncology*. 2016;25(3):266–274.

77. Romito F, Goldzweig G, Cormio C, Hagedoorn M, Andersen BL. Informal caregiving for cancer patients. *Cancer*. 2013;119:2160–2169.

78. Chen M-L, Chu L, Chen H-C. Impact of cancer patients' quality of life on that of spouse caregivers. *Support Care Cancer*. 2004;12(7):469–475.

79. Cassileth BR, Lusk EJ, Strouse TB, Miller DS, Brown LL, Cross PA. A psychological analysis of cancer patients and their next-of-kin. *Cancer*. 1985;55(1):72–76.

80. Nijboer C, Triemstra M, Tempelaar R, Sanderman R, van den Bos GAM. Determinants of caregiving experiences and mental health of partners of cancer patients. *Cancer*. 1999;86(4):577–588.

81. Williamson GM, Shaffer DR. Relationship quality and potentially harmful behaviors by spousal caregivers: how we were then, how we are now. The Family Relationships in Late Life Project. *Psychol Aging*. 2001;16(2):217–226.

82. Robinson-Whelen S, Tada Y, MacCallum RC, McGuire L, Kiecolt-Glaser JK. Long-term caregiving: what happens when it ends? *J Abnorm Psychol*. 2001;110(4):573–584.

83. Blum K, Sherman DW. Understanding the experience of caregivers: a focus on transitions. *Semin Oncol Nurs*. 2010;26(4):243–258.

84. Kim Y, Schulz R. Family caregivers' strains: comparative analysis of cancer caregiving with dementia, diabetes, and frail elderly caregiving. *J Aging Health*. 2008;20(5):483–503.

85. Flórez KR, Aguirre AN, Viladrich A, Céspedes A, De La Cruz AA, Abraído-Lanza AF. Fatalism or destiny? A qualitative study and interpretative framework on Dominican women's breast cancer beliefs. *J Immigr Minor Health*. 2009;11(4):291–301.

CHAPTER 6

Measurement of Caregiver Burden

State of the Science and

Future Directions

LAURIE ANDERSON, LAURA C. POLACEK,
AND KIMBERSON TANCO

Caregiver burden is described by Given et al. as a "multidimensional biopsychosocial reaction resulting from an imbalance of care demands relative to caregivers' personal time, social roles, physical and emotional states, financial resources, and formal care resources given the other multiple roles they fulfill."[1,2] Burden may be categorized as either objective (the stress and requirements imposed by the caregiving role) or subjective (the resulting distress experienced by caregivers).[3,4] In the 2015 AARP report of caregiving in the United States, of 1,248 caregivers assessed, cancer was listed as the fourth most common illness of the care recipient, but that which resulted in the highest level of burden.[5] Cancer caregivers generally spend more time providing care than caregivers of patients with other chronic or life-limiting illnesses.[6,7] Among their many responsibilities, caregivers assume medical and financial decision-making and advocate on behalf of patients. This is often without formal training and occurs concurrently with other responsibilities, including caring for other family members. Importantly, the demands of caregiving often continue as patients transition into survivorship. The caregiving role, therefore, has the potential to compromise caregivers' ability to carry out full-time employment and other life goals. Together, these factors contribute to the experience of caregiver burden detailed in previous chapters. As such, the timely detection of caregiver burden can be profoundly beneficial. Here, our aim is to highlight instruments that have been developed and used to assess cancer caregiver burden broadly, as well as specific risk factors for burden.

Caregiver *strain* has often been used interchangeably with caregiver *burden* and refers to factors that may threaten caregiver well-being, their role, and their relationship with the patient.[8,9] Early studies informed the development of the Caregiver Strain Index (CSI),[8-10] one of the earliest tools used to measure strain, originally developed with caregivers of cardiac patients and those recovering from hip surgery.[8] The CSI is a self-report instrument composed of 13 yes/no items that measure employment, financial, physical, social, and temporal factors associated with strain. Scores range from 0 to 13, with higher scores indicating greater strain. The measure was modified into a three-tier response scale (yes, sometimes, no) after long-term caregivers (i.e., providing care from 3 months to 30 years) expressed an interest in having a middle response category to better reflect their extended caregiving experiences. This modified scale demonstrated internal and test-retest reliability.[11] The CSI has been used with caregivers of patients who suffered a stroke, those with advanced heart failure, and patients with cancer in a community palliative care setting.[12-15]

A variety of instruments that assess caregiver burden exists for both clinical and research purposes. Many of these, such as the Zarit Burden Interview (ZBI) and Bakas Caregiving Outcomes Scale, were developed initially for use among caregivers of dementia and stroke patients, respectively.[16-18] They were subsequently validated in the oncology setting.[19,20] In their review, Deeken et al. illustrated the increase in complexity and psychometric testing of caregiver burden assessments over time.[3] These instruments initially measured emotional strain as a unidimensional construct, with later measures developed to distinguish between objective and subjective burden. More recently, Tanco et al. reviewed instruments that were used to evaluate burden among caregivers of adult and pediatric cancer patients.[3,15,21-23] They found that 35% of the 26 instruments reviewed were considered appropriate for delivery in clinical settings, and among those, 56% were validated and reliable self-report tools.[15] In Tables 6.1 and 6.2, we summarize the validated measures most commonly used to evaluate burden among caregivers of adult and pediatric patients with cancer, respectively. Next, we briefly describe several of the instruments listed.

Table 6.1 INSTRUMENTS USED TO ASSESS BURDEN IN CAREGIVERS OF ADULT CANCER PATIENTS

Instrument	Domains Assessed	Original Test Population	Items	Reliability/Validity
Appraisal of Caregiving Scale (ACS)[24]	Harm/loss, threat, challenge, benign	Family members of cancer patients receiving radiotherapy	53 (original version), 27 (revised version)	α = .72–.91/content, construct
Bakas Caregiving Outcomes Scale[18]	None identified	Caregivers of stroke survivors and patients in rehabilitation hospital and support groups	10	α = .77/content, criterion, construct
Brief Assessment Scale for Caregivers (BASC)[25]	Positive and negative personal impact, other family members, medical issues, concern about loved one	Caregivers of patients with chronic illness (cancer, neurological, psychiatric)	14	α = .58–.80/construct
Burden Assessment Scale[26]	Subjective: personal distress, time perspective, guilt Objective: disrupted activities, social functioning	Caregivers of patients with mental illness	19	α = .89–.91/construct
Burden Index of Caregivers[27]	Time dependent, emotional, existential, physical, service related, total burden	Family caregivers of patients with stroke or intractable neurological disease	11	α = .68–.91; test-retest (ICC .83)/construct
Care Task Scale—Cancer (CTS-C)[28]	Accompany patient and monitor care, substitutive care for social and general affairs, communication and emotional care, mobility maintenance care	Spouse caregivers of patients with cancer	37	α = .83–.88; test-retest (r = .92–.94)/construct
Caregiver Burden Inventory[29]	Time dependence, developmental, physical, social, emotional	Caregivers of patients with dementia or organic brain disease	24	α = .73–.86/construct

(continued)

Table 6.1 CONTINUED

Instrument	Domains Assessed	Original Test Population	Items	Reliability/Validity
Caregiver Burden Scale (CBS-E)[30]	General strain, isolation, disappointment, emotional involvement, environment	Caregivers of stroke patients 3 years after primary stroke	22	α = .53–.87/construct
Caregiver Burden Scale (CBS-G)[31]	Relationship with care recipient, personal limitations	Caregivers of psychogeriatric patients	13	α = .77–.84/construct
Caregiver Experience Assessment[32]	Emotional well-being, family environment, carer role, care recipient disability, help needed, help provided, behavior problems	Caregivers of elderly, chronically ill, or disabled patients	75	α = .59–.78/construct
Caregiver Reaction Assessment[33]	Caregiver esteem, lack of family support, impact on finances, impact on schedule, impact on health	Caregivers of elderly patients with dementia/Alzheimer's disease or various physical impairments and cancer patients	24	α = .91 (whole); .80–.90 (subscales)/construct
Caregiver Strain Index (CSI)[8]	Perception of caregiving, care recipient characteristics, emotional status	Family caregivers of elderly hip surgery and heart disease patients	13	α = .86/construct
Caregiver Self-Efficacy Scale (CaSES)[34]	Resilience, self-maintenance, emotional connectivity, instrumental caregiving	Caregivers of patients with advanced cancer	21	α = .73–.94/convergent, divergent
Caregiver's Burden Scale in End-of-Life Care[35]	None identified	Family caregivers of patients receiving palliative care	16	α = .91–.94/construct, convergent
Caregiving Consequences Inventory (CCI)[36]	Mastery, appreciation for others, meaning in life, reprioritization, perceived burden	Bereaved family members of cancer patients	16	α = .78–.93/construct

Measure	Content/dimensions	Population	N	Reliability/Validity
Demand-of-Illness Inventory (DOII)[37]	Physical symptoms, personal meaning, family functioning, social relationships, self-image, monitoring symptoms, treatment issues	Family of mothers with breast cancer, diabetes, and fibrocystic breast changes	125	α = .96/construct, discriminant
Family Appraisal of Caregiving Questionnaire for Palliative Care (FACQ-PC)[38]	Caregiver strain, positive caregiving appraisals, caregiver distress, family well-being	Family caregivers of a relative with cancer	25	α = .73–.86/construct
Family Decision-Making Self-Efficacy Scale[39]	Being a surrogate, choosing treatments, accepting palliative care, meeting spiritual needs, maintaining family harmony, communicating with health professionals	Caregivers to patients with amyotrophic lateral sclerosis (*gradual decline*) and pancreatic cancer (*rapid decline*)	26	α = .91–.95; test-retest r = .96/content
Family's Difficulty Scale (FDS)[40]	Burden of care, concerns about home-care doctor, balance of work and care, patient's pain and condition, concerns about visiting nurse, concerns about home-care service, relationship between family caregivers and their families, funeral preparations	Families caring for cancer patients at end-of-life at home	29	α = .73–.75; test-retest (ICC) r = .75–.85/ convergent, divergent
Parental Cancer Questionnaire[41]	Parental cancer benefits, emotional experiences, caregiver strain	Adult children of parents with cancer	53	α = .87–.91/convergent, discriminant
Perceived Burden Measure[42]	Walking, transportation, housekeeping, farming/yard work, house repairs, cooking, shopping, decision-making, financial record-keeping, eating, administering medication, bathing, dressing, toileting, leaving patient unattended	Caregivers of patients with dementia	15	α = .87/construct

(continued)

Table 6.1 CONTINUED

Instrument	Domains Assessed	Original Test Population	Items	Reliability/Validity
Perceived Burden Scale[43]	Impact on finances, feelings of abandonment, impact on schedule, impact on health, sense of entrapment	Family caregivers of dependent elderly relatives	31	α = .72–.88/criterion
Perceived Family Burden Scale[44]	None identified	Family caregivers of adults with schizophrenia	24	α = .83; test-retest r = .54/ construct
Prostate Care Questionnaire for Carers (PCQ-C)[45]	Carer experience during patient testing, diagnosis, treatment decision-making, treatment administration and monitoring	Caregivers of men with prostate cancer	64	α = .80–.89; test-retest (ICC .52–.83)/content
Screen for Caregiver Burden[46]	Objective burden, subjective burden	Caregivers of patients with Alzheimer's disease	25	α = .85–.88; test-retest r = .70/construct, criterion
Zarit Burden Inventory[16,17]	None identified	Caregivers of patients with senile dementia	29 (original version), 22	α = .93; test-retest r = .89/ construct (based on 22-item version)

ICC = intraclass correlation coefficient

Table 6.2 INSTRUMENTS USED TO ASSESS BURDEN IN CAREGIVERS OF PEDIATRIC CANCER PATIENTS

Instrument	Domains/Sections	Original Test Population	Items	Reliability/Validity
Care of My Child With Cancer (CMCC)[47]	None identified	Primary caregivers of children with cancer	28	α = .93; test-retest r = .90/ content, construct
Parental Coping Strategy Inventory (PCSI)[48]	Learning; struggling; interaction with patient, spouse, and healthy sibling; emotion, information, and actual support; maintaining stability; maintaining an optimistic state of mind; searching for spiritual meaning; increasing religious activities	Parents of children with cancer	48	α = .69–.88/construct
Parental Worry and Attitudes Toward Childhood Cancer[49]	Perseveration of parental worry, psychosocial losses	Parents of childhood cancer survivors	11	α = .91 [Factor 1]; α=.76 [Factor 2]/content
Pediatric Inventory for Parents (PIP)[50]	Medical care, communication, role functioning, emotional functioning	Parents of children with a critical illness, childhood cancer	42	α = .80–.96/construct
Psychosocial Assessment Tool[51]	Family structure, social support, family resources, family problems, stress reaction, family beliefs, child problems, sibling problems	Families of newly diagnosed pediatric oncology patients	20	α = .81; test-retest r = .78–.87/ content

COMPREHENSIVE MEASURES
OF CAREGIVER BURDEN

One of the most commonly used instruments is the ZBI, a self-report measure of various domains of burden, including caregiver health, psychosocial and financial well-being, and the quality of the patient-caregiver relationship.[16,17,23,52] The ZBI was originally developed as a 29-item instrument to measure subjective burden, with scores ranging from 0 (never) to 4 (always), where higher scores indicate greater burden.[17] It was further refined into its most widely used version consisting of 22 items (ZBI-22). Several additional abbreviated versions of the ZBI have been developed, and the original measure has been translated into other languages, including Spanish, Portuguese, Persian, and Burmese.[19,52–58]

Six short-form versions of the ZBI exist (consisting of 12, 8, 7, 6, 4, and 1 items), all of which have demonstrated good correlations with the 22-item instrument, with the exception of the 1-item version, which consists of a global question: *Overall, how burdened do you feel?* Among these, the 12-, 8-, and 4-item versions are the most commonly used, with ZBI-12 achieving the highest level of validity as compared to the ZBI-22.[19] A secondary analysis conducted among caregivers of patients with advanced cancer, dementia, and acquired brain injury highlighted the need to tailor the choice of ZBI version to particular situations; the ZBI-12 was suitable in most situations, while the 6- and 7-item versions were most appropriate in palliative care settings, and 1- and 4-item versions were useful when rapid screening was needed.[19] The ZBI-22 has displayed predictive validity in identifying caregivers at risk for depression[53] and may be most appropriate when investigating the role burden plays in caregiver outcomes. Other examples of self-report measures include the Caregiver Reaction Assessment (CRA),[33] Appraisal of Caregiving Scale (ACS),[24] Perceived Burden Measure,[42] Caregiver Burden Scale (CBS-E),[24] Caregiver Experience Assessment (CEA),[30] Bakas Caregiving Outcomes Scale (BCOS),[18] and the Burden Assessment Scale (BAS).[26] Several of these are described in detail next.

The CRA was originally developed to assess burden in caregivers of patients with Alzheimer disease, cancer, and physical impairments and evaluates multiple social and emotional domains of burden, as well as potential benefits (e.g., sense of competence, self-efficacy) of caregiving.[33] The CRA has demonstrated good reliability and construct validity and consists of 24 items rated on a 5-point Likert scale ranging from "strongly agree" to "strongly disagree." An overall score and five subscale scores (Disrupted Schedule, Financial Problems, Lack of Family Support, Health Problems, and the Impact of Caregiving on Self-Esteem) are generated.[33,59,60]

The ACS is a 27-item instrument measuring positive and negative appraisals of caregiving across three domains (threat, general stress, and benefit). It was originally developed and revised among family caregivers of cancer patients receiving radiotherapy and later psychometrically tested in family caregivers of patients with various advanced cancers.[24,61] Caregivers answer questions related to their caregiving responsibilities, support systems, and effects on their psychosocial, physical, and personal functioning. Items are rated on a 5-point Likert scale ranging from 1 ("very untrue") to 5 ("very true"), with higher scores representing greater intensity of the specific domain.[24,61]

The BCOS was originally developed for family caregivers of stroke patients and subsequently used among caregivers of patients with hematologic and lung cancers.[18,62] The initial version of the BCOS consisted of 10 items that measured life changes associated with caregiving.[18] It was further revised to 15 items and adapted for Greek caregivers of advanced cancer patients receiving palliative radiation.[20,63]

MEASURES THAT ASSESS UNIQUE DOMAINS OF CAREGIVER BURDEN

In addition to comprehensive measures that address the multidimensional nature of burden, assessments of distinct elements of burden have also been widely used to describe the experience of caregivers. We summarize these in Table 6.3. For example, the Edmonton Symptom Assessment System (ESAS) and the Rotterdam Symptom Checklist have been used to evaluate symptom burden among cancer caergivers.[70,82] The Distress Thermometer is a visual analog scale that has been increasingly used to evaluate distress among cancer caregivers, with scores of 4 or greater indicating potentially clinically significant distress.[83,84] The Hospital Anxiety and Depression Scale measures both anxious and depressive symptomatology in clinical and non-clinical populations and has been widely used with cancer patients.[78] The Herth Hope Index measures positive readiness and expectancy for experience, temporality, and future-oriented attitudes and interconnectedness.[77]

Additional instruments used to measure distinct areas of caregiver distress include the Positive and Negative Affect Schedule (PANAS) and the Beck Depression Inventory (BDI).[64,81,85] The PANAS is a brief self-report measure that captures caregivers' positive and negative mood dimensions and can be adapted to measure affect in a number of time frames depending on the given instructions, including the current moment, today, over the past week, over the past year, and generally.[81] The BDI is composed of 21

Instrument	Domains Assessed	Original Test Population	Items	Reliability/Validity
Beck Depression Inventory (BDI)[64]	Depression	Inpatient and outpatient psychiatric patients	21	$\alpha = .91$, test-retest $r = .93$/content, construct, concurrent
Caregiver Well-Being Scale[65,66]	Basic needs, activities of daily living	Family caregivers of adults with dementia, healthy children, and children with severe developmental disabilities	45	$\alpha = .94$/criterion, construct
Distress Thermometer[67,68]	General distress; physical, family, emotional, and spiritual concerns	Patients with prostate cancer	36 (thermometer and 35-item problem list)	Sensitivity = 80.9%, specificity = 60.2%
Duke-UNC Functional Social Support Questionnaire (DUFSS)[69]	General, confidant, and affective support	Primary care patients	14	Item-remainder correlations $r = .62$ (confidant), $r = .64$ (affective); test-retest $r = .66$/construct, concurrent, discriminant
Edmonton Symptom Assessment System (ESAS)[70,71]	Not specified	Patients with advanced cancer	10	$\alpha = .68$–0.80; test-retest $r = .35$–$.80$/ convergent, divergent
Financial Impact Scale[72]	Not specified	Informal long-term caregivers	20	$\alpha = .93$/convergent
Finding Meaning Through Caregiving Scale[73]	Loss/powerlessness, provisional meaning, ultimate meaning	Caregivers of patients with Alzheimer's disease	43	$\alpha = .88$–$.95$, test-retest $r = .80$–$.89$/ convergent, discriminant

Instrument	Domains	Population	Items	Reliability/Validity
Functional Assessment of Chronic Illness Therapy—Spiritual Well-Being (FACIT-Sp)[74]	Meaning/peace, faith	Patients with cancer	12	α = .81–.88/convergent
Health Care Needs Survey (HCN)[75,76]	Information; household, personal, spiritual, psychological care; patient care	Patients with cancer and their caregivers	90	α = .93–.98/content, concurrent
Herth Hope Index[77]	Positive readiness and expectancy for experience, temporality and future-oriented attitudes, interconnectedness	Adults with acute, chronic, and terminal physical illnesses	12	α = .97, test-retest r = .91/criterion, convergent, divergent, construct
Hospital Anxiety and Depression Scale[78]	Anxiety, depression	General health clinic adult outpatients	14	α = .84–.89 (among caregivers)
Multidimensional Scale of Perceived Social Support (MSPSS)[79]	Perceived social support from family, friends, and significant others	University undergraduates	12	α = .81–.98/construct, convergent, discriminant
Needs Assessment of Family Caregivers-Cancer (NAFC-C)[80]	Psychosocial, medical, financial, and daily living needs	Caregivers of cancer survivors	27	α = .56–.86/predictive
Positive and Negative Affect Schedule (PANAS)[81]	Positive and negative affect	Undergraduate college students	10	α = .85–.90
Rotterdam Symptom Checklist[82]	Physical and psychological quality of life	Patients with cancer participating in clinical research	39	α = .82–.95/construct, predictive

items that ask caregivers to evaluate their depressive symptoms over the past week. Responses are scored on a 4-point scale and range from 0 to 63, with higher scores indicating more severe depressive symptomatology.[64]

Measures have also been developed to assess functional well-being among caregivers more generally. The Caregiver Well-Being Scale[65,66,85] assesses functioning across two domains, basic needs and activities of living. Basic needs encompass physical needs, expression of emotion, and self-security, while activities of living include time for self and leisure, family support, household maintenance, household tasks, and participation in social activities outside the home. Originally developed for use with caregivers of healthy and chronically ill adults and children, it has since been used with caregivers of patients with leukemia, among whom it demonstrated strong internal consistency.[86]

As caregivers spend more time providing care, activities and time normally spent for socializing, hobbies, travel, or self-care become limited. This often leads to isolation and strain in their interpersonal relationships, which in turn contribute to caregiver burden.[87-89] Therefore, social support is another important correlate of burden that warrants assessment. The Duke-UNC Functional Social Support Questionnaire (DUFSS) is a 14-item multidimensional measure of social support that provides a general score of overall support and two subscale scores that address confidant support and affective support.[69] Originally developed for use among primary care patients, the DUFSS has since been used with caregivers of children with brain tumors.[90-93] The Multidimensional Scale of Perceived Social Support (MSPSS) is a 12-item measure of perceived social support from family, friends, and significant others that was originally developed for use with university undergraduates.[79] Responses are scored on a seven-interval scale, with higher scores indicating greater perceived social support. The MSPSS has been used with caregivers of patients in the inpatient and outpatient settings and has been translated for use with Turkish-speaking individuals.[94-96]

Financial and temporal burden is also common among caregivers.[87,97,98] With the time, emotional, and physical commitments involved in caring for a patient with cancer, some caregivers are unable to work or are required to reduce their paid employment hours. Therefore, financial strain can be significant. Several of the measures discussed have subscales that address financial strain,[85] while a small number of scales were developed specifically to evaluate financial burden. For example, the Financial Impact Scale, which is composed of 20 items, measures the financial impact of long-term informal caregiving and has demonstrated reliability and validity.[72]

As part of the growing literature surrounding cancer caregiver burden, a number of measures have been used to identify caregivers' unmet needs.[99] For example, the Health Care Needs (HCN) Survey assesses needs across six domains (information, household, personal, spiritual, psychological, and patient care) by asking caregivers to rate the importance of each need and whether or not they are being satisfied.[75] The HCN has demonstrated high internal consistency and concurrent validity among cancer caregivers.[100,101] Similarly, the Needs Assessment of Family Caregivers–Cancer (NAFC-C) rates the importance of psychosocial, medical, financial, and daily living needs and how well they are being met.[80] It was designed for use throughout the cancer trajectory and has shown to have good internal consistency.[66]

Religiosity and spirituality have been shown to promote caregivers' overall well-being.[102] For example, personal faith has been associated with positive coping skills and lowered negative emotions among caregivers both pre- and postbereavement,[102,103] while spiritual distress or negative religious coping has been associated with increased distress, worse physical and emotional well-being, and diminished quality of life.[104] Furthermore, spiritual well-being has been found to be as strongly correlated with quality of life as physical well-being.[105] Therefore, assessing spirituality/religiosity in caregivers can be of great benefit. The Functional Assessment of Chronic Illness Therapy—Spiritual Well-Being (FACIT-Sp) measures spiritual well-being and was developed for and widely used in the cancer setting.[74] Its 12 items measure two main domains of spirituality: sense of meaning and peace in one's life and sense of strength from one's faith.

One of the only measures developed specifically to evaluate existential distress in caregivers is the Finding Meaning Through Caregiving Scale, which is composed of three subscales: Loss/Powerlessness, Provisional Meaning, and Ultimate Meaning. These subscales assess caregivers' feelings of loss for the patient and themselves, powerlessness over the situation, day-to-day meaning of caregiving, and spiritual/religious associations with caregiving.[73] This measure can be used to understand how caregivers find positive meaning in the caregiving role.

MEASUREMENT OF BURDEN IN CAREGIVERS OF PEDIATRIC CANCER PATIENTS

The experience of caregivers of pediatric patients is described as a uniquely challenging one.[106,107] There are a variety of instruments that have been developed specifically to measure various domains of burden, ranging from assessments of the demands of caregiving to the availability of support and resources. For example, the Care of My Child With Cancer (CMCC) is a 28-item instrument that assesses the demands of caregiving in parents of children with cancer.[34] The Psychosocial Assessment Tool (PAT) assesses psychosocial risks of families of children with recently diagnosed cancer and screens for social support and resources, child knowledge and behavioral concerns, family beliefs, and marital and family problems. Higher scores indicate higher psychosocial risk.[51] This instrument was further modified into the PAT 2.0 for better comprehension and usabilty.[108]

The Parental Worry and Attitudes Toward Childhood Cancer instrument was developed to examine parents' attitude toward pediatric cancer survivors[49] and examines two factors, perseveration of parental worry (i.e., concerns about cancer recurrence and survival) and psychosocial losses (i.e., change in the parent's life after coping with their child's cancer).

CONCLUSIONS AND FUTURE DIRECTIONS

Numerous instruments have been developed to assess caregiver burden across a variety of disease settings, some of which have been modified for use with caregivers of cancer patients. More recently, a handful of measures have been developed for use in this population specifically, and many have abbreviated versions for faster and easier administration and translations for use among non-English speakers. While these tools are useful in assessing the presence and severity of burden, they do not consider risk factors for its development. Fortunately, a number of measures targeting risk factors such as depression, anxiety, and general distress have been adapted for use with caregivers and may be particularly useful in predicting or preventing the experience of burden. Moving forward, our primary challenge is incorporating the assessment of both risk factors for and the presence of caregiver burden into routine clinical practice, with the ultimate goal of reducing and preventing burden among caregivers of patients with cancer.

REFERENCES

1. Given B, Kozachik S, Collins C, et al. Caregiver role strain. In Maas M, Buckwalter K, Hardy M, Tripp-Reimer T, Title M., eds., *Nursing Care of Older Adult Diagnoses: Outcome and Interventions*. St. Louis, MO: Mosby; 2001:679–695.
2. Given B, Wyatt G, Given C, et al. Burden and depression among caregivers of patients with cancer at the end-of-life. *Oncol Nurs Forum*. 2004;31(6):1105–1117.

3. Deeken JF, Taylor KL, Mangan P, Yabroff KR, Ingham JM. Care for the caregivers: a review of self-report instruments developed to measure the burden, needs, and quality of life of informal caregivers. *J Pain Symptom Manage*. 2003;26(4):922–953.
4. Hoenig J, Hamilton MW. The schizophrenic patient in the community and his effect on the household. *Int J Soc Psychiatry*. 1966;12:165–176.
5. National Alliance for Caregiving (NAC) and the AARP Public Policy Institute. Caregiving in the US. 2015. https://www.aarp.org/content/dam/aarp/ppi/2015/caregiving-in-the-united-states-2015-report-revised.pdf. Published June 2015. Last Accessed March 23, 2018.
6. Hayman JA, Langa KM, Kabeto MU, et al. Estimating the cost of informal caregiving for elderly patients with cancer. *J Clin Oncol*. 2001;19:3219–3225.
7. Yabroff KR, Kim Y. Time costs associated with informal caregiving for cancer survivors. *Cancer*. 2009;115:4362–4373.
8. Robinson BC. Validation of a Caregiver Strain Index. *J Gerontol*. 1983;38:344–348.
9. Robinson B, Thurnher M. Taking care of aged parents: a family cycle transition. *Gerontologist*. 1979;19(6):586–593.
10. Pearlin LI, Schooler C. The structure of coping. *J Health Soc Behav*. 1978;19(1):2–21.
11. Thornton M, Travis SS. Analysis of the reliability of the modified Caregiver Strain Index. *J Gerontol B Psychol Sci Soc Sci*. 2003;58(2):S127–S132.
12. Akosile CO, Banjo TO, Okoye EC, Ibikunle PO, Odole AC. Informal caregiving burden and perceived social support in an acute stroke care facility. *Health Qual Life Outcomes*. 2018;16(1):57.
13. Bidwell JT, Lyons KS, Mudd JO, et al. Patient and caregiver determinants of patient quality of life and caregiver strain in left ventricular assist device therapy. *J Am Heart Assoc*. 2018;7(6):e008080.
14. Payne S, Smith P, Dean S. Identifying the concerns of informal carers in palliative care. *Palliat Med*. 1999;13(1):37–44.
15. Tanco K, Park JC, Cerana A, Sisson A, Sobti N, Bruera E. A systematic review of instruments assessing dimensions of distress among caregivers of adult and pediatric cancer patients. *Palliat Support Care*. 2017;15(1):110–124.
16. Zarit S, Reever K, Bach-Peterson J. Relatives of the impaired elderly: correlates of feelings of burden. *Gerontologist*. 1980;20:649–655.
17. Seng BK, Luo N, Ng WY, et al. Validity and reliability of the Zarit Burden Interview in assessing caregiver burden. *Ann Acad Med Singapore*. 2010;39(10):758–763.
18. Bakas T, Champion V. Development and psychometric testing of the Bakas Caregiving Outcomes Scale. *Nurs Res*. 1999;48:250–259.
19. Higginson IJ, Gao W, Jackson D, Murray J, Harding R. Short-form Zarit Caregiver Burden Interviews were valid in advanced conditions. *J Clin Epidemiol*. 2010;63(5):535–542.
20. Govina O, Kotronoulas G, Mystakidou K, Giannakopoulou M, Galanos A, Patiraki E. Validation of the revised Bakas Caregiving Outcomes Scale in Greek caregivers of patients with advanced cancer receiving palliative radiotherapy. *Support Care Cancer*. 2013;21(5):1395–1404.
21. Hudson PL, Trauer T, Graham S, et al. A systematic review of instruments related to family caregivers of palliative care. *Palliat Med*. 2010;24(7):656–668.
22. Van Durme T, Macq J, Jeanmart C, Gobert M. Tools for measuring the impact of informal caregiving of the elderly: a literature review. *Int J Nurs Stud*. 2012;49:490–504.
23. Shilling V, Matthews L, Jenkins V, Fallowfield L. Patient-reported outcome measures for cancer caregivers: a systematic review. *Qual Life Res*. 2016;25:1859–1876.

24. Oberst MT, Thomas SE, Gass KA, Ward SE. Caregiving demands and appraisal of stress among family caregivers. *Cancer Nurs.* 1989;12:209–215.
25. Glajchen M. Role of family caregivers in cancer pain management. In: Bruera ED, Portenoy RK, eds. *Cancer Pain: Assessment and Management.* 2nd ed. New York, NY: Cambridge University Press; 2009:597–607.
26. Reinhard SC, Gubman GD, Horwitz AV, Minsky S. Burden assessment scale for families of the seriously mental ill. *Eval Progr Plan.* 1994;17:261–269.
27. Miyashita M, Yamaguchi A, Kayama M, et al. Validation of the Burden Index of Caregivers (BIC), a multidimensional short care burden scale from Japan. *Health Qual Life Outcomes.* 2006;4:52.
28. Chen HC, Chen ML, Lotus Shyu YI, Tang WR. Development and testing of a scale to measure caregiving load in caregivers of cancer patients in Taiwan, the care task scale-cancer. *Cancer Nurs.* 2007;30(3):223–231.
29. Novak M, Guest C. Application of a multidimensional caregiver burden inventory. *Gerontologist.* 1989;29:798–803.
30. Elmstahl S, Mainberg B, Annerstedt L. Caregiver's burden of patients 3 years after stroke assessed by a novel caregiver burden scale. *Arch Phys Med Rehabil.* 1996;77:177–182.
31. Gerritsen JC, van der Ende PC. The development of a care-giving burden scale. *Age Ageing.* 1994;23:483–491.
32. Schofield HL, Murphy B, Herrman HE, Bloch S, Singh B. Family caregiving: measurement of emotional well-being and various aspects of the caregiving role. *Psychol Med.* 1997;27(3):647–657.
33. Given CW, Given B, Stommel M, Collins C, King S, Franklin S. The Caregiver Reaction Assessment (CRA) for caregivers to persons with chronic physical and mental impairments. *Res NursHealth.* 1992;15:271–283.
34. Ugalde A, Krishnasamy M, Schofield P. Development of an instrument to self-efficacy in caregivers of people with advanced cancer. *Psychooncology.* 2013;22(6):1428–1434.
35. Dumont S, Fillion L, Gagnon P, Bernier N. A new tool to assess family caregiver's burden during end-of-life care. *J Palliat Care.* 2008;24:151–161.
36. Sanjo M, Morita T, Miyashita M. Caregiving Consequences Inventory: a measure for evaluating caregiving consequences from the bereaved family member's perspective. *Psychooncology.* 2009;18(6):657–666.
37. Haberman MR, Woods NF, Packard NJ. Demands of chronic illness: reliability and validity assessment of a demands-of-illness inventory. *Holist Nurs Pract.* 1990;5:25–35.
38. Cooper B, Kinsella GJ, Picton C. Development and initial validation of a family appraisal of caregiving questionnaire for palliative care. *Psychooncology.* 2006;15(7):613–622.
39. Nolan MT, Hughes MT, Kub J, et al. Development and validation of the Family Decision-Making Self-Efficacy Scale. *Palliat Support Care.* 2009;7:315–321.
40. Ishii Y, Miyashita M, Sato K, Ozawa T. Family's difficulty scale in end-of-life home care: a new measure of the family's difficulties in caring for patients with cancer at the end of life at home from bereaved family's perspective. *J Palliat Med.* 2012;15(2):210–215.
41. Levesque JV, Maybery DJ. The Parental Cancer Questionnaire: scale structure, reliability, and validity. *Support Care Cancer.* 2014;22(1):23–32.
42. Macera CA, Eaker ED, Jannarone RJ, Davis DR, Stoskopf CH. A measure of perceived burden among caregivers. *Eval Health Prof.* 1993;16(2):204–211.

43. Stommel M, Given CW, Given B. Depression as an overriding variable explaining caregiver burdens. *J Aging Health*. 1990;2:81–102.
44. Levene JE, Lancee WJ, Seeman MV. The perceived family burden scale: measurement and validation. *Schizophr Res*. 1996;22:151–157.
45. Sinfield P, Baker R, Tarrant C, et al. The Prostate Care Questionnaire for Carers (PCQ-C): reliability, validity and acceptability. *BMC Health Serv Res*. 2009;9:229.
46. Vitaliano PP, Russo J, Young HM, Becker J, Maiuro RD. The screen for caregiver burden. *Gerontologist*. 1991;31(1):76–83.
47. Wells DK, James K, Stewart J, et al. The Care of My Child With Cancer: a new instrument to measure caregiving demand in parents of children with cancer. *J Pediatr Nurs*. 2002;17:201–210.
48. Yeh CH. Development and testing of the parental coping strategy inventory (PCSI) with children with cancer in Taiwan. *J Adv Nurs*. 2001;36:78–88.
49. Duran B. Developing a scale to measure parental worry and their attitudes toward childhood cancer after successful completion of treatment: a pilot study. *J Pediatr Oncol Nurs*. 2011;28:154–168.
50. Streisand R, Braniecki S, Tercyak KP, Kazak AE. Childhood illness-related parenting stress: the pediatric inventory for parents. *Pediatr Psychol*. 2001;26:155–162.
51. Kazak AE, Prusak A, McSherry M, et al. The Psychosocial Assessment Tool (PAT): pilot data on a brief screening instrument for identifying high risk families in pediatric oncology. *Fam SystHealth*. 2001;19:303–317.
52. Ankri J, Andrieu S, Beaufils B, Grand A, Henrard JC. Beyond the global score of the Zarit Burden Interview: useful dimensions for clinicians. *Int J Geriatr Psychiatry*. 2005;20:254–260.
53. Schreiner AS, Morimoto T, Arai Y, Zarit S. Assessing family caregiver's mental health using a statistically derived cut-off score for the Zarit Burden Interview. *Aging Ment Health*. 2006;10:107–111.
54. Bedard M, Molloy DW, Squire L, Dubois S, Lever JA, O'Donnell M. The Zarit Burden Interview: a new short version and screening version. *Gerontologist*. 2001;41:652–657.
55. Stevens LF, Arango-Lasprilla JC, Deng X, et al. Factors associated with depression and burden in Spanish speaking caregivers of individuals with traumatic brain injury. *NeuroRehabilitation*. 2012;31(4):443–452.
56. Goncalves-Pereira M, Zarit SH. The Zarit Burden Interview in Portugal: validity and recommendations in dementia and palliative care. *Acta Med Port*. 2014;27(2):163–165.
57. Rajabi-Mashhadi MT, Mashhadinejad H, Ebrahimzadeh MH, et al. The Zarit Caregiver Burden Interview Short Form (ZBI-12) in spouses of veterans with chronic spinal cord injury, validity and reliability of the Persian version. *Arch Bone Jt Surg*. 2015;3(1):56–63.
58. Ha NHL, Chong MS, Choo RWM, Tam WJ, Yap PLK. Caregiving burden in foreign domestic workers caring for frail older adults in Singapore. *Int Psychogeriatr*. 2018 Mar 21:1–9.
59. Nijboer C, Triemstra M, Tempelaar R, Sandman R, van den Bos GA. Determinants of caregiving experiences and mental health of partners of cancer patients. *Cancer*. 1999;86:577–588.
60. Nijboer C, Triemstra M, Tempelaar R, Sanderman R, van den Bos G. Measuring both negative and positive reactions to giving care to cancer

patients: psychometric qualities of the Caregiver Reaction Assessment (CRA). *Soc Sci Med.* 1999;48(9):1259–1269.

61. Lambert SD, Yoon H, Ellis KR, Northouse L. Measuring appraisal during advanced cancer: psychometric testing of the appraisal of caregiving scale. *Patient Educ Couns.* 2015;98(5):633–639.

62. Creedle C, Leak A, Deal AM, et al. The impact of education on caregiver burden on two inpatient oncology units. *J Cancer Educ.* 2012;27(2):250–256.

63. Bakas T, Champion V, Perkins SM, Farran CJ, Williams LS. Psychometric testing of the revised 15-item Bakas Caregiving Outcomes Scale. *Nurs Res.* 2006;55(5):346–355.

64. Beck AT, Ward CH, Mendelson M, Mock J, Erbaugh J. An inventory for measuring depression. *Arch Gen Psychiatry.* 1961;4:561–571.

65. Tebb SS. (1995). An aid to empowerment: a caregiver well-being scale. *Health Soc Work.* 20:87–92.

66. Berg-Weger M, McGartland Rubio D, Steiger Tebb S. The Caregiver Well-Being Scale revisited. *Health Soc Work.* 2000;25(4):255–263. https://doi.org/10.1093/hsw/25.4.255

67. Mitchell AJ. Pooled results from 38 analyses of the accuracy of Distress Thermometer and other ultra-short methods of detecting cancer-related mood disorders. *J Clin Oncol.* 2007;25(29):4670–4681.

68. Roth AJ, Kornblith AB, Batel-Copel L, Peabody E, Scher HI, Holland JC. Rapid screening for psychologic distress in men with prostate carcinoma: a pilot study. *Cancer.* 1998;82:1904–1908.

69. Broadhead WE, Gehlbach SH, DeGruy FV, Kaplan BH. The Duke-UNC Functional Social Support Questionnaire: measurement of social support in family medicine patients. *Med Care.* 1988;26:709–723.

70. Tanco K, Vidal M, Arthur J, et al. Testing the feasibility of using the Edmonton Symptom Assessment System (ESAS) to assess caregiver symptom burden. *Palliat Support Care.* 2017;16(1):14–22.

71. Richardson AL, Jones G. A review of the reliability and validity of the Edmonton Symptom Assessment System. *Curr Oncol (Toronto, Ont.).* 2009;16:55. doi:10.3747/co.v16i1.261

72. Todtman K, Gustafson AW. The financial impact scale: an instrument for assessing informal long-term caregivers. *J Gerontol Soc Work.* 1991;18:135–150.

73. Farran CJ, Miller BH, Kaufman JE, Donner E, Fogg L. Finding meaning through caregiving: development of an instrument for family caregivers of persons with Alzheimer's disease. *J Clin Psychol.* 1999;55(9):1107–1125.

74. Peterman AH, Fitchett G, Brady MJ, Hernandez L, Cella D. Measuring spiritual well-being in people with cancer: the Functional Assessment of Chronic Illness Therapy—Spiritual Well-Being Scale (FACIT-Sp). *Ann Behav Med.* 2002;24(1):49–58. https://doi.org/10.1207/S15324796ABM2401_06

75. Wingate AL, Lackey NR. A description of the needs of noninstitutionalized cancer patients and their primary caregivers. *Cancer Nurs.* 1989;12:216–225.

76. Prue G, Santin O, Porter S. Assessing the needs of informal caregivers to cancer survivors: a review of the instruments. *Psychooncology.* 2015;24:121–129. doi:10.1002/pon.3609

77. Herth K. Abbreviated instrument to measure hope: development and psychometric evaluation. *J Adv Nurs.* 1992;17:1251–1259. doi:10.1111/j.1365-2648.1992.tb01843.x

78. Gough K, Hudson P. Psychometric properties of the Hospital Anxiety and Depression Scale in family caregivers of palliative care patients. *J Pain Symptom Manage.* 2009;37:797–806.
79. Zimet GD, Dahlen NW, Zimet SG, Farley GK. The Multidimensional Scale of Perceived Social Support. *J Pers Assess.* 1988;52:30–41.
80. Kim Y, Kashy DA, Spillers RL, Evans TV. Needs assessment of family caregivers of cancer survivors: three cohorts comparison. *Psychooncology.* 2010;19:573–582.
81. Watson D, Clark LA, Tellegen A. Development and validation of brief measures of positive and negative affect: the PANAS scales. *J Pers Soc Psychol.* 1988;54:1063–1070.
82. Hardy JR, Edmonds P, Turner R, Rees E, A'Hern R. The use of the Rotterdam Symptom Checklist in palliative care. *J Pain Symptom Manage.* 1999;18(2):79–84.
83. Badr H, Gupta B, Sikora A, Posner M. Psychological distress in patients and caregivers over the course of radiotherapy for head and neck cancer. *Oral Oncol.* 2014;50:1005–1011.
84. Fujinami R, Sun V, Zachariah F, Uman G, Grant M, Ferrell B. Family caregivers' distress levels related to quality of life, burden and preparedness. *Psychooncology.* 2015;24:54–62.
85. Family Caregiver Alliance and Benjamin Rose Institute on Aging. Selected caregiver assessment measures: a resource inventory for practioners. 2nd edition. https://www.caregiver.org/sites/caregiver.org/files/pdfs/SelCGAssmtMeas_ResInv_FINAL_12.10.12.pdf. Published December 2012. Accessed April 2, 2018.
86. Tamayo GJ, Broxson A, Munsell M, Cohen MZ. Caring for the caregiver. *Oncol Nurs Forum.* 2010;37(1):E50–E57. doi:10.1188/10.ONF.E50-E57
87. Girgis A, Lambert S, Johnson C, Waller A, Currow D. Physical, psychosocial, relationship, and economic burden of caring for people with cancer: a review. *J Oncol Pract.* 2013;9(4):197–202.
88. Goldstein NE, Concato J, Fried TR, Kasl SV, Johnson-Hurzeler R, Bradley EH. Factors associated with caregiver burden among caregivers of terminally ill patients with cancer. *J Palliat Care.* 2004;20(1):38–43.
89. Edwards B, Ung L. Quality of life instruments for caregivers of patients with cancer: a review of their psychometric properties. *Cancer Nurs.* 2002;25(5):342–349.
90. Choi KE, Yoon JS, Kim, JH, Park JH, Kim YJ, Yu ES. Depression and distress in caregivers of children with brain tumors undergoing treatment: Psychosocial factors as moderators. *Psychooncology.* 2015;25. doi:10.1002/pon.3962
91. Meca-Lallana J, Mendibe M, Hernández-Clares R, ocío et al. Predictors of burden and depression among caregivers of relapsing-remitting MS patients in Spain: MS Feeling study. *Neurodegener Dis Manage.* 2016;6(4):277–287. doi:10.2217/nmt-2016-0014
92. Delgado J, Almenar L, Crespo-Leiro MG, et al. Health-related quality of life, social support, and caregiver burden between six and 120 months after heart transplantation: a Spanish multicenter cross-sectional study. *Clin Transplant.* 2015;29(9):771–780. doi:10.1111/ctr.12578
93. Godoy-Ramírez MA, Pérez-Verdún ÁM, Doménech-Del Rio A, Prunera-Pardell JM. 2014[Caregiver burden and social support perceived by patients with chronic obstructive pulmonary disease.]. *Rev Calid Asist.* 2014;29(6):320–324.
94. Kuscu MK, Dural U, Önen P, et al. The association between individual attachment patterns, the perceived social support, and the psychological well-being of Turkish informal caregivers. *Psychooncology.* 2009;18:927–935. doi:10.1002/pon.1441

95. Kahriman F, Zaybak A. 2015Caregiver burden and perceived social support among caregivers of patients with cancer. *Asian Pac J Cancer Prev*. 2015;16:3313–3317. doi:10.7314/APJCP.2015.16.8.3313

96. Demirtepe-Saygılı D, Bozo Ö. Perceived social support as a moderator of the relationship between caregiver well-being indicators and psychological symptoms. *J Health Psychol*. 2011;16:1091–1100. doi:10.1177/1359105311399486

97. Yabroff KR, Kim Y. Time costs associated with informal caregiving for cancer survivors. *Cancer*. 2009;115:4362–4373.

98. Siegel K, Raveis VH, Houts P, Mor V. Caregiver burden and unmet patient needs. *Cancer*.1991;68(5):1131–1140.

99. Hileman JC, Lackey NR. Self-identified needs of patients with cancer at home and their home caregivers: a descriptive study. *Oncol Nurs Forum*. 1990;17:907–912.

100. Hileman JW, Lackey NR, Hassanein RS. Identifying the needs of home caregivers of patients with cancer. *Oncol Nurs Forum*. 1992;19:771–777.

101. Vroom VH. Some personality determinants of the effects of participation. *J Abnorm Soc Psychol*. 1959;59:322–327.

102. Bialon LN, Coke S. A study on caregiver burden: stressors, challenges, and possible solutions. *Am J Hosp Palliat Care*. 2012;29(3):210–218.

103. Lai C, Luciani, M, Di Mario C. Psychological impairments burden and spirituality in caregivers of terminally ill cancer patients. *Eur J Cancer Care (Engl)*. 2018;27(1). doi:10.1111/ecc.12674

104. Hills J, Paice JA, Cameron JR, Shott S. Spirituality and distress in palliative care consultation. *J Palliat Med*. 2005;8(4):782–788.

105. Brady MJ, Peterman AH, Fitchett G, Mo M, Cella D. A case for including spirituality in quality of life measurement in oncology. *Psychooncology*. 1999;8:417–428.

106. LeSeure P, Chongkham-ang S. The experience of caregivers living with cancer patients: a systematic review and meta-synthesis. *J Pers Med*. 2015;5(4):406–439. http://doi.org/10.3390/jpm5040406

107. Jones BL. The challenge of quality care for family caregivers in pediatric cancer care. *Semin Oncol Nurs*. 2012;28(4):213–220.

108. Pai A, Patino-Fernandez AM, McSherry M, et al. The Psychosocial Assessment Tool (PAT2.0): psychometric properties of a screener for psychosocial distress in families of children newly diagnosed with cancer. *J Pediatr Psychol*. 2008;33:50–62.

Addressing the Needs of Cancer Caregivers

Empirically Supported Treatments

CHAPTER 7

Psychoeducational Interventions for Cancer Family Caregivers

J. NICHOLAS DIONNE-ODOM, MARIE A. BAKITAS,
AND BETTY FERRELL

Nearly all family members who assume a caregiving role already have coping habits that they have developed over a lifetime. When their loved ones are first diagnosed with cancer, however, skills to manage stressful situations are often exceeded and many do not have an existing repertoire of coping strategies to counterbalance the sudden upheaval of their normal day-to-day life. Because general feelings of distress and fear are never completely new to most individuals, a certain level of adaptive coping is at least possible during the initial cancer diagnosis period.

Yet, this initial period can also be a completely alien experience. The caregiver may be faced with completely unfamiliar tasks, such as regulating the distressing emotions that result when learning that someone close to them is under mortal threat, learning about the cancer and its treatments, coordinating care and healthcare appointments, and managing medications, all while balancing work and caregiving responsibilities. Consequently, many family members react to their loved one's new cancer diagnosis with feelings of desperation and disbelief and assume their caregiving role in a disorganized and frantic manner.

Ideally, psychoeducation for cancer caregivers should start near the time of diagnosis and encompass content that facilitates a basic comprehension of performing in the cancer caregiving role. The primary aim of psychoeducation is to heighten empowerment and stimulate self-help behavioral activation through greater self-awareness of one's affliction.[1] In family caregiving, psychoeducation empowers caregivers by facilitating basic comprehension of cancer, its treatments, and its implications for day-to-day life. Without a basic understanding of the cancer affecting their loved one and the resulting insight, enhancement in caregiving skills, and promotion of adaptive coping that follows, caregivers are suboptimally positioned for long-term tenure and resilience in a role that can consume up to 8 hours per day of care over a period of several years.[2-4] It is only from an informed position that caregivers are able to fully leverage their self-help potential to maximize their ability to acquire skills in delivering complex home-based medical care, extend their repertoire of coping and stress management strategies, and cultivate a social support network that diffuses the caregiving workload.

KEY ELEMENTS OF PSYCHOEDUCATION IN CANCER FAMILY CAREGIVING

Psychoeducation is a composite of numerous therapeutic counseling techniques that stresses (1) establishing a strong therapeutic alliance between the practitioner and the family caregiver; (2) promoting cancer disease, cancer treatment, and technical "how-to" caregiving knowledge; and (3) enhancing adaptive coping.[1]

Establishing the Therapeutic Alliance

The basis for nearly all forms of psychotherapy, including psychoeducation, is establishing a strong, trusting practitioner-client relationship, where for the purposes here, the "client" is the family caregiver. This therapeutic alliance is a necessary bridge to reach caregivers to communicate that they are highly valued, that the practitioner empathizes with their experiences, that the caregiver is held in unconditional positive regard, and that the relationship with the practitioner is a partnership where goals and content are caregiver driven and mutually agreed on. While therapeutic alliance has been understudied in psychoeducational interventions to support cancer caregiving, systematic reviews examining therapeutic alliance in psychotherapies for other illness populations reported that this variable has a moderate and reliable impact on psychotherapy outcomes.[5,6] It has been suggested that the therapeutic alliance influences the outcomes of psychotherapy not because the alliance is helpful in its own right, but because it facilitates engagement with the topical content, the setting and following through of goals, and adaptive coping strategies. While full treatment of establishing a therapeutic alliance is beyond the scope of this chapter, practitioners are referred to additional references.[7]

Promoting Cancer Family Caregiver Knowledge and Skills

Transmitting information that is basic and universal to the cancer caregiving role is perhaps the most obvious and salient component of psychoeducation for cancer caregivers. Basic background information on cancer and how it impacts the family must be effectively conveyed. Fundamentally, the goal is to help caregivers have greater understanding of the cancer illness and a cause-and-effect framework that helps them better reason through how cancer impacts their loved one's health and, as a consequence, their role and actions as a caregiver. For example, understanding the basic pathophysiologic causes of chemotherapy-induced nausea and vomiting helps a caregiver understand at an elementary level what makes this symptom better and worse, how to help the patient manage this symptom, and when it is appropriate to contact a professional for additional guidance and assistance.

Admittedly, there is a wide range of individual situations that require one-on-one customizing of topics, yet there are many common elements to the caregiving experience that are generalizable and applicable to most cancer caregiving situations. Table 7.1 outlines common psychoeducational program topics for cancer family caregivers. Teaching this information is often accompanied by brochures, guidebooks, and videos to help consolidate topical content. However, using these various forms of media never substitutes for one-on-one dialogue between the clinician and caregiver to help associate the topical content with the caregiver's individual situation.

Enhancing Adaptive Coping

In close concert with instilling basic cancer and supportive care knowledge, psychoeducation for cancer family caregivers also includes promoting adaptive coping skills. Adaptive coping includes ways of framing and behaviorally reacting to a problem or situation that alleviate distress, promote psychological well-being and resilience, and facilitate positive, constructive outcomes. Adaptive coping is enhanced in part by increasing a caregiver's topical knowledge of potential future stressors to expect and prepare for (e.g., by providing information on future decision-making)

Table 7.1 COMMON TOPICS IN PSYCHOEDUCATIONAL PROGRAMS
FOR CANCER CAREGIVERS

Care Coordination

- Transportation
- Scheduling doctor and medical appointments
- Accompanying patients to medical appointments and therapy
- Finances
- Respite
- Hospice
- Transitions in care (e.g., hospital to home)
- Managing medications (including purchase and administration)
- Balancing paid work and family caregiving
- Assisting with personal care
- Domestic responsibilities (e.g., cooking, cleaning)
- Arranging funeral services

Skills in Interpersonal Communication

- Interacting with care recipient
- Interacting with children
- Interacting with spouse or partner
- Interacting with other family members (local and long distance)
- Interacting with healthcare providers and other professionals

Self-Care, Spirituality/Faith, Emotions, and Coping

- Exercise
- Nutrition
- Stress management
- Sleep
- Maintaining a healthy social life
- Finding time for solitude and self-reflection
- Finding time for meditation and prayer
- Impact of cancer on spirituality/faith
- Feeling overwhelmed
- Anxiety
- Depression
- Anger
- Grief and loss
- Detachment
- Resentment
- Loneliness
- Shame
- Neglect
- Guilt
- Empathetic distress (e.g., from witnessing someone close to you suffer)

Managing Physical Side Effects of Cancer and Cancer Treatment

- Patient symptoms and how to help
- Anemia
- Appetite loss
- Bleeding, bruising
- Constipation
- Confusion and seizures
- Delirium
- Diarrhea
- Edema
- End-of-life and dying
- Fatigue
- Fertility
- Fever and infections
- Hair loss
- Infection, neutropenia
- Lymphedema
- Memory, poor concentration
- Mobility problems and falls
- Mouth and throat problems
- Nausea and vomiting
- Pain
- Sexual health issues
- Skin and nail issues
- Sleep problems
- Urinary and bladder problems

Table 7.1 CONTINUED

Decisional	
• Decision aids	• Partnering with patients to help them make
• Advance care planning	medical decisions
• Durable power of attorney for	• When to seek a second opinion
healthcare	• "The right time" for accessing various services
• Care transition decisions	(e.g., respite)
• Deciding to take patients to the hospital or emergency department	

Cancer Treatments and Clinical Trials	
• Surgery	• Targeted therapy
• Radiation therapy	• Hormone therapy
• Chemotherapy	• Stem cell transplantation
• Immunotherapy	• Precision medicine
	• What are clinical trials?

and potentially neutralize before ever occurring. In contrast, maladaptive coping exacerbates distress and typically worsens the conditions of a situation. Maladaptive coping can include behaviors such as avoidance and distancing, escape (e.g., through use of drugs or alcohol), and self-blaming.

When problems arise, the psychotherapeutic effect of adaptive coping is in moving the locus of control from an external source beyond the control of the individual to one that is more internal and intentional. This can be challenging in the context of cancer family caregiving when what happens with the patient's cancer is in many ways outside of anyone's control. This perhaps is why psychoeducation for cancer caregivers has often employed problem-solving education, where practitioners teach caregivers that much of how we react to stressful situations is by how we frame a problem or stressor. The goal is to help family caregivers reframe problems in a way that allows them to see that they can do something about them. More detailed discussion of problem-solving education is presented in the ENABLE (Educate, Nurture, Advise, Before Life Ends), case example and in the work of Dionne-Odom et al.[8]

SUMMARY OF TESTED PSYCHOEDUCATIONAL INTERVENTIONS IN CANCER FAMILY CAREGIVING

In the prior section, the underlying conceptual basis of psychoeducation for cancer caregivers was described. This section summarizes the state of the science of evidence-based psychoeducational interventions that have undergone randomized clinical trials testing for cancer caregivers. This summary is based on a secondary analysis of psychoeducational interventions identified in a recent seminal systematic review of cancer caregiver interventions by Ferrell and Wittenberg.[9] This review identified 50 articles reporting results from randomized controlled trials (RCTs) of cancer family caregiver interventions between 2010 and 2016; of these, 36 reported on one or more psychoeducational intervention.[10-45] Readers interested in further details of the methods for this review are referred to the original source. In the following, to promote translation of these interventions into practice, readers are familiarized with the dose, format, content, caregiver characteristics, measured outcomes, and effectiveness of the psychoeducational interventions cited in the Ferrell and Wittenberg review.

Dose and Format

Based on the Ferrell and Wittenberg review,[9] there were 44 discrete psychoeducational interventions tested in the identified articles, noting that, in some cases, articles reported more than one psychoeducational intervention, and in others, two articles may have reported data on the same intervention (Table 7.2). Of those interventions that reported clinician-caregiver one-on-one sessions (excluding monthly or periodic "check-in" calls), intervention sessions/contacts ranged from 1 to 14, with the average of 4.5 sessions. Sessions ranged from 23 to 120 minutes, and the average was approximately 51 minutes for studies reporting this information. The duration of programs varied greatly, from 1 day to over 2 years. Most interventions were between 4 and 8 weeks. Of those interventions reporting clinician-caregiver session length and number of sessions, about half had a total time involvement of 2 hours or less.

Sixteen interventions (39%) included both the caregiver and the patient in the intervention, and 25 (61%) targeted only the caregiver. Interventions were conducted by telephone alone (22%), face to face alone (20%), or a mix of both (20%). Only two included a group format.[14,41] Most interventions included some form of educational materials, including print guidebooks, booklets, or manuals (n = 27, 66%); CDs or DVDs (n = 7, 17%); or web-based content (n = 6, 15%). The interventionist was a nurse in 16 interventions (39%) and a mental health professional (e.g., psychologist) in 3; 10 (24%) interventions had limited or no interventionist involvement as they were self-directed (e.g., web-based intervention).

Table 7.2 RANDOMIZED TRIALS OF PSYCHOEDUCATIONAL INTERVENTIONS FOR CANCER CAREGIVERS, 2010–2016

Study	# Sessions/ Structured Contacts With Intervener	Average Minutes per Session	Duration	Intervener	Face to Face	Telephone	Web Based	CG Only?	Educational Materials: DVD/CD (V) Print (P) Website (W)	Learning Content: CG Tasks (CT) Marital/ Family (MF) Self-Care (SC)	Significant Findings
Badger, 2011[11]	4	28	8 weeks	Paraprofessional		X			P	CT, SC	Improvements in depression, fatigue, social support from family, social well-being, and spiritual well-being.
Badger, 2013[12]	4	29	8 weeks	Paraprofessional		X			P	CT, SC	Within-group improvement in quality of life.
Badger, 2013[12]	4	30	8 weeks	Information specialist	X	X				CT	Within-group improvement in quality of life.
Badr, 2015[13]	6	30	6 weeks	Master's-trained mental health counselor		X			P	CT, MF, SC	Improvements in depression, anxiety, and caregiver burden.
Caserta, 2013[14]	NR	NR	14 weeks	Support group facilitator				X		SC	Lower depression, grief, and loneliness over time in partners of patients who died expectedly from causes other than cancer. Cancer bereavement was equal in distress to unexpected death.

(continued)

Table 7.2 CONTINUED

Study	# Sessions/ Structured Contacts With Intervener	Average Minutes per Session	Duration	Intervener	Face to face	Telephone	Web Based	CG Only?	Educational Materials: DVD/CD (V) Print (P) Website (W)	Learning Content: CG Tasks (CT) Marital/Family (MF) Self-Care (SC)	Significant Findings
Chambers, 2015[15]	14	29	22 weeks	Peer-support volunteer		X			P	CT, MF	None.
Chambers, 2014[16]: Arm 1	1	46	NR	Oncology nurse		X			V, P	CT	Caregivers in both the single-session, nurse-led, self-management intervention group and the five-session psychologist telephone intervention had decreased distress and improved post-traumatic growth.
Chambers, 2014[16]: Arm 2	5	49	NR	Psychologist		X			P	CT	
Chih, 2012[17]: Arm 1	NR	NR	12 months	NR			X		W	CT, MF, SC	Caregivers in the interactive cancer communication (ICC) system combined with clinician report of symptom distress reported less negative mood than those in the ICC-alone group.
Chih, 2012[17]: Arm 2	NR	NR	12 months	NR			X		W	CT, MF, SC	

Collinge, 2013[18]	NR	NR	4 weeks	Massage therapist					V, P	CT, MF	Patients in both the caregiver massage group and the caregiver reading group reported reduced symptoms, and caregiver massage group had increased confidence and self-efficacy.
Dionne-Odom, 2015[19]	3	23	2 years	Advanced practice nurse		X		X	V, P	CT, MF, SC	Early group (vs. delayed group) caregivers had lower depression and stress burden.
Dubenske, 2014[21]	NR	NR	2 years	NR			X	X	W	CT, MF, SC	Caregivers assigned to a web-based support system (Comprehensive Health Enhancement Support System [CHESS]) reported lower burden and negative mood.
Heinrichs, 2012[22]	1	120	8 weeks	Therapist	X				P	CT	Patients in the couples skills group had reduced fear of progression, and couples had less avoidance, more post-traumatic growth and better relationship skills.

(continued)

Table 7.2 CONTINUED

Study	# Sessions/ Structured Contacts With Intervener	Average Minutes per Session	Duration	Intervener	Face to face	Telephone	Web Based	CG Only?	Educational Materials: DVD/CD (V) Print (P) Website (W)	Learning Content: CG Tasks (CT) Marital/ Family (MF) Self-Care (SC)	Significant Findings
Hendrix, 2016[23]	1	56.5	1-time session	Social worker or nurse	X			X	P	CT, SC	Greater caregiver self-efficacy for symptom management and stress management and preparation for caregiving at post-training assessment but not at 2- and 4-week follow-up.
Holtslander et al., 2016[24]	3	NR	2 weeks	Nurse				X	P	SC	Significant improvement in restoration-oriented coping and higher oscillation activity.
Hudson, 2013[25]: Arm 1	4	NR	4 weeks	Nurse	X	X		X	P	SC	The two-visit intervention group had improvement in levels of preparedness and competence from baseline to 1 week postintervention.
Hudson, 2013[25]: Arm 2	4	NR	4 weeks	Nurse	X	X		X	P	SC	

Hudson, 2015[26]: Arm 1	4	NR	4 weeks	Nurse	X	X	X	P	SC	FCG in the one-visit intervention had less worsening in distress compared to the control group between baseline and 8 weeks' postdeath.
Hudson, 2015[26]: Arm 2	4	NR	4 weeks	Nurse	X	X	X	P	SC	
Laudenslager, 2015[27]	8	67.5	8 weeks	MSW	X	X	X	P	MF, SC	Lower caregiver stress at 3 months.
Leow, 2015[28]	3	60	6 weeks	Nurse	X	X	X	V, W	MF, SC	Improvement in quality of life, social support satisfaction, and number of supported persons; closeness with patient; self-efficacy in self-care; rewards of caregiving; knowledge; and lower stress and depression.
Manne, 2013[29]: Arm 1	NR	NR	1 week	NR				P	CT	No significant benefit on cancer screening, yet increase in screening intention.
Manne, 2013[29]: Arm 2	NR	NR	1 week	NR				P	CT, MF	Significant increase in husbands' support of wives' screening; significant increase in screening benefits.
Mitchell, 2013[30]	NR	NR	3 months	NR	X		X	P	CT, SC	No significant differences in number or intensity of needs at 6 months.

(continued)

Table 7.2 CONTINUED

Study	# Sessions/ Structured Contacts With Intervener	Average Minutes per Session	Duration	Intervener	Face to face	Telephone	Web Based	CG Only?	Educational Materials: DVD/CD (V) Print (P) Website (W)	Learning Content: CG Tasks (CT) Marital/ Family (MF) Self-Care (SC)	Significant Findings
Namkoong, 2012[31]	NR	NR	6 months	NR			X	X	W	CT, MF, SC	Improvement in caregivers' perceived bonding; perceived bonding was positively associated with caregivers' appraisal and problem-based coping strategies at 6 months.
Northouse, 2013[33]. Arm 1	3	40	10 weeks	Nurse (master's degree)	X					CT, MF, SC	Significant group-by-time interactions showed improvement in dyads' social and emotional quality of life at 3 months.
Northouse, 2013[33]. Arm 2	6	70	10 weeks	Nurse (master's degree)	X	X				CT, MF, SC	
Northouse, 2014[32]	3	NR	6 weeks	NR			X		W	CT, MF, SC	Significant decrease in emotional distress; increase in quality of life.
Perz, 2015[34]: Arm 1	NR	NR	2 weeks	NR	X				P	MF, SC	No significant improvements in quality of life.
Perz, 2015[34]: Arm 2	1	60	2 weeks	Health professional	X				P	MF, SC	

Porter, 2011[35]	14	45	8 months	Nurse	X		P	CT, MF, SC	Improvement in anxiety at 4 months; significant main effects of time for anxiety.
Segrin, 2012[36]	4	28	8 weeks	Master's-prepared nurse or social worker	X		P	CT	Patient's prostate-specific function was associated with partner's psychological QOL. The better the patient's QOL, the better the caregiver's reported QOL.
Shaw, 2016[37]	4	NR	10 weeks	Clinical psychologist	X	X	P	CT, MF, SC	Mental health score was improved at 3 months, but not statistically significant; no significant differences in physical health at 3 or 6 months.
Sherwood, 2012[38]	3	NR	8 weeks	Research staff member	X	X	P	CT	No significant effects for caregiver emotional health; caregivers with lower depressive symptoms were more likely to provide assistance at 10 weeks for nurse-delivered intervention.

(continued)

Table 7.2 CONTINUED

Study	# Sessions/ Structured Contacts With Intervener	Average Minutes per Session	Duration	Intervener	Face to face	Telephone	Web Based	CG Only?	Educational Materials: DVD/CD (V) Print (P) Website (W)	Learning Content: CG Tasks (CT) Marital/ Family (MF) Self-Care (SC)	Significant Findings
Silveira, 2010[39]: Arm 1	8	NR	8 weeks	Nurse		X		X	W	CT, SC	No statistically significant findings on agreement between patient and caregiver perception of symptom severity.
Silveira, 2010[39]: Arm 2	8	NR	8 weeks	Nonnurse coach		X		X	P	CT, SC	
Song, 2012[40]	3	90	13 weeks	Nurse (master's degree)	X	X				CT, MF, SC	Communication decreased over time; phase of illness affected couples' open communication, with no patterns of change over time; couples' perceived communication increased as they reported social support; demographic factors and symptoms did not affect levels of open communication.

Study				Delivered by					Findings
Tsianakas, 2015[41]	1	60	1-time session	Nurse		X	V, P	CT, SC	Significant improvement in understanding symptoms and side effects; information needs more frequently met.
Valeberg, 2013[42]	6	NR	5 weeks	Nurse	X	X	P	CT	Significantly higher knowledge scores on single items, but not total FPQ score; significant group-by-time interactions for the family pain questionnaire (FPQ) scores except "cancer pain can be relieved."
Van den Hurk, 2015[43]	NR	NR	8 weeks	Health professionals and qualified mindfulness trainers	X		V, P	SC	No significant changes found for psychological distress.
Walker, 2013[44]	1	60	2 weeks	Male and female researcher	X		P	CT, MF	No statistically significant differences in intimacy; couples maintained sexual activity.
Yun, 2013[45]: Arm 1	NR	NR	NR	NR		X	V	CT, MF	No difference in changes in the decision to discuss terminal prognosis.
Yun, 2013[45]: Arm 2	NR	NR	NR	NR		X	V	CT, MF	

Source: From Ferrell and Wittenburg, 2017.[9]

CG, caregiver; NR, not reported or unable to ascertain; QOL, quality of life; FCG, family caregiver.

Content

In the parent systematic review, the topical content of sessions was assigned to one or more of the following three categories: (1) care tasks related to providing health and medical support to the patient; (2) caregiver self-care and stress management; and (3) marital/family care related to relationship skills and coping. Most interventions (n = 33, 75%) included care task content, particularly around managing patient symptoms. This was closely followed by content on caregiver self-care (n = 30, 68%), where frequent topics included emotional support and accessing resources. Half (n = 22) of the interventions included content on marital/family care, with communication between caregiver and care recipient the most commonly presented topic.

Outcomes Measured and Effectiveness

The most commonly measured primary outcomes were quality of life (n = 8 studies) and distress, including anxiety and depressive symptoms (n = 10). Most studies measuring these outcomes found a significant effect favoring the intervention group.

PSYCHOEDUCATIONAL INTERVENTION EXAMPLE: THE ENABLE CAREGIVER MODEL

The final section of this chapter details ENABLE (Educate, Nurture, Advise, Before Life Ends), an evidenced-based telehealth psychoeducational intervention for family caregivers. The ENABLE caregiver model comprises an advanced practice, nurse-led, manualized, psychoeducational curriculum that is targeted toward the needs and circumstances of family caregivers of newly diagnosed loved ones with advanced metastatic or recurrent cancers who have life span prognoses of 1–2 years. The telehealth format makes it particularly well suited for those who live in remote rural locations.

The caregiver model was based on the successful ENABLE patient intervention and curriculum[46] that was first developed in 1999 and had demonstrated marked benefit to patients in the ENABLE II RCT (2003–2008).[47] In the ENABLE II trial, family caregivers completed measures of burden, but unlike their care recipients, did not receive an intervention. ENABLE II family caregivers did not demonstrate any improvement or differences in burden compared to the usual care group,[48] hence serving as impetus for development of the ENABLE caregiver model. The ENABLE

III waitlist randomized trial (2010–2013) tested the ENABLE caregiver model and found that caregiver participants randomized to the early group compared to the delayed group (12 weeks later) had lower depressive symptom and burden scores at 12 weeks (when the delayed group was just starting the intervention) and looking backward 36 weeks prior to the patients' deaths.[19] Current work with the ENABLE caregiver model is focused on scalability and implementation[49] and adaptation to different cultures and underserved US populations.

Basic Elements of the ENABLE Caregiver Model

The basic dose, format, and delivery elements of the ENABLE caregiver model include the following:

- ENABLE caregiver and patient participants each have their own separate nurse coach. The rationale for this separation is so that caregivers can freely express their own thoughts and issues, which often relate to their relationship and interaction with their patients.
- The program is introduced to family caregivers within 2 months of their loved one being diagnosed with a metastatic or recurrent advanced cancer and continues through bereavement as this is a time period that caregivers typically experience heightened distress and high levels of unmet needs.[50]
- The program is led by an advanced practice nurse coach who undergoes approximately 30 hours of training and role-play and who preferably has some background in palliative or hospice care. Nurse coaches are convened on a weekly basis to debrief and review their past week's cases with a board-certified hospice and palliative care clinician.
- Caregivers receive three initial telephone sessions that cover specific educational topics. These sessions are delivered every 1–2 weeks and are typically 30–60 minutes in length. After these three base sessions, family caregivers are contacted monthly by the coach to follow up with any ongoing or new issues and to reinforce prior educational content. Caregivers of patients who die receive an after-death bereavement call where condolences are offered, the need for additional grief resources are assessed, and the coaching relationship is brought to a close.
- To facilitate the educational component of the three base telephone sessions, fundamental cancer caregiving concepts are conveyed in a study team–developed curriculum and guidebook called *Charting Your Course—Caregiver* (CYC-C). CYC-C topical content is further detailed in Table 7.3.

Table 7.3 ENABLE CAREGIVER INTERVENTION: CHARTING YOUR COURSE
SESSION CONTENT

Session # and Title	Topical Content
1. Problem-Solving and the COPE Attitude	• Introduction to being a caregiver • Introduction to problem-solving • COPE: The problem-solving attitude • Six steps of problem-solving (1. Identify the problem; 2. Set a SMART (specific, measurable, achievable, relevant, time-bound) goal; 3. Brainstorm solutions; 4. Choose a solution; 5. Write down a weekly action plan; 6. Review your progress) • Problem-solving worksheet • ACTIVITY: Identify common problems of serious illness • Problem-solving examples: (a) Difficulty with sleep; (b) Balancing family responsibilities and illness
2. Symptom Management	• Introduction to taking care of yourself • Healthy eating • Exercise • Relaxation • Relaxed breathing • Muscle relaxation • Body scan • Imagery/visualization • Meditation • Being a partner in managing symptoms • Helping patients to assess and prioritize symptoms • Distress Thermometer • Communication with clinicians about symptoms • Common symptoms for patients and caregivers • Energy-conserving strategies • Emotional effects of illness • Types of grief • ACTIVITY: Identify your strengths and resources in coping with loss • Spiritual issues • ACTIVTY: Identify and manage symptoms
3. Communication, Decision-Making, and Advance Care Planning	• Tips for effective communication • Building a support network • ACTIVITY: Identifying your support team • Designating your support team • Communicating with your healthcare team • Medical decision-making • ACTIVITY: Viewing the shared decision-making program • Ottawa personal decision guide tool • Advance care planning

- In order to integrate and customize the educational content of the CYC-C curriculum with the unique circumstances and challenges of individual caregivers, a problem-solving support approach is introduced by coaches in CYC-C Session 1 and includes a 5-step process for dealing with stressful life problems encountered by cancer caregivers (see Table 7.3, CYC-C Session 1). ENABLE caregiver investigators developed problem-solving support as a variant of problem-solving treatment[51,52] and COPE (Creativity, Optimism,

Planning, Expert Information) problem-solving education.[53,54] After CYC-C Session 1, all coach-caregiver encounters begin with the coach inviting the family caregiver participant to discuss active problems they are facing using this approach. Readers with further interest in the development and steps of this problem-solving support approach are directed to further reading.[8]

ENABLE Caregiver Case Example

To demonstrate the ENABLE caregiver model, a fictional case example is presented next that mirrors a typical ENABLE caregiver participant. Brianne is the 62-year-old primary family caregiver to her husband, Cecil, who was diagnosed 5 weeks ago with stage IV non–small cell lung cancer. The nurse coach called Brianne on a Tuesday afternoon to briefly introduce herself and the ENABLE service. Brianne sounded hurried, noting that she works part-time at a public library, and a bit despondent but readily agreed to schedule a first session with the nurse coach on the following Thursday afternoon. The nurse coach verified that Brianne had received her CYC-C guidebook in the mail and encouraged Brianne to review Chapter 1 if possible before their appointment.

In Session 1, the nurse coach began by asking Brianne to tell her a little bit about who she was, what she does for a living, and what she understood about her husband's cancer and his treatment. The nurse coach learned that Brianne and Cecil had been married for 38 years and currently lived by themselves in a small rural town of 6,000 residents, where they had lived for most of their lives. Brianne and Cecil have two adult sons, one who lives about 20 minutes away and another who lives 4 hours away in the city. The son living close by has two children that Brianne regularly helps take care of a few days a week. Brianne talked about Cecil's cancer, describing it as "one of those nightmares that just came true." Cecil had "a lot of blood tests done," and they "took some of his lung" about a week after he was diagnosed to see if he was a candidate for targeted therapy. He started chemotherapy 2 weeks ago and would receive one additional treatment the next week. The nurse coach asked Brianne how she had been coping with all this. Brianne said that she and Cecil have a strong faith, and that they "trust that God will get us through this." She said she has felt overwhelmed and anxious when she thinks about how uncertain the future seems: "I'm just living one day at a time." The nurse coach then spent about 5 minutes highlighting key points of the CYC-C Chapter 1 content on problem-solving. After asking Brianne what she thought about the content, Brianne seemed intrigued by the problem-solving activity. She decided she wanted to try to use the problem-solving steps to set limits with how often she watches her grandchildren during the week as she felt the need to focus on Cecil's care. The nurse coach helped Brianne develop a goal concerning her grandchild care commitments, brainstorm options for reaching this goal, and set a plan for the week to work toward implementing one of her solutions. Before ending the call, the nurse coach asked Brianne to review the content for CYC-C Chapter 2. They set a time and date for an appointment the following week.

Session 2 was held the following Wednesday afternoon. After asking how Brianne's past week was, the nurse coach began the session by asking how Brianne's plan was going regarding her problem-solving goal of setting limits on the time spent watching her grandchildren each week. Brianne encountered some challenges with care of her grandchildren. She was having a difficult time scheduling a time to have a conversation with her son and daughter-in-law, who were constantly "running in and out of the house to work" before she ever got an opportunity to have a discussion with them. The coach helped Brianne think through and develop a strategy to overcome this barrier for the following week. The coach then briefly highlighted key points of each of the main sections of CYC-C Chapter 2, including partnering in self-care and symptom management, communicating with clinicians, discussing strategies to manage common physical and emotional symptoms and spirituality. After highlighting each of these individual sections, the coach checked in with Brianne to see what she thought of each section's content. Brianne really liked the section on self-care, expressing that she really needed to start taking better care of herself as she felt she had neglected her own health since Cecil was diagnosed. Brianne also talked about some of the grief she has experienced with not being able to do the same things with Cecil that they used to really enjoy, most especially horseback riding. When asked about how this experience has affected her spirituality, Brianne expressed that their faith in God was strong, and that she had many people from her church praying for her and Cecil. She and the coach agreed on a time for Session 3 the following week.

The beginning of Session 3 started with Brianne excitedly sharing with the nurse coach her progress on setting limits with care of her grandchildren. Brianne was able to have a conversation with her son about how much strain it was putting on her to watch her grandchildren each week, especially given all the travel for Cecil's appointments that were an hour's drive away. She was delightfully surprised at how accommodating her son was to find some other ways to help with the grandkids. As with prior chapters, the nurse coach then briefly highlighted each of the main sections of the third chapter, including effective communication, building a support network, medical decision-making, and advance care planning. Brianne talked a lot during this session about how hard it was to get Cecil to have a conversation about what kind of medical care he would want if he got really ill. "He just shuts down and won't talk about it. With my mom, she was the same way and never wanted to talk about dying. We ended up putting her in a nursing home, which she hated and I've always felt guilty about that." The nurse coach asked Brianne if anything from the chapter gave her ideas about what she could do to try to initiate a conversation with Cecil. Brianne liked what she read about how advanced care planning not only is about having your wishes honored, but also is an expression of love and caring because it protects family members from any anxiety and guilt that might arise from not knowing how to advocate and make decisions for a loved one's care. Brianne said she would present that point to Cecil to see if it would help him open up a bit more and perhaps consider completing an advance directive. Brianne and the nurse coach were at the end of their weekly sessions but set up a time to touch base in a month to see how things were going.

CONCLUSIONS

Psychoeducation is one of the most commonly cited psychotherapeutic approaches and tested interventions to support family carers of individuals with cancer.[9] The goals of psychoeducation in the context of cancer caregiving are to communicate information about performing in the caregiving role, have caregivers react to and synthesize this information as it relates to their own individual circumstances, and have them empowered with self-help skills and coping strategies to perform optimally in this role. Psychoeducational interventions tested to date may be delivered individually or in groups, by different clinicians, and conducted in person, telephonically, or they may be self-directed, such as through a web-based program. These interventions also vary greatly in their topical content, format, delivery, and frequency. While many of these interventions appear to be efficacious, more research is needed to further specify what combination of content, format, and delivery is optimal for specific caregiving settings and circumstances.

REFERENCES

1. Walsh J. *Psychoeducation in Mental Health.* New York, NY: Oxford University Press; 2010.
2. National Alliance for Caregiving. *Cancer Caregiving in the US: An Intense, Episodic, and Challenging Care Experience.* Bethesda, MD: National Alliance for Caregiving; 2016.
3. Yabroff KR, Kim Y. Time costs associated with informal caregiving for cancer survivors. *Cancer.* 2009;115:4362–4373.
4. Dionne-Odom JN, Demark-Wahnefried W, Taylor RA, et al. The self-care practices of family caregivers of persons with poor prognosis cancer: differences by varying levels of caregiver well-being and preparedness. *Support Care Cancer.* 2017;25:2437–2444.
5. Schnur J, Montgomery G. A systematic review of therapeutic alliance, group cohesion, empathy, and goal consensus/collaboration in psychotherapeutic interventions in cancer: uncommon factors? *Clin Psychol Rev.* 2010;30:238–247.
6. Barber J, Shabad-Ratan K, Sharpless B. The validity of the alliance as a predictor of psychotherapy outcome. In: Muran J, Barber J, eds. *The Therapeutic Alliance: An Evidence-Based Guide to Practice.* New York, NY: Guilford Press; 2010:29–43.
7. Muran J, Barber J, eds. *The Therapeutic Alliance: An Evidence-Based Guide to Practice.* New York, NY: Guilford Press; 2010.
8. Dionne-Odom JN, Lyons KD, Akyar I, Bakitas MA. Coaching family caregivers to become better problem solvers when caring for persons with advanced cancer. *J Soc Work End Life Palliat Care.* 2016;12:63–81.
9. Ferrell B, Wittenberg E. A review of family caregiving intervention trials in oncology. *CA Cancer J Clin.* 2017;67:318–325.
10. Badger T, Segrin C, Pasvogel A, Lopez AM. The effect of psychosocial interventions delivered by telephone and videophone on quality of life in early-stage breast cancer survivors and their supportive partners. *J Telemed Telecare.* 2013;19:260–265.
11. Badger TA, Segrin C, Figueredo AJ, et al. Psychosocial interventions to improve quality of life in prostate cancer survivors and their intimate or family partners. *Qual Life Res.* 2011;20:833–844.
12. Badger TA, Segrin C, Hepworth JT, Pasvogel A, Weihs K, Lopez AM. Telephone-delivered health education and interpersonal counseling improve quality of life for Latinas with breast cancer and their supportive partners. *Psychooncology.* 2013;22:1035–1042.
13. Badr H, Smith CB, Goldstein NE, Gomez JE, Redd WH. Dyadic psychosocial intervention for advanced lung cancer patients and their family caregivers: results of a randomized pilot trial. *Cancer.* 2015;121:150–158.
14. Caserta MS, Utz RL, Lund DA. Spousal Bereavement Following Cancer Death. *Illn Crises Loss.* 2013;21:185–202.
15. Chambers SK, Occhipinti S, Schover L, et al. A randomised controlled trial of a couples-based sexuality intervention for men with localised prostate cancer and their female partners. *Psychooncology.* 2015;24:748–756.
16. Chambers SK, Girgis A, Occhipinti S, et al. A randomized trial comparing two low-intensity psychological interventions for distressed patients with cancer and their caregivers. *Oncol Nurs Forum.* 2014;41:E256–E266.

17. Chih MY, DuBenske LL, Hawkins RP, et al. Communicating advanced cancer patients' symptoms via the Internet: a pooled analysis of two randomized trials examining caregiver preparedness, physical burden, and negative mood. *Palliat Med.* 2013;27:533–543.
18. Collinge W, Kahn J, Walton T, et al. Touch, Caring, and Cancer: randomized controlled trial of a multimedia caregiver education program. *Support Care Cancer.* 2013;21:1405–1414.
19. Dionne-Odom JN, Azuero A, Lyons KD, et al. Benefits of early versus delayed palliative care to informal family caregivers of patients with advanced cancer: outcomes from the ENABLE III randomized controlled trial. *J Clin Oncol.* 2015;33:1446–1452.
20. Dionne-Odom JN, Hull JG, Martin MY, et al. Associations between advanced cancer patients' survival and family caregiver presence and burden. *Cancer Med.* 2016;5:853–862.
21. DuBenske LL, Gustafson DH, Namkoong K, et al. CHESS improves cancer caregivers' burden and mood: results of an eHealth RCT. *Health Psychol.* 2014;33:1261–1272.
22. Heinrichs N, Zimmermann T, Huber B, Herschbach P, Russell DW, Baucom DH. Cancer distress reduction with a couple-based skills training: a randomized controlled trial. *Ann Behav Med.* 2012;43:239–252.
23. Hendrix CC, Bailey DE, Steinhauser KE, et al. Effects of enhanced caregiver training program on cancer caregiver's self-efficacy, preparedness, and psychological well-being. *Support Care Cancer.* 2016;24:327–336.
24. Holtslander L, Duggleby W, Teucher U, et al. Developing and pilot-testing a Finding Balance Intervention for older adult bereaved family caregivers: a randomized feasibility trial. *Eur J Oncol Nurs.* 2016;21:66–74.
25. Hudson P, Trauer T, Kelly B, et al. Reducing the psychological distress of family caregivers of home-based palliative care patients: short-term effects from a randomised controlled trial. *Psychooncology.* 2013;22:1987–1993.
26. Hudson P, Trauer T, Kelly B, et al. Reducing the psychological distress of family caregivers of home based palliative care patients: longer term effects from a randomised controlled trial. *Psychooncology.* 2015;24:19–24.
27. Laudenslager ML, Simoneau TL, Kilbourn K, et al. A randomized control trial of a psychosocial intervention for caregivers of allogeneic hematopoietic stem cell transplant patients: effects on distress. *Bone Marrow Transplant.* 2015;50:1110–1118.
28. Leow M, Chan S, Chan M. A pilot randomized, controlled trial of the effectiveness of a psychoeducational intervention on family caregivers of patients with advanced cancer. *Oncol Nurs Forum.* 2015;42:E63–E72.
29. Manne SL, Kashy DA, Weinberg DS, Boscarino JA, Bowen DJ, Worhach S. A pilot evaluation of the efficacy of a couple-tailored print intervention on colorectal cancer screening practices among non-adherent couples. *Psychol Health.* 2013;28:1046–1065.
30. Mitchell GK, Girgis A, Jiwa M, Sibbritt D, Burridge LH, Senior HE. Providing general practice needs-based care for carers of people with advanced cancer: a randomised controlled trial. *Br J Gen Pract.* 2013;63:e683–e690.
31. Namkoong K, DuBenske LL, Shaw BR, et al. Creating a bond between caregivers online: effect on caregivers' coping strategies. *J Health Commun.* 2012;17:125–140.
32. Northouse L, Schafenacker A, Barr KL, et al. A tailored web-based psychoeducational intervention for cancer patients and their family caregivers. *Cancer Nurs.* 2014;37:321–330.

33. Northouse LL, Mood DW, Schafenacker A, et al. Randomized clinical trial of a brief and extensive dyadic intervention for advanced cancer patients and their family caregivers. *Psychooncology.* 2013;22:555–563.

34. Perz J, Ussher JM, Team ACaSS. A randomized trial of a minimal intervention for sexual concerns after cancer: a comparison of self-help and professionally delivered modalities. *BMC Cancer* 2015;15:629.

35. Porter LS, Keefe FJ, Garst J, et al. Caregiver-assisted coping skills training for lung cancer: results of a randomized clinical trial. *J Pain Symptom Manage.* 2011;41:1–13.

36. Segrin C, Badger TA, Harrington J. Interdependent psychological quality of life in dyads adjusting to prostate cancer. *Health Psychol.* 2012;31:70–79.

37. Shaw JM, Young JM, Butow PN, et al. Improving psychosocial outcomes for caregivers of people with poor prognosis gastrointestinal cancers: a randomized controlled trial (Family Connect). *Support Care Cancer.* 2016;24:585–595.

38. Sherwood PR, Given BA, Given CW, Sikorskii A, You M, Prince J. The impact of a problem-solving intervention on increasing caregiver assistance and improving caregiver health. *Support Care Cancer.* 2012;20:1937–1947.

39. Silveira MJ, Given CW, Given B, Rosland AM, Piette JD. Patient-caregiver concordance in symptom assessment and improvement in outcomes for patients undergoing cancer chemotherapy. *Chronic Illn.* 2010;6:46–56.

40. Song L, Northouse LL, Zhang L, et al. Study of dyadic communication in couples managing prostate cancer: a longitudinal perspective. *Psychooncology.* 2012;21:72–81.

41. Tsianakas V, Robert G, Richardson A, et al. Enhancing the experience of carers in the chemotherapy outpatient setting: an exploratory randomised controlled trial to test impact, acceptability and feasibility of a complex intervention co-designed by carers and staff. *Support Care Cancer.* 2015;23:3069–3080.

42. Valeberg BT, Kolstad E, Småstuen MC, Miaskowski C, Rustøen T. The PRO-SELF pain control program improves family caregivers' knowledge of cancer pain management. *Cancer Nurs.* 2013;36:429–435.

43. van den Hurk DG, Schellekens MP, Molema J, Speckens AE, van der Drift MA. Mindfulness-based stress reduction for lung cancer patients and their partners: results of a mixed methods pilot study. *Palliat Med.* 2015;29:652–660.

44. Walker LM, Hampton AJ, Wassersug RJ, Thomas BC, Robinson JW. Androgen deprivation therapy and maintenance of intimacy: a randomized controlled pilot study of an educational intervention for patients and their partners. *Contemp Clin Trials.* 2013;34:227–231.

45. Yun YH, Lee MK, Bae Y, et al. Efficacy of a training program for long-term disease-free cancer survivors as health partners: a randomized controlled trial in Korea. *Asian Pac J Cancer Prev.* 2013;14:7229–7235.

46. Maloney C, Lyons KD, Li Z, Hegel M, Ahles TA, Bakitas M. Patient perspectives on participation in the ENABLE II randomized controlled trial of a concurrent oncology palliative care intervention: benefits and burdens. *Palliat Med.* 2013;27:375–383.

47. Bakitas M, Lyons K, Hegel M, et al. Effects of a palliative care intervention on clinical outcomes in patients with advanced cancer: the Project ENABLE II randomized controlled trial. *JAMA.* 2009;302:741–749.

48. O'Hara RE, Hull JG, Lyons KD, et al. Impact on caregiver burden of a patient-focused palliative care intervention for patients with advanced cancer. *Palliat Support Care.* 2010;8:395–404.

49. Zubkoff L, Dionne-Odom JN, Pisu M, et al. Developing a "toolkit" to measure implementation of concurrent palliative care in rural community cancer centers. *Palliat Support Care.* 2018;16:60–72.

50. Dionne-Odom JN, Applebaum AJ, Ornstein KA, et al. Participation and interest in support services among family caregivers of older adults with cancer. *Psychooncology.* 2018;27:969–976.

51. Hegel MT, Dietrich AJ, Seville JL, Jordan CB. Training residents in problem-solving treatment of depression: a pilot feasibility and impact study. *Fam Med.* 2004;36:204–208.

52. Unützer J, Katon W, Callahan CM, et al. Collaborative care management of late-life depression in the primary care setting: a randomized controlled trial. *JAMA.* 2002;288:2836–2845.

53. McMillan S, Small B. Using the COPE intervention for family caregivers to improve symptoms of hospice homecare patients: a clinical trial. *Oncol Nurs Forum.* 2007;34:313–321.

54. McMillan S, Small B, Weitzner M, et al. Impact of coping skills intervention with family caregivers of hospice patients with cancer. *Cancer.* 2005;106:214–222.

CHAPTER 8

FOCUS

A Psychoeducational Program for Cancer
Patients and Their Family Caregivers

LAUREL NORTHOUSE, CLAYTON SHUMAN,
MOIRA VISOVATTI, BONNIE DOCKHAM,
AND MARITA TITLER

BACKGROUND

FOCUS is a psychoeducational program that was developed in 2002 with funding from the American Cancer Society to provide information and support to cancer patients and their family caregivers.[1] FOCUS was based on a series of descriptive and exploratory studies that reported that family members experienced as much emotional distress as patients, received little support from others, and felt unprepared to provide complex care at home.

Stress and coping theory[2,3] and family stress theory[4] provided the theoretical foundation for the FOCUS program. These theories contend that personal and environmental factors can affect how people appraise and cope with a stressful event such as cancer. They provided the theoretical basis for developing interventions to reduce negative appraisals (e.g., uncertainty, hopelessness, symptom distress); to enhance coping resources (e.g., active coping, family communication, social support, self-efficacy); and to improve the quality of life (QOL) of both patients and their family caregivers. Furthermore, the theories contend patients' and caregivers' responses to illness (e.g., QOL) are interdependent[4] (Figure 8.1).

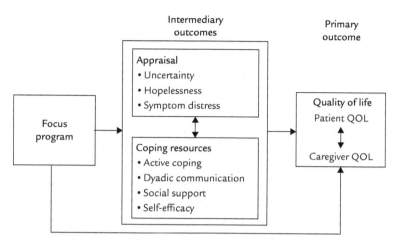

Figure 8.1: Theoretical framework and examples of study variables.

We designed the FOCUS program to address five content areas that form the acronym F-O-C-U-S. *Family involvement* (**F**) is the central component of the program because it promotes effective interpersonal relationships between patients and their family caregivers to help manage the demands associated with both the illness and caregiving. *Optimistic attitude* (**O**) helps patients and their family caregivers maintain hope, find meaning and purpose, focus on the present, and set realistic goals for the future. *Coping effectiveness* (**C**) assists patients and family caregivers to use active coping strategies (e.g., problem-solving) rather than avoidant coping strategies (e.g., denial) and encourages them to engage in healthy lifestyle behaviors (nutrition and exercise) to combat stress. *Uncertainty reduction* (**U**) provides patients and caregivers with information about the illness and treatments. It also includes helping them to learn to live with the pervasive uncertainty that typically accompanies a cancer diagnosis. Finally, *symptom management* (**S**) addresses any physical or emotional symptoms patients and their family caregivers experience and teaches ways to manage them.

EFFICACY STUDIES WITH THE FOCUS PROGRAM

Three longitudinal randomized controlled trials (RCTs) were conducted to determine the efficacy of the FOCUS program in improving outcomes for cancer patients and their family caregivers.[5-7] Efficacy was demonstrated for three adult cancer populations: women with recurrent breast cancer (*N* = 134 dyads), men with localized or advanced prostate cancer (*N* = 235 dyads), and people with advanced cancer (lung, colorectal, breast, prostate)

(N = 302 dyads) (Table 8.1).[5-7] Participants' satisfaction with the FOCUS program was high across these studies (Table 8.1).[1,8]

In the first two studies, FOCUS consisted of three home visits (90 minutes per session) and two telephone calls (30 minutes per session) offered over 10 weeks.[5,6] The third study examined the effect of program dose: a brief three-session FOCUS program (two home visits, one phone call) and an extensive six-session FOCUS program (four home visits, two phone calls).[7] FOCUS was delivered by licensed nurses who received 40 hours of training and used the FOCUS Program Manual, which contained a checklist of interventions for each session to ensure program fidelity. The type of outcomes assessed following receipt of FOCUS varied somewhat across studies, as detailed in Table 8.1.

In the first RCT, recurrent breast cancer patients who received FOCUS reported significantly less hopelessness and less negative appraisal of illness, and their family caregivers reported less negative appraisal of caregiving as compared to the control group (Table 8.1). In the second RCT, prostate cancer patients who received FOCUS reported significant improvement in their communication with their partners and less uncertainty about the illness (Table 8.1). Interestingly, partners reported a greater number of positive outcomes than the prostate cancer patients, including less negative appraisal of caregiving, uncertainty, hopelessness, avoidant coping, better communication with their husbands, higher self-efficacy, and better physical and mental QOL (Table 8.1). Some intervention effects (e.g., improved communication, physical QOL) were still evident at the 12-month follow-up (Table 8.1). The third RCT with dyads facing advanced cancer of various types demonstrated no difference in efficacy by *program dose* (Brief vs. Extensive), regardless of baseline risk status (low vs. high distress scores) or type of cancer. However, dyads in both the Brief and Extensive FOCUS programs used significantly less avoidant coping strategies, maintained their social QOL, and had higher emotional QOL (caregivers only) than controls. In addition, dyads in the Brief program engaged in a greater number of healthy lifestyle behaviors (e.g., good nutrition), whereas dyads in the Extensive program reported greater self-efficacy (Table 8.1).

Together, findings from the three RCTs provide empirical support for the efficacy of the FOCUS program when delivered to cancer patients and family caregivers facing different types of cancer (breast, prostate, lung, colorectal) and stages of cancer (localized, advanced). The program was also efficacious for different types of caregivers (spousal, nonspousal) and when offered as a three-, five-, or six-session program. Participants' satisfaction with the program remained high even when the program dose varied (Table 8.1).

Table 8.1 FOCUS PROGRAM EFFICACY AND EFFECTIVENESS STUDIES

Reference	Study Design	Intervention	Outcomes	Main Findings
Northouse,[1,5] 2002, 2005	Longitudinal RCT at three time points: 0, 3, & 6 months. Sample included 134 recurrent breast cancer patient-caregiver dyads (69 intervention, 65 usual care).	The program included the five FOCUS components and was delivered to a dyad by a nurse. The dose was 5.5 hours (three 90-min HVs and two 30-min PCs over 10 weeks).	Appraisal of illness/caregiving Uncertainty Hopelessness Coping strategies Quality of life	*Baseline to 3-month findings* • Intervention patients showed a significant decrease in negative appraisal of illness ($p = .008$), and control patients did not ($p = .68$). • Intervention patients showed a significant decrease in hopelessness ($p = .03$), while control patients showed a significant increase in hopelessness ($p = .03$). • Caregivers in the intervention group showed a significant decrease in negative appraisal of caregiving ($p = .004$), but control caregivers did not ($p = .89$). *Satisfaction* • Satisfaction scores were 4.7 for patients and 4.3 for caregivers (range 1–5).
Northouse,[6,8] 2007, 2009	Longitudinal RCT at four time points: 0, 4, 8, & 12 months. Sample included 235 prostate cancer patient-spouse dyads (112 intervention, 123 usual care).	The program included the five FOCUS components and was delivered to a dyad by a nurse. The dose was 5.5 hours (three 90-min HVs and two 30-min PCs over 10 weeks).	Appraisal of illness/caregiving Uncertainty Hopelessness Coping strategies Self-efficacy Communication Symptoms Quality of life	*Findings at 4 months* • Intervention patients reported significantly less uncertainty about their illness ($p < .05$) and more communication about their illness with spouses ($p < .05$) than control patients. • Intervention spouses reported significantly better mental QOL ($p < .05$); better overall QOL ($p < .01$); less negative appraisal of caregiving ($p < .01$); less hopelessness ($p < .05$); less uncertainty ($p < .01$); higher self-efficacy ($p < .05$); better communication ($p < .01$), and less symptom distress ($p < .01$) than control spouses.

(continued)

Table 8.1 CONTINUED

Reference	Study Design	Intervention	Outcomes	Main Findings
				Findings at 8 months
				• Intervention spouses reported significantly better physical QOL ($p < .01$); better communication with patients ($p < .05$); and less distress about patients' urinary symptoms ($p < .01$) than control spouses.
				Findings at 12 months
				• Intervention spouses reported significantly better physical QOL ($p < .05$); higher self-efficacy ($p < .05$); better communication with patients ($p < .01$); and more active coping at 12 months ($p < .05$).
				Satisfaction.
				• Mean satisfaction score for both patients and spouses was 4.5 (range 1–5).
Northouse,[7] 2013	Longitudinal RCT at three time points: 0, 3, & 6 months. Sample included 302 advanced prostate, lung, or colorectal cancer patient–caregiver dyads (99 extensive, 99 brief, 104 usual care).	The program included the five FOCUS components and was delivered to a dyad by a nurse. The dose was 7 hours for the extensive group (four 90-min HVs and two 30-min PCs over 10 weeks). The dose was 3.5 hours for the brief group (two 90-min HVs and one 30-min PC over 10 weeks).	Appraisal of illness/caregiving Uncertainty Hopelessness Coping strategies Self-efficacy Communication Healthy behaviors Dyadic support Quality of life	*Baseline to 3-month findings*
				• Dyads in the extensive group ($p < .001$) and brief group ($p = .033$) showed a significant decrease in avoidant coping at 3 months, but dyads in control group did not.
				• Dyads in the brief and extensive interventions maintained their social QOL at 3 months, while control dyads had a significant decline ($p < .01$).
				• Caregivers in brief and extensive interventions had higher emotional QOL ($p < .01$) than control caregivers.
				• Dyads in the brief group ($p = .001$) showed a significant increase in use of healthy behaviors, but control or extensive group did not.
				• Dyads in the extensive group ($p = .041$) showed a significant increase in self-efficacy, but dyads in the control or brief group

Northouse,[13] 2014	Translation to web-based format with pre-post design.

Sample included 38 breast, prostate, lung, or colorectal cancer patient-caregiver dyads. | The program included the family involvement component of FOCUS only and was delivered to a dyad through the web.

The dose included three online sessions and three tailored emails over 6 weeks. | Appraisal of illness/ caregiving

Self-efficacy

Communication

Dyadic support

Emotional distress

Quality of life

Satisfaction | *Baseline to 6-months findings*
- Dyads in the extensive and brief interventions maintained their social QOL, while control dyads had lower social QOL.
- Caregivers in brief and extensive interventions had higher emotional QOL ($p < .05$) than control caregivers.
- Dyads in the brief group ($p = .045$) had a decrease in avoidant coping at 6 months, but dyads in the control or extensive groups did not.

Satisfaction
- Mean patient satisfaction scores for both the brief and extensive groups was 4.6 (range 1–5).
- Mean caregiver satisfaction score for both the brief and extensive groups was 4.4 (range 1–5).

Pre-post findings
- Dyads reported decreased emotional distress ($p < .05$); increased overall total QOL ($p < .05$), physical QOL ($p < .05$), and functional QOL ($p < .01$); and greater benefits of illness/ caregiving ($p < .01$).
- Caregivers reported higher self-efficacy ($p < .05$).

Feasibility findings
- Enrollment and retention rates were 51% and 86%, respectively.
- Mean satisfaction scores were 6.0 for usability, 4.4 for usefulness, and 4.8 for general satisfaction (range 1–7). |

(continued)

Table 8.1 CONTINUED

Reference	Study Design	Intervention	Outcomes	Main Findings
Dockham,[9] 2016	Implementation & effectiveness study with pre-post design. Sample included 37 patient-caregiver dyads with any type of cancer.	The program included the five FOCUS components and was delivered to a small group (3–4 dyads) by a social worker. The dose was 12 hours (six weekly 120-min sessions).	Appraisal of illness/ caregiving Self-efficacy Communication Dyadic support Quality of life Satisfaction	*Pre-post findings* • Dyads reported an increase in overall QOL ($p = .002$), physical QOL ($p = .019$), emotional QOL ($p = .004$), and functional QOL ($p = .003$); perceived benefits of illness ($p = .032$); and self-efficacy ($p = .002$). *Feasibility findings* • Enrollment and retention rates were 60% and 92%, respectively. • Fidelity rate was 94%. • Mean satisfaction score for both patients and caregivers was 4.3 (range 1–5).
Titler,[10] 2017	Implementation & effectiveness study with pre-post design. Sample included 36 patient-caregiver dyads with any type of cancer.	The program included the five FOCUS components and was delivered to a small group (3–4 dyads) by a social worker/therapist. The dose was 10 hours (five weekly 120-min sessions).	Appraisal of illness/ caregiving Self-efficacy Communication Emotional distress Satisfaction	*Pre-post findings* • Dyads reported increased total QOL ($p = .014$), emotional QOL ($p = .012$), and functional QOL ($p = .049$); benefits of illness ($p = .013$); and self-efficacy ($p = .001$), as well as a decrease in emotional distress ($p = .002$). *Feasibility findings* • Enrollment and retention rates were 71% and 90%, respectively. • Fidelity rate was 85%. • Mean satisfaction scores were 4.0 for patients and 4.5 for caregivers (range 1–5).

HV, home visit; min, minute; PC, phone call; RCT, randomized control trial.
Instruments used to measure outcomes: appraisal of illness/caregiving by Appraisal of Illness Scale and Appraisal of Caregiving Scale or the Benefits of Illness Scale; uncertainty by the Mishel Uncertainty in Illness Scale; hopelessness by the Beck Hopelessness Scale; coping by the Brief Cope; quality of life by the Functional Assessment of Cancer Treatment (version 4), the Short Form (36) Health Survey, or Medical Outcomes Study 12-item Short Form; self-efficacy by the Lewis Cancer Self-efficacy Scale; communication by the Lewis Mutuality and Interpersonal Sensitivity Scale; healthy behaviors by researcher-developed scale; dyadic support by a modified version of the Social Support Questionnaire; emotional distress by the Profile of Mood States—

IMPLEMENTATION AND EFFECTIVENESS STUDIES WITH THE FOCUS PROGRAM

Although the dyadic FOCUS program has demonstrated efficacy, too often efficacious programs are not moved into practice and evaluated for effectiveness. (Table 8.2 describes differences between FOCUS efficacy and effectiveness studies). Our team was dedicated to moving FOCUS into practice so that patients and caregivers could benefit from it. We chose the Cancer Support Community (CSC) as the ideal location for conducting an effectiveness study with FOCUS. The CSC is a large network of community agencies in the United States that provide professional psychosocial care at no cost to cancer patients and their caregivers who reside in the community. All programs at CSC are offered by licensed oncology social workers/therapists in a small-group format to facilitate support among participants and to reduce resource expenditures.

Considerations for Implementing FOCUS in CSC

The first consideration was how to deliver FOCUS and who would deliver it. When implementing an evidence-based program, it is important to understand the workflow in the practice setting and how the agency could integrate the program into its philosophy and structure. For example, CSCs deliver group-based interventions in six small-group sessions facilitated by licensed social workers. Since licensed nurses delivered the FOCUS efficacy trials to individual dyads, we had to convert the FOCUS program into a group format and train the facilitators. A second consideration was determining how to evaluate the effectiveness of FOCUS, what measures to use, and if a comparison/nonintervention group was needed. Third, we discussed how to recruit and enroll potential participants for the FOCUS program. Fourth, we considered how to ensure fidelity to the FOCUS intervention now that social workers/therapists were delivering it.

Conversion of FOCUS to Group Delivery Format

Research staff who delivered FOCUS in the efficacy trials met with the program director at the Ann Arbor, Michigan, CSC to translate FOCUS into a group format that would be delivered over 6 weeks. An intervention grid

Table 8.2 COMPARISON OF FOCUS EFFICACY AND EFFECTIVENESS STUDIES

Elements	FOCUS Efficacy Trials	Effectiveness and Implementation Studies
Design	Longitudinal randomized control trial.	Pre-post intervention (no control group).
Setting	Delivered in patients' home with additional phone calls.	Delivered face to face at CSC affiliate sites.
Recipients of the intervention (sample)	More homogeneous. Included breast, prostate, lung, and colorectal cancer patient-caregiver dyads.	More heterogeneous. Less stringent inclusion criteria. Included patient-caregiver dyads with any type of cancer.
How FOCUS was delivered	Delivered to individual patient-caregiver dyads.	Delivered to small groups of patient-caregiver dyads (3–4 dyads per group).
	Delivered by a trained research assistant (licensed nurse).	Delivered by trained facilitators employed by the CSC (licensed social worker/family therapist).
Intervention dose	Tested various intervention doses on outcomes over 10 weeks.	Tested similar dose and administration over 5–6 weeks: weekly 120-min group sessions (10–12 hours).
	Initial two trials (5.5 hours): 3 home visits and 2 phone calls.	
	Brief (3.5 hours): 2 home visits and 1 phone call.	
	Extensive (7 hours): 4 home visits and 2 phone calls.	
	Third trial: Brief (3.5hours): 2 home visits and 1 phone call.	
	Extensive (7 hours): 4 home visits and 2 phone calls.	
Training	Research assistants trained 40 hours on how to deliver the FOCUS intervention.	Facilitators trained 8 hours on how to recruit participants, deliver the FOCUS intervention (fidelity), and collect data, as well as implementation steps.
Intervention fidelity	Fidelity assessed in multiple ways.	Fidelity checklist completed by the facilitator.
	Fidelity checklist completed by research assistant.	
	Research assistant audiotaped one intervention session per month that was reviewed by intervention coordinator.	
	Research assistant presented one case study per month at intervention staff meetings.	
Data collection	Collected by trained data collector, blind to participants' group assignment (i.e., treatment vs. control).	Collected by trained CSC staff.

was developed to ensure that the content in the small-group format included the same five core areas as in the original home-based program (F-O-C-U-S) but was spread out over six group intervention sessions. The detailed content of the original FOCUS program was not changed, but ground rules about effective group processes were added. As a result, a modified program protocol was created. Our research team decided that the group would consist of three to four dyads to ensure intimacy, facilitate participation by each member, and provide time to cover the content itemized in each of the five components. The FOCUS program inventor (Northouse) reviewed and approved the final translation of FOCUS to the group delivery format. Because staff at the CSC affiliates are licensed social workers, there was consensus that they could effectively deliver the program following training. People with different types and stages of cancer were allowed to participate as this was consistent with the CSC philosophy and model of program delivery.

Following implementation at the Ann Arbor site, the FOCUS program expanded to include two additional CSC affiliates. Research staff developed a training program and FOCUS Implementation Training Manual in collaboration with the Ann Arbor CSC affiliate to educate the staff of the affiliates joining the project about the benefits of FOCUS (as found in the efficacy trials), the components of FOCUS, emphasis of each FOCUS component by week, and use of educational materials incorporated into the program. Facilitators and project managers from the two new CSC affiliates (California and Ohio) attended a 1-day, in-person training session. In addition to the training manual, we developed a FOCUS Intervention Manual designed for use by the facilitator to guide delivery of the program each week and to ensure intervention fidelity.

At the beginning of implementation, the team held weekly conference calls with the facilitators to discuss challenges and share successes. Topics included recruitment of participants, fidelity to the program, problems or concerns that arose from the groups (e.g., one group member dominating), and use of educational materials. After initial implementation, calls were scheduled every other week.

Implementation, Feasibility, and Effectiveness

We decided a pre-post intervention design (no control group) was appropriate for implementation and to evaluate effectiveness because three prior randomized trials demonstrated the efficacy of the FOCUS program with significant findings across studies. Outcome measures were collected prior to delivery of the FOCUS program and on completion. For implementation, it is important that outcome measures are parsimonious, will detect change (i.e., effectiveness), and are derived from the efficacy trials. We decided to measure some of the same outcomes that the FOCUS efficacy trials assessed (Table 8.1). In addition, we believed it was important to measure participants' satisfaction with the FOCUS program delivered in a group format and to use these data to refine the program.

The implementation of FOCUS was first piloted at a local CSC site, the CSC of greater Ann Arbor,[9] followed by implementation at two CSC affiliate sites outside our local geographic area (Ohio and California).[10] At the first site, we implemented a six-session small-group program but modified it to a five-session small-group program in the other two sites because it seemed sufficient to cover program content and required less time from participants and the interventionist. When FOCUS was implemented at these sites in a small-group format by agency staff using either the five- or six-session program, patients and caregivers who participated in the program reported significant improvement in their overall QOL, emotional and functional well-being, emotional distress, perceived benefits of experiencing cancer, and self-efficacy managing the illness.[9,10] Participants were highly satisfied with the program (Table 8.1).

To determine if it was feasible to deliver FOCUS at these three CSC sites, we also examined enrollment and retention rates and intervention fidelity. Data demonstrated that it was feasible to enroll and retain dyads and deliver the program with high intervention fidelity[9,10] (Table 8.1).

We also assessed the cost of delivering FOCUS, which had not been assessed in prior studies. We estimated costs based on the mean total time to provide oversight and delivery for one 5-session FOCUS program multiplied by the median hourly wage of staff. Average cost estimates for oversight and delivery of one 5-session FOCUS program was $669.45 or $168.00 per dyad, assuming four dyads per group.[10]

The case example that follows describes a couple's experience who participated in the FOCUS program, delivered as a small group, at one of the CSC sites. As indicated in the case example and study findings (Table 8.1), FOCUS was feasible to deliver in a group format in CSC affiliate sites with positive effects on patients and their caregivers. Fidelity to the program and participant satisfaction were both high.

Case Example

Introduction

Rebecca and John had just celebrated their 12th wedding anniversary. Rebecca was a stay-at-home mother caring for their two young children, Samantha (age 9) and Ethan (age 7). John worked in the maintenance department at the local hospital and was paid an hourly wage. Extended family was moderately supportive, although there was some conflict. Financial problems persisted before Rebecca was diagnosed with advanced colon cancer at the age of 38. Rebecca was initially diagnosed with stage III disease and was treated successfully. After a short remission (<1 year), her cancer had spread to her bones, liver, and brain. Rebecca was heartbroken that she was facing the end of her life with two young children, and John refused to admit that her death was a possibility. Rebecca was in a lot of pain that was not being well controlled by her healthcare team. Her depression escalated, resulting in Rebecca's withdrawal from her family and increased irritability with them.

Money was tight, and although Rebecca recognized the need for emotional support for their entire family, they could not afford the additional copays for mental health services required by their insurance. John was hesitant to see an individual therapist because he thought he was "strong enough" to cope on his own. The FOCUS program provided a viable option for the support they needed and was a reasonable cost-free alternative. The group format also appealed to John, who thought that his participation could be beneficial to others (his wife in particular).

The FOCUS Program: Rebecca and John's Group

The group that Rebecca and John joined consisted of three other heterosexual couples, all married, with children ranging in age from 5 to 12 years. Two of the other patients were facing advanced illness; one was not. The content design of the FOCUS program aligned well with the presenting problems for Rebecca and John. In particular, the program allowed them to incorporate their children in the process of treatment, learn ways to manage symptoms, and discuss death and dying concerns. Despite John's initial discomfort and resistance, as he heard other couples in the group admit to their fears and reservations about the end of life, he became more willing to admit his own feelings and fears. His willingness to explore these discussions in the group setting translated into more work being done at home between Rebecca and John. They set a goal to have a "date" to talk about these issues weekly throughout the program. This opened communication between the couple and reduced Rebecca's sense of isolation.

The program also enabled Rebecca and John to reframe their sense of hope. Throughout the program, Rebecca was able to feel more hopeful, whereas before she was unable to hope for anything. Initially, her perception of hope was limited to cure, which was a known impossibility. Hearing others share their hopes and fears allowed her to change her mindset and recognize multiple types of hope. Now, she was hoping for a peaceful death.

Benefits

Because of her involvement in the FOCUS program, Rebecca was able to achieve a peaceful death. She and John incorporated strategies learned in the group to talk with their children and prepare them for her death and the grief around it. The group also provided a lasting benefit: belief in the power of professional assistance. The stigma once held by John that asking for help was "weak" had dissipated. The primary aims of the FOCUS program were parallel to the needs of Rebecca and John and other members of the group. Additionally, learning that other dyads shared these concerns allowed for normalization of their feelings and the exploration of other coping and support strategies. After the completion of the FOCUS program, both John and Rebecca joined other support groups at the CSC and enrolled their children in their Children's Program. Following her death, the family remained involved in bereavement support through community organizations.

PLANNING FOR BROADER IMPLEMENTATION AND DISSEMINATION

The FOCUS Program has demonstrated efficacy or effectiveness in a variety of contexts (i.e., home, community agency); delivery formats (i.e., individual, small group); and with different types of trained facilitators (i.e., registered nurses, social workers). An important next step for FOCUS involves planning and preparing for broader dissemination so that more people with cancer and their caregivers have the opportunity to participate in the program and benefit from it. Existing implementation and dissemination frameworks, like the RE-AIM framework, can guide efforts for broader dissemination of FOCUS. RE-AIM stands for reach, effectiveness, adoption, implementation, and maintenance.[11] Table 8.3 includes questions to consider for each of the RE-AIM dimensions.

Table 8.3 BROADER IMPLEMENTATION AND DISSEMINATION OF THE FOCUS
PROGRAM USING THE RE-AIM FRAMEWORK AS A GUIDE

RE-AIM Dimension	Questions to Consider[a]
Reach	• What is the target population?
	• What are their characteristics (e.g., cancer diagnosis, type of dyad)?
	• Where does target population live (e.g., rural United States, Europe)?
Effectiveness	• Is the FOCUS program likely to benefit the target population?
	• Do stakeholders (e.g., potential FOCUS participants or facilitators, clinic or community leaders) find it beneficial and appropriate?
	• How should the success of the FOCUS program be measured (e.g., satisfaction ratings and feedback, quality-of-life measures, etc.)?
Adoption	• What are the barriers (e.g., lack of time, funding) and facilitators (e.g., supportive leadership, stakeholder interest) to adoption by staff, leadership, and potential participants?
	• How should facilitators be trained to deliver the FOCUS program? How much training is needed?
	• Do facilitators need ongoing support?
Implementation	• How should the FOCUS program be branded, packaged, and marketed?
	• How should fidelity to the program be monitored? Should it be reported?
	• Can the FOCUS program be adapted for different practice settings?
Maintenance	• What is needed to sustain the FOCUS program in organizations?
	• What is needed to keep participants engaged in the program?

[a] Based on RE-AIM Planning Tool.[11,12]

Reach

Reach refers to the identified audience for the FOCUS program and includes its demographic and medical characteristics. Future target populations for FOCUS could include international audiences, lower socioeconomic groups, or people with cancer diagnoses (e.g., ovarian cancer) not previously reached during the efficacy and effectiveness studies.

Effectiveness

Organizations and stakeholders interested in the FOCUS program must determine its effectiveness; they need to know how the program will benefit their target population and have a way to measure this benefit. Outcome measures from our previous studies may be helpful, such as QOL, perceived benefits of illness, dyadic communication, emotional distress, self-efficacy in managing cancer, and participant satisfaction.[9,10]

Adoption

Adoption refers to the organizations or stakeholders that plan to deliver the FOCUS program. Identifying barriers and facilitators to adoption is crucial. Ideal characteristics and minimum requirements for potential facilitators need to be identified and described. Facilitators must receive sufficient training to ensure that the FOCUS program is adopted and delivered as intended to achieve the same level of benefit demonstrated in previous research. Training must take into account facilitator availability, associated training costs, and format (e.g., web based, self-directed, train the trainer). Facilitators in previous studies reported that training and ongoing support during implementation were beneficial.

Implementation

Implementation of the FOCUS program refers to the delivery of the FOCUS program as intended. Branding, packaging, marketing, and implementation costs are important considerations. Branding involves the identification of program components, the language used to describe the program and its components, and the logos and slogans designed to communicate and market the program in order to make FOCUS consistently recognizable and relatable to consumers. Program components and materials need to be packaged in an organized, accessible, and usable way. Lack of attention to packaging may result in poor uptake, inconsistent delivery, or threats to program sustainability. Included in the packaging should be implementation guides and fidelity checklists to help organizations and facilitators implement the program and monitor its fidelity.

Marketing the program to stakeholders and potential participants improves brand recognition while encouraging participation of members from the target population. Marketing may include printed or web-based postings, direct email invitations, or use of mass media outlets (e.g., newspapers, television, social media). Understanding the cost of the program allows program managers to make appropriate budget allocations ahead of time. This planning should include identification of a revenue stream that will ensure the program is sustainable long term.

Maintenance

The sustainability of the FOCUS program over time is referred to as *maintenance* and involves oversight by both the organizations and stakeholders delivering FOCUS. Embedding the FOCUS program in community and clinical settings requires acquisition or reallocation of resources to support ongoing delivery. Additionally, oversight and support from the FOCUS program research team are critical for addressing concerns, providing materials, and ensuring program fidelity.

TRANSLATION AND DISSEMINATION OF FOCUS PROGRAM COMPONENTS

We translated FOCUS to a tailored web-based program in order to increase patients' and caregivers' access to the program and to facilitate broader dissemination.[13] (See Zulman et al.[14] for details on the translation process). The central module of the program was the Family Involvement component of FOCUS. The program was designed for patients and caregivers to work together on the program (i.e., sitting side by side in front of the computer screen) and to facilitate interactions among the dyad in a manner similar to the dyadic format of the original nurse-delivered FOCUS program. The web-based program was delivered in three sessions over a 6-week period. The program was tested in a pre- and postintervention study (no control) with 38 dyads (Table 8.1). Findings indicated significant improvement in dyads' emotional distress; overall, physical, and functional QOL; and perceived benefits of illness/caregiving, as well as in patients' physical health and caregivers' self-efficacy.

The web-based program needs further refinement before broad dissemination. Additional modules need to be developed that address other components of the FOCUS acronym (i.e., optimistic attitude, coping effectiveness, uncertainty reduction, and symptom management). In addition, the platform used for delivering the dyadic program needs to be updated regularly to incorporate the latest technology. Nevertheless, we have demonstrated that the FOCUS program can be translated to a web-based format and have positive effects on patient and caregiver outcomes.

Dissemination of FOCUS on the National Cancer Institute's Research-Tested Intervention Program Website

In an effort to begin disseminating information about the FOCUS program, we submitted an application for the FOCUS program (prostate cancer version) to be included in the National Cancer Institute's (NCI's) searchable database on Research-Tested Intervention Programs (RTIPS). Research coordinators for RTIPS reviewed the program and rated it for its research integrity, intervention impact, and dissemination impact and in 2009 accepted it for inclusion on the RTIPs website.[15] The RTIPs website provides an evaluation of the FOCUS program as well as downloadable program content, including FOCUS program handouts, manuals, and other supplementary materials.

Dissemination by Michigan Department of Community Health

To meet the need of the growing number of prostate cancer survivors and their partners, the Michigan Department of Community Health requested that FOCUS program symptom management and psychosocial handouts (i.e., communication, coping, and optimism) be made available on the state's Michigan Cancer Consortium Prostate Cancer website for survivors, family members, and professionals. With funding from the Centers for Disease Control and Prevention, the original FOCUS educational materials used in the prostate RCT were updated and made available in three languages (English, Spanish, Arabic) on the Michigan Cancer Consortium (MCC) website.[16-17]

The Michigan Department of Community Health examined the 5-year utilization (downloads) of these educational materials (i.e., guides) between January 2011 and December 2015 and reported that nearly 90,000 guides were downloaded during that period of time,[16-17] suggesting that the symptom management and psychosocial handouts continued to meet important needs of survivors, family members, and others.

CONCLUSIONS

The FOCUS program was developed to address the educational and support needs of both cancer patients and their family caregivers. The program has produced positive outcomes for patients and caregivers when delivered by nurses at home, by agency staff in small-group sessions, and via the web. It is essential to continue to find ways to implement and disseminate efficacious programs such as FOCUS to help meet the needs of the growing number of families living with the stressful effects of cancer.

REFERENCES

1. Northouse LL, Walker J, Schafenacker A, et al. A family-based program of care for women with recurrent breast cancer and their family members. *Oncol Nurs Forum.* 2002;29(10):1411–1419.
2. Lazarus RS. Toward better research on stress and coping. *Am Psychol.* 2000;55(6):665–673.
3. Lazarus RS, Folkman S. *Stress, Coping and Appraisal.* New York, NY: Springer; 1984.
4. McCubbin MA, McCubbin HI. Resiliency in families: a conceptual model of family adjustment and adaptation in response to stress and crises. In McCubbin HI, Thompson AI, McCubbin MA, eds. *Family Assessment: Resiliency, Coping, and Adaptation: Inventories for Research and Practice.* Madison, WI: University of Wisconsin System; 1996:1–64.
5. Northouse L, Kershaw T, Mood D, Schafenacker A. Effects of a family intervention on the quality of life of women with recurrent breast cancer and their family caregivers. *Psychooncology.* 2005;14(6):478–491.
6. Northouse LL, Mood DW, Schafenacker A, et al. Randomized clinical trial of a family intervention for prostate cancer patients and their spouses. *Cancer.* 2007;110(12):2809–2818.
7. Northouse LL, Mood DW, Schafenacker A, et al. Randomized clinical trial of a brief and extensive dyadic intervention for advanced cancer patients and their family caregivers. *Psychooncology.* 2013;22(3):555–563.
8. Harden J, Falahee M, Bickes J, et al. Factors associated with prostate cancer patients' and their spouses' satisfaction with a family-based intervention. *Cancer Nurs.* 2009;32(6):482–492.
9. Dockham B, Schafenacker A, Yoon H, et al. Implementation of a psychoeducational program for cancer survivors and family caregivers at a cancer support community affiliate: a pilot effectiveness study. *Cancer Nurs.* 2016;39(3):169–180.
10. Titler MG, Visovatti MA, Shuman C, et al. Effectiveness of implementing a dyadic psychoeducational intervention for cancer patients and family caregivers. *Support Care Cancer.* 2017;25(11):3395–3406.
11. Glasgow RE, Vogt TM, Boles SM. Evaluating the public health impact of health promotion interventions: the RE-AIM framework. *Am J Public Health.* 1999;89(9):1322–1327.
12. RE-AIM. Re-Aim Planning Tool. http://www.re-aim.org/resources-and-tools/self-rating-quiz/. Accessed February 12, 2018.
13. Northouse L, Schafenacker A, Barr KL, et al. A tailored web-based psychoeducational intervention for cancer patients and their family caregivers. *Cancer Nurs.* 2014;37(5):321–330.
14. Zulman DM, Schafenacker A, Barr KL, et al. Adapting an in-person patient-caregiver communication intervention to a tailored web-based format. *Psychooncology.* 2012;21(3):336–341.

15. National Cancer Institute. Family-based interventions (The FOCUS Program) for men with prostate cancer and their spouses/partners. https://rtips.cancer. gov/rtips/programDetails.do?programId=102766. Updated October 29, 2013. Accessed February 12, 2018.
16. Skolarus TA, Ragnoni JA, Garlinghouse C, et al. Multilingual self-management resources for prostate cancer survivors and their partners: results of a long-term academic-state health department partnership to promote survivorship care. *Urology*. 2017;110:92–97.
17. Michigan Cancer Consortium. Prostate cancer survivorship guides—help after treatment. http://www.prostatecancerdecision.org/helpAfterTreatmentEnglish. htm. Accessed February 12, 2018.

CHAPTER 9

Cognitive Behavioral Therapy for Informal Cancer Caregivers

JAMIE M. JACOBS, LARA TRAEGER,
EMILY A. WALSH, AND JOSEPH A. GREER

Informal family and friend caregivers for patients with cancer play a crucial role throughout the course of illness, handling a multitude of responsibilities related to the patient's care. These include coordinating healthcare visits, treatments and medication management, decision-making, daily responsibilities, and communicating with family and friends. In addition, caregivers must manage prognosis-related uncertainty and possible end-of-life issues.[1,2] Given the tremendous needs of patients along the continuum of cancer care, it is not uncommon for informal caregivers to become burdened and overwhelmed by the volume of their tasks and responsibilities. In addition to vast needs of the patient, caregivers must continue to attend to their own needs and potentially those of other dependents. This immense stress and caregiver burden can have substantial negative effects on a caregiver's mental, emotional, and physical health,[3,4] with up to 50% of caregivers of patients with cancer reporting elevated anxiety or depression.[1,5] Caregivers may also suffer stress-related physical morbidities both acutely and chronically. This burden among cancer caregivers has been well documented and previously described in Section 1 of this textbook.

A growing body of literature documents the positive impact of empirically supported interventions on the psychosocial needs of burdened caregivers. One such intervention is cognitive behavioral therapy (CBT). CBT is a psychotherapeutic intervention initially deemed effective among caregivers of patients with dementia[6] and more recently is finding significance within the context of cancer caregiving.[7] CBT is an evidence-based therapy used to treat anxiety, depression, substance use disorders, insomnia, and stress management, among others.[8] Initially introduced by Ellis[9] and Beck,[10] CBT focuses on altering an individual's interpretation of a stressor to influence the emotional response in the presence of that stressor, thus promoting problem-solving skills. Within the field of oncology, growing evidence for CBT supports its efficacy for use with patients and caregivers. The use of CBT with patients with cancer has been shown to decrease fatigue, anxiety, depression, and functional impairment and improve symptom management and quality of life (QOL).[11,12] Preliminary studies indicated that CBT improved symptoms of insomnia, moderated negative reactions to the burdens of caregiving, and decreased psychological distress in caregivers of patients with cancer.[13] Although more research is still needed, the efficacy of CBT with caregivers of patients with cancer is encouraging as it can be optimized to best fit the needs of the cancer caregiver population.

ELEMENTS OF COGNITIVE BEHAVIORAL THERAPY INTERVENTIONS

Cognitive behavioral therapy practitioners in cancer care may integrate multiple interventions to meet a range of patient and caregiver needs.[14] Caregiver interventions typically begin with education about CBT structure and goals, with emphasis on the importance of the caregiver's interpretations of their current stressors as they relate to their emotions and coping responses. The descriptions that follow underscore how CBT can be used to help caregivers value and prioritize self-care. Interventions can also be adapted to co-target the concerns of caregiver-patient dyads.

Behavioral activation (BA). This evidence-based treatment was designed to help patients with depression reduce inertia and avoidance of enjoyable or meaningful activities, thereby increasing positive reinforcement.[15] BA may be adapted carefully for caregivers, given their often reduced or halted engagement in such activities due to caregiver burden, lack of time, depression-related anhedonia, or a combination of these. We recommend that CBT practitioners and caregivers work together to identify and problem-solve practical ways for caregivers to engage in activities that maintain or boost their well-being. Some caregivers may be amenable to activities that they also can frame as benefitting the patient (e.g., afternoon walks together). Caregivers also might experience social isolation;

therefore, meeting and connecting with other caregivers in their community may be a particularly powerful BA intervention.

Cognitive restructuring. This established CBT strategy involves identifying thoughts that arise automatically during a stressful moment; challenging such thoughts to identify those that are unrealistic or unhelpful; and replacing these with more realistic or helpful thoughts. The CBT practitioner uses open-ended questions to help patients challenge their thoughts, rather than directly identifying errors in thinking. For caregivers, the goals of reducing negative self-talk may be to manage distress and make more effective coping decisions. Yet, the cancer care setting can involve realistic concerns or confusion related to diagnosis, treatment, and prognosis. Therefore, the CBT practitioner and caregiver will need to work carefully to differentiate negative self-talk that may be realistic (i.e., "Our daughter lives too far away to drive my loved one to his next oncology visit"); unhelpful (i.e., "Our friend might be able to drive my loved one to the clinic, but I would never burden him"); or unclear (i.e., "I don't think our community has transportation services"). This exercise may help the caregiver make choices between coping options that are acceptance oriented (for concerns that are uncontrollable) versus action oriented (for concerns that are controllable or actionable) or to work on finding more information.[14] Figure 9.1 illustrates a helpful exercise for use with caregivers to determine whether to take an acceptance-oriented or action-oriented approach based on the controllability of the concern at hand.

Exposure. A range of exposure-based CBT interventions have been developed to treat anxiety-related conditions in the general population.[16-18] These interventions involve graded exposure to feared situations in parallel with use of specific coping strategies to manage anxiety and reduce avoidance. Exposure may be adapted to help caregivers reduce avoidance of activities that cause intolerable anxiety. For instance, a caregiver may have developed anxiety and avoidance of certain objects, sights, or sounds at the patient's oncology clinic due to prior experiences with illness. By learning to pair a relaxation response with the feared stimuli, the caregiver may reduce his or her own suffering while also increasing his or her ability to provide care and support to the patient.

Motivational interviewing (MI). MI is a specific counseling style in which practitioners use open-ended questions to help patients elicit their motivation for working toward therapeutic goals.[19] CBT practitioners may integrate MI techniques throughout an intervention to assist caregivers in first identifying motivation to initiate therapy and then maintaining motivation to work toward their identified goals. As an intervention target,

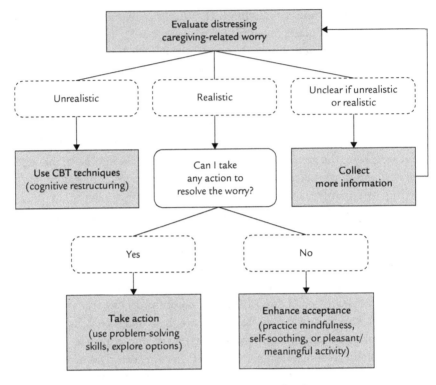

Figure 9.1: Decisional model for coping with caregiving-related worry.
Adapted from Greer JA, Graham JS, Safren SA. Resolving treatment complications associated with comorbid medical conditions. In: Otto M, Hofmann S, eds. *Avoiding Treatment Failure in Anxiety Disorders.* New York, NY: Springer; 2009.

motivation may be especially critical for caregivers who have disengaged from self-care as they increasingly attend to the evolving needs of the patient or increasingly lose sight of their own needs or the needs of other dependents.

Mindfulness. As a practice, mindfulness involves cultivating awareness of present thoughts and feelings using a nonjudgmental stance. Individuals can foster "nonjudgmental awareness" through daily mindfulness exercises that anchor their attention, such as a walking meditation. Mindfulness has been incorporated into some integrative, evidence-based protocols for mental health disorders in the general population.[20,21] In cancer care, CBT practitioners may integrate mindfulness to help caregivers acknowledge and label stressful thoughts and feelings before engaging in automatic unhelpful coping reactions. For instance, in the moment of experiencing uncontrollable worry about the future, mindfulness may be a critical first step that helps caregivers validate their own painful emotions while making space to decide whether/how to act on them.

Relaxation. A diverse range of relaxation exercises, such as diaphragmatic breathing or guided visual imagery, can be used to help calm the mind and reduce elevated physiologic tension.[22] CBT practitioners in cancer care commonly integrate relaxation training into therapy. Practitioners can assist caregivers, particularly those who are managing busy schedules, to problem-solve strategies for making relaxation practice a daily habit so that such strategies—and their stress management benefits—are available during stressful situations.

INTEGRATION OF CBT AND CONSIDERATIONS

Cognitive behavioral therapy interventions can be integrated with other feasible evidence-based strategies to help caregivers increase motivation and self-efficacy for enhancing self-care and managing caregiver burden and related distress. Use of CBT within this population may differ primarily due to the context in which a patient or caregiver is in need of support.[23] When working with a caregiver of a patient with cancer, one must recognize the validity and context of automatic thoughts.[7] The traditional cognitive behavioral model emphasizes the existence of an individual's unrealistic or unhelpful automatic thoughts and the benefit of CBT to reframe these cognitions to be more realistic or accurate. In the oncology setting, these methods may lack appropriate validation of the lived experience of caregivers who are coping with patients' changing needs and prognoses. Thus, consideration of and sensitivity to the validity (i.e., grains of truth) of caregivers' thoughts must be accounted for when implementing CBT with this population.

CASE EXAMPLE

Carla is a 50-year-old sales manager, wife, and mother of two adult sons whose husband was diagnosed with lymphoma and had undergone a hematopoietic stem cell transplantation (HSCT). She has high personal satisfaction from her ability to be a supportive wife and mother while managing extensive work demands. She finds significant meaning and purpose in her job; she is successful at managing a large team with effective communication and decision-making skills.

However, with the increasing demands of providing care for her husband and spending time with him in the hospital throughout the transplantation process, she has had to take time off from work and is having difficulty preparing for his discharge from the hospital. Carla and her husband live 5 hours from the hospital where he is receiving his care; therefore, she has rented an apartment in closer proximity, with a 1-hour commute each way. Both Carla's and her husband's family have offered to help, yet Carla has had difficulty accepting their support as she is accustomed to being in charge and fully in control. While she excels at organizing, planning, and problem-solving, she struggles to manage the uncertainties surrounding the transplant process, distress related to her husband's physical symptoms, and fears about a cancer recurrence or post-transplant complications. She attempts to hide her emotions and worries from her husband, but he has noticed an increase in her anxiety and worsening mood. He mentions his concerns to his nurse, who suggests a referral to the hospital's outpatient psychosocial oncology service. The nurse normalizes the referral, noting that she often recommends that the caregiver meet with a mental health practitioner during this highly stressful time.

At Carla's initial CBT evaluation, the practitioner encourages Carla to share her story and challenges related to being a caregiver for her husband during this time. The practitioner notes her thoughts, feelings, and coping behaviors, and the relationships among them. He then provides brief psychoeducation about the rationale for CBT to cope with caregiver-related stress and burden during chronic illness and normalizes her experience with the complex demands of caregiving for someone with cancer. He uses motivational interviewing to elicit Carla's own motivation for engaging in CBT and commitment to enhancing her coping and stress management skills. The practitioner and Carla agree to begin CBT, meeting weekly in person when Carla comes to the hospital to visit her husband and by videoconference after he is discharged to their rental apartment. They discuss and identify Carla's goals for treatment, including reducing symptoms of depression, effectively managing worries and concerns about the transplant process and outcome, expanding strategies for coping with difficult emotions, and managing stressors such as family involvement and her frustrations around the commute to their temporary rental apartment. They formulate an 8-week treatment plan using specific CBT strategies and continuous goal monitoring with validated self-report measures at each session to monitor progress.

CBT begins with the practitioner conveying the importance of between-session exercises and instilling hope and optimism for achieving goals. In the first session, discussions of coping strategies lead Carla to recognize that she feels equipped to problem-solve difficult situations when there are active tasks that she can do to reach a resolution; however, she lacks tools to cope with situations and stressors that are not within her control. The practitioner introduces coping effectiveness and the importance of choosing a coping strategy based on the controllability of the stressor. Together, they identify acceptance-oriented coping strategies that Carla can engage in to help tolerate her distress when her worries are high and controllability is low (e.g., physical side effects that her husband is experiencing as his blood counts return to normal), such as taking a walk, talking to a friend, or listening to relaxing music. Carla practices these before the next session and expands on this list, adding "playing games on smartphone" to her acceptance-oriented coping strategies. She expresses to the practitioner that she noticed how she previously had minimal tools to cope with emotional distress, and that these activities were helpful in calming her body down when she could not immediately resolve the problem.

Carla's daily thought-monitoring logs show that she has high and somewhat rigid expectations for herself and her ability to care for her husband, continue in her role as manager at work, and be the primary point person for all caregiving responsibilities. Her automatic thoughts consist of language such as "I should . . . " and "I must be able to . . . " and an all-or-nothing thinking style, where she insists on spending all day at the hospital while working remotely and hesitates to ask for or accept help from others. The practitioner uses Socratic questioning to help Carla identify negative self-talk and rigid cognitive beliefs that are increasing her irritability, depression, and physiological stress level, leading to interference with her ability to function optimally daily when she cannot meet the demands she has set for herself.

Over the next few sessions, Carla learns to challenge these unhelpful thoughts and generate more helpful and accurate self-talk that results in desired behavior. She comes to recognize that while her husband is in the hospital, he has a full-time medical team caring for him, and she can use some of this time to accomplish chores and other tasks for herself at home. She also begins to be more flexible in her thinking, allowing others to contribute and assist with small tasks that help relieve some of the burden, such as allowing her sister-in-law to clean the rental unit to prepare for her husband's discharge.

Finally, the hour-long drive and unpredictable traffic from the rental unit to the hospital had been causing Carla significant anxiety and stress. After conversations with the practitioner around acceptance of situations that are unmodifiable and cultivating mindful awareness of the present moment, Carla began to use her skills to reframe how she appraises the car ride and begins to view it as a time to be mindful or to listen to a book on tape for enjoyment. With additional learned skills in communication and assertiveness during subsequent sessions, she speaks with her employer about temporarily reducing her hours and working remotely while her husband transitions from the hospital to home. The practitioner continues to work with Carla to hone skills of cognitive reframing, employing acceptance-oriented coping skills, mindfulness and acceptance, and problem-solving. Carla continues to apply these skills once her husband has been discharged and her demands of caregiving at home increase. She feels more equipped to manage difficult emotions and the challenges of adjusting to life post-transplant.

EVIDENCE FOR COGNITIVE BEHAVIORAL THERAPY WITH CANCER CAREGIVERS

Historically, caregivers were often included in observational and interventional studies that focused primarily on improving patient outcomes and less on the impact of such interventions on caregiver outcomes. More recently, attention has now been directed to address the psychosocial needs of caregivers throughout the cancer treatment trajectory.[7] CBT interventions for cancer caregivers have targeted several outcomes. For example, a brief cognitive behavioral intervention that included stimulus control, relaxation, cognitive therapy, and sleep hygiene components for cancer caregivers showed improvements in sleep quality and reductions in depressive symptoms.[24] A coping skills training program for cancer caregivers resulted in improvements in caregiver QOL, less burden from patient symptoms, and lower caregiving task burden.[25] In addition, a nine-session cognitive behavioral intervention resulted in caregivers exhibiting lower scores on the Brief Symptom Inventory and better psychological adjustment to illness than those in the control condition. Caregivers in this study also reported fewer sleep difficulties and higher perceived support.[26] An example of a structured cognitive behavioral therapy intervention for caregivers is illustrated in Table 9.1.

In general, psychosocial interventions for caregivers of patients with cancer have been found to be somewhat beneficial, but only a minority of these interventions are cognitive behavioral in nature.[27] In a recent meta-analysis of cognitive behavioral therapies for informal caregivers of both patients with cancer and cancer survivors, CBT for caregivers had a negligible effect, with some evidence suggesting that CBT may be more effective for caregivers who were younger and female.[28] It is notable that most studies in this review were open pilot trials rather than randomized controlled trials, and those that employed a randomized

Table 9.1 BRIEF STRUCTURED CBT INTERVENTION FOR CANCER CAREGIVERS

Module	No. of Sessions	Techniques	Description
1	1	Psychoeducation Goal setting	- Establish goals and expectations for CBT - Explore expectations around cancer treatment trajectory and caregiving responsibilities - Normalize and emphasize the importance of caring for oneself while caring for others - Explore awareness of stressors and associated thoughts, feelings, and behaviors - Elicit motivation for behavior change and skill acquisition
2	1	Coping	- Explore caregiving role, burden, and stressors - Explore caregiver's coping style and effectiveness - Introduce acceptance-oriented vs. action-oriented coping strategies - Discuss importance of matching coping strategy to controllability of the stressor - Expand list of available coping strategies and assign at-home practice
3	1–2	Mindfulness and acceptance	- Review ongoing caregiving responsibilities and strategies for coping or minimizing burden - Introduce themes and strategies for cultivating acceptance and mindfulness - Discuss formal and informal mindfulness practices - Conduct in-session relaxation or mindfulness exercise (i.e., body scan, visual imagery) and audio-record exercise - Assign practice of recorded relaxation or mindfulness exercise to caregiver
4	2–3	Managing worry, uncertainty, and fears of recurrence	- Identify unhelpful thoughts or belief patterns - Differentiate realistic worries from unrealistic or exaggerated worries - Challenge accuracy of unrealistic worries - Generate more accurate and realistic statements and self-talk to replace unhelpful beliefs and thoughts - Assign thought monitoring and practice for homework

(continued)

Table 9.1 CONTINUED

Module	No. of Sessions	Techniques	Description
5	1	Social support	- Discuss comfort with asking for and receiving support from others - Introduce types of support (i.e., tangible, informational, emotional) - Review skills for asking for support and reframing barriers for receiving support to offset caregiving demands
6	1	Communication	- Introduce interpersonal styles of communication (i.e., aggressive, passive, passive-aggressive, and assertiveness) - Discuss skills for formulating an assertiveness statement (e.g., statement of fact, statement of feeling, statement of fair request) - Practice and role-play assertive statements that the caregiver may make with the healthcare team, employer, or care recipient
7	1	Self-care and maintenance	- Normalize difficulties around adjustment to different phases of treatment and corresponding caregiving tasks - Discuss strategies for and barriers to self-care (e.g., physical activity, diet, sleep, etc.) - Strategize plan for skill practice, implementation, and maintenance after therapy

controlled design compared CBT to a nonactive control condition. Additionally, the studies evaluated in this review employed various theoretical frameworks and therefore may not have all been designed based on a true CBT model. Most CBT studies for caregivers were delivered face to face versus via telephone or other telehealth modality, targeting either the individual caregiver or the patient-caregiver dyad, and included patients of mixed cancer stages. The interventions employed skills and techniques used across various CBT interventions, with the most common treatment components including coping skills training, problem-solving, cognitive restructuring, structured homework, and relaxation.[28] The authors concluded that interventions focusing on affective and emotion regulation should be investigated in addition to traditional CBT methods.

In a previous meta-analysis, Northouse and colleagues[29] reviewed interventions aimed at providing information or skills to caregivers to carry out patient-related tasks, to help couples manage family and marital concerns, and to manage their own physical and emotional health needs through self-care. Individual CBT skills were employed in these studies, such as enhancing coping behavior by promoting active coping in the form of problem-solving or reducing ineffective coping, such as avoidance or denial. These interventions had small-to-medium effects on reducing caregiver burden, improving caregivers' ability to cope, increasing caregivers' self-efficacy, and improving QOL. However, the sustainability of the intervention effects were not established, as many of these trials assessed caregiver-reported outcomes during the first 3 months following the intervention, with only approximately one-quarter assessing longer term outcomes.[7]

Many of the aforementioned studies focused on psychological distress and caregiver adjustment during the acute phase of treatment, from diagnosis to 1–2 years postdiagnosis. In fact, psychological distress and problems with role adjustment have been found among spousal caregivers approximately 1 year after cancer treatment, and fears of recurrence and existential concerns are often persistent even if an individual is disease free.[30] Kim and Given[30] called attention to the importance of considering caregivers' needs at various points across the cancer trajectory, including middle- to long-term survivorship for caregivers of individuals who no longer need consistent care; middle- to long-term survivorship for caregivers who continue to provide care due to recurrence, secondary cancer, or late/long-term side effects and those who are providing care to a loved one at the end of life. Very few interventions are tailored to address challenges during this later phase of caregiving, and fewer studies have addressed topics of bereavement in family caregivers using cognitive behavioral theory or interventions.

CHALLENGES, OPPORTUNITIES, AND FUTURE DIRECTIONS

Innovations in cancer screening and treatment, as well as the evolving needs and demographics of caregivers, present a number of unique challenges and opportunities for future intervention development. Novel cancer therapeutics, such as targeted therapies and immunotherapies, will continue to transform the landscape of cancer care and prolong survival. Although such medical breakthroughs confer numerous benefits for improving cancer outcomes, they often come with a host of new challenges for patients and caregivers, such as difficulties with understanding prognosis and preparing for the future, managing debilitating side effects from treatment, and coping with cancer as a chronic, long-term illness.[31,32]

Moreover, our understanding of who caregivers are must also continue to evolve. As the population ages and those diagnosed with cancer live longer, so do caregivers. Caregiving responsibilities will increasingly fall on adult children, siblings, other relatives, friends, as well as formal hired aides, whose caregiving capacities and supportive care needs vary considerably.[33] This complexity is further compounded by the lack of data on how best to serve families from diverse racial, cultural, and socioeconomic backgrounds.[30] Across this spectrum of caregivers, further research is needed to identify the characteristics and subpopulations of caregivers who are more or less able to provide support and promote positive engagement with treatment versus those who are at risk for heightened distress and poorer outcomes, requiring additional intervention.[7,28,34]

Other challenges in considering the needs of caregivers include defining the content and format of delivering supportive care interventions.[20] For example, evidence-based CBT for treating psychological conditions typically involves 12–15 weekly hour-long sessions that most often take place in person in a clinic to learn skills and adopt new behaviors. Such a model of care is generally prohibitive for caregivers, given the burden of time and resources, high costs, and limited access to therapists with the requisite training and expertise. When designing supportive care interventions for caregivers, much more research is needed to determine the optimal target population (e.g., individual, dyad, or family); intervention focus (e.g., informational, pragmatic/logistical, social, and/or emotional or psychological); and medium of delivery (e.g., in person, telehealth, or online). Adapting evidence-based CBT interventions, in both content and delivery format, to alleviate distress in this population certainly represents one promising avenue to pursue in follow-up study. Investigators may also consider alternative approaches that promote positive affect and resilience, especially as evidence suggests that potential benefits of caregiving may be derived through greater appreciation of others and acquiring a sense of meaning in life.[28]

Finally, while using innovative technology such as mobile apps and smartphones to deliver supportive care interventions may facilitate broader dissemination, patient adherence to such interventions has traditionally been poor, averaging approximately 50% across studies.[35] Further work is needed to determine if uptake of this technology would be greater among caregivers, as studies are lacking on the use of web-based approaches in this population.[7,33] Nonetheless, investigators seeking to develop such novel interventions should incorporate features that encourage active engagement of caregivers, such as through personalization, persuasive messages, rewards, and other design elements to create a positive affective experience with the technology.[36]

Intervention development and research on how best to support the caregivers of patients with cancer must keep pace with the rapid shifts in emerging cancer therapeutics along with changing trends in who caregivers represent. As a result, as this field continues to grow, caregiver interventions will likely be as diverse as the needs and populations they target through a range of modalities and approaches that help to alleviate distress, reduce burden, foster resilience, and enhance access to care.

REFERENCES

1. Girgis A, Lambert S, Johnson C, Waller A, Currow D. Physical, psychosocial, relationship, and economic burden of caring for people with cancer: a review. *J Oncol Pract.* 2012;9(4):197–202.
2. Given B, Kozachik S, Collins C, Devoss D, and Given CW. Caregiver Role Strain. In *Nursing care of older adults diagnosis: Outcome and interventions*, Eds. M. Maas, K. Buckwalter, M. Hardy, T. Tripp-Reimer, and M. Titler, 679–695. St Louis, Missouri: Mosby; 2001.
3. Haley WE, LaMonde LA, Han B, Narramore S, Schonwetter R. Family caregiving in hospice: Effects on psychological and health functioning among spousal caregivers of hospice patients with lung cancer or dementia. *Hosp J* 2001;15(4):1–18.
4. Kim Y, Carver CS, Shaffer KM, Gansler T, Cannady RS. Cancer caregiving predicts physical impairments: Roles of earlier caregiving stress and being a spousal caregiver. *Cancer* 2015;121(2):302–310.
5. Pitceathly C, Maguire P. The psychological impact of cancer on patients' partners and other key relatives: A review. *Eur J Cancer* 2003;39(11):1517–1524.
6. Schulz R, O'Brien A, Czaja S, et al. Dementia caregiver intervention research: in search of clinical significance. *Gerontologist.* 2002;42(5):589–602.
7. Northouse LL, Katapodi MC, Song L, Zhang L, Mood DW. Interventions with family caregivers of cancer patients: meta-analysis of randomized trials. *CA Cancer J Clin.* 2010;60(5):317–339.
8. Hofmann SG, Asnaani A, Vonk IJ, Sawyer AT, Fang A. The efficacy of cognitive behavioral therapy: a review of meta-analyses. *Cognit Ther Res.* 2012;36(5):427–440.
9. Ellis A. *Reason and Emotion in Psychotherapy.* Oxford, UK: Lyle Stuart; 1962.
10. Beck AT. Cognitive therapy: nature and relation to behavior therapy. *Behav Ther.* 1970;1(2):184–200.
11. Greer JA, Traeger L, Bemis H, et al. A pilot randomized controlled trial of brief cognitive-behavioral therapy for anxiety in patients with terminal cancer. *Oncologist.* 2012;17(10):1337–1345.
12. Osborn RL, Demoncada AC, Feuerstein M. Psychosocial interventions for depression, anxiety, and quality of life in cancer survivors: meta-analyses. *Int J Psychiatry Med.* 2006;36(1):13–34.

13. Applebaum AJ, Breitbart W. Care for the cancer caregiver: a systematic review. *Palliat Support Care*. 2013;11(3):231–252.
14. Greer JA, Park ER, Prigerson HG, Safren SA. Tailoring cognitive-behavioral therapy to treat anxiety comorbid with advanced cancer. *J Cogn Psychother*. 2010;24(4):294–313.
15. Martell CR, Dimidjian S, Herman-Dunn R. *Behavioral Activation for Depression: A Clinician's Guide*. Reprint edition. New York, NY: Guilford Press; 2010.
16. Wolitzky-Taylor KB, Horowitz JD, Powers MB, Telch MJ. Psychological approaches in the treatment of specific phobias: a meta-analysis. *Clin Psychol Rev*. 2008;28(6):1021–1037.
17. Craske MG, Antony MM, Barlow DH. *Mastery of Your Fears and Phobias: Therapist Guide*. 2nd ed. New York, NY: Oxford University Press; 2006.
18. Foa E, Hembree E, Rothbaum B. *Prolonged Exposure Therapy for PTSD: Emotional Processing of Traumatic Experiences (Therapist Guide)*. 2nd ed. New York, NY: Oxford University Press; 2010.
19. Emmons KM, Rollnick S. Motivational interviewing in health care settings. Opportunities and limitations. *Am J Prev Med*. 2001;20(1):68–74.
20. Linehan M. *Cognitive-Behavioral Treatment of Borderline Personality Disorder*. New York, NY: Guilford Press; 1993.
21. Segal ZV, Williams JMG, Teasdale JD. *Mindfulness-Based Cognitive Therapy for Depression*. 2nd ed. New York, NY: Guilford Press; 2012.
22. Wallace RK, Benson H, Wilson AF. A wakeful hypometabolic physiologic state. *Am J Physiol*. 1971;221(3):795–799.
23. Levin TT, Applebaum AJ. Acute cancer cognitive therapy. *Cognit Behav Pract*. 2014;21(4):404–415.
24. Carter PA. A brief behavioral sleep intervention for family caregivers of persons with cancer. *Cancer Nurs*. 2006;29(2):95–103.
25. McMillan SC, Small BJ, Weitzner M, et al. Impact of coping skills intervention with family caregivers of hospice patients with cancer: a randomized clinical trial. *Cancer*. 2006;106(1):214–222.
26. Cohen M, Kuten A. Cognitive-behavior group intervention for relatives of cancer patients: a controlled study. *J Psychosom Res*. 2006;61(2):187–196.
27. Manne S, Badr H. Intimacy and relationship processes in couples' psychosocial adaptation to cancer. *Cancer*. 2008;112(11)(suppl):2541–2555.
28. O'Toole MS, Zachariae R, Renna ME, Mennin DS, Applebaum A. Cognitive behavioral therapies for informal caregivers of patients with cancer and cancer survivors: a systematic review and meta-analysis. *Psychooncology*. 2017;26(4):428–437.
29. Given B, Wyatt G, Given C, et al. Burden and depression among caregivers of patients with cancer at the end of life. *Oncol Nurs Forum*. 2004;31(6):1105–1117.
30. Kim Y, Given BA. Quality of life of family caregivers of cancer survivors: across the trajectory of the illness. *Cancer*. 2008;112(11)(suppl):2556–2568.
31. Temel JS, Shaw AT, Greer JA. Challenge of prognostic uncertainty in the modern era of cancer therapeutics. *J Clin Oncol*. 2016;34(30):3605–3608.
32. Temel JS, Gainor JF, Sullivan RJ, Greer JA. Keeping expectations in check with immune checkpoint inhibitors. *J Clin Oncol*. 2018;36(17):1654–1657. doi:JCO.2017.76.146
33. Northouse L, Williams AL, Given B, McCorkle R. Psychosocial care for family caregivers of patients with cancer. *J Clin Oncol*. 2012;30(11):1227–1234.

34. Shaffer KM, Jacobs JM, Nipp RD, et al. Mental and physical health correlates among family caregivers of patients with newly-diagnosed incurable cancer: a hierarchical linear regression analysis. *Support Care Cancer.* 2017;25(3):965–971.
35. Kelders SM, Kok RN, Ossebaard HC, Van Gemert-Pijnen JE. Persuasive system design does matter: a systematic review of adherence to web-based interventions. *J Med Internet Res.* 2012;14(6):e152.
36. Ludden GD, van Rompay TJ, Kelders SM, van Gemert-Pijnen JE. How to increase reach and adherence of web-based interventions: a design research viewpoint. *J Med Internet Res.* 2015;17(7):e172.

CHAPTER 10

Problem-Solving Interventions

ARTHUR M. NEZU, CHRISTINE MAGUTH NEZU, AND LAUREN B. JOHNSON

INTRODUCTION

It is estimated that the number of cancer survivors worldwide who are within 5 years of initial diagnosis is close to 29 million.[1] In addition to the myriad healthcare professionals involved in the treatment of such individuals, informal caregivers of these patients, including spouses, partners, family members, and friends, provide essential support and care throughout the cancer experience. Such help can be practical as well as provide psychological and emotional support. As evidenced throughout this volume, the burden of caregiving for a cancer patient can be substantial, with negative effects on caregivers seen in their physical health, quality of life, and emotional well-being.

The incidence of high levels of emotional distress, such as depression, among cancer caregivers has been estimated to be approximately 20%.[2,3] This rate appears to increase when patients themselves are experiencing high levels of distress, poor physical functioning, and advanced disease.[4] Difficulties in caregiving often lead to significant "unmet needs" and problems.[5] These include fatigue, depression, difficulties making decisions or coordinating the care of various professionals, fear of the future, reduced income, and physical pain.[6]

Such negative effects have been found to be reciprocal between cancer patients and their family caregivers. For example, in a meta-analysis of 21 investigations involving over 1,000 patient-caregiver dyads, a significant relationship was found between their distress scores, indicating that their emotional responses to cancer were interrelated.[7] A second meta-analysis involving 46 studies focused on couples coping with cancer also found a significant association between patients' and their spousal caregivers' level of distress (this time controlling for illness-related factors, including disease stage).[8] Both meta-analyses strongly suggest that as patient distress increases, so does caregiver distress.

The other side of this coin posits that as caregiver distress increases, so does patient distress.[9] Given this framework, the intention to minimize caregiver distress and improve their overall quality of life is obvious. More specifically, interventions geared to help caregivers cope more effectively might alleviate the burden associated with the caregiver role and improve patient outcomes.[10] The present chapter depicts one type of psychosocial intervention for cancer caregivers: problem-solving therapy (PST).

PROBLEM-SOLVING THERAPY

Problem-solving therapy is a psychosocial intervention developed within a social learning framework and is based on a biopsychosocial, diathesis-stress model of psychopathology.[11] In general, this intervention involves training individuals in a set of skills aimed at enhancing their ability to cope effectively with a variety of life stressors that have the potential to generate negative medical and mental health outcomes, including chronic medical conditions, depression, and anxiety. Life stressors can include major negative life events, such as cancer and its treatment, as well as chronic daily problems (e.g., the responsibilities and difficulties associated with caregiving). PST assumes that much of what is conceptualized as psychopathology and behavioral difficulties, including significant emotional problems, is a function of continuous ineffective coping with life stressors. Consequently, it is hypothesized that teaching individuals to become better problem-solvers can serve to reduce extant physical and mental health difficulties. The overarching goal of PST is to promote the successful adoption of adaptive problem-solving attitudes (i.e., optimism, enhanced self-efficacy) and the effective implementation of certain behaviors (i.e., adaptive emotional regulation, planful problem-solving) as means of coping with stressors and thereby attenuating the negative effects of stress on physical and mental health.

The origins of PST from a social learning perspective can be traced back to the seminal article by D'Zurilla and Goldfried, who developed a prescriptive model of training to enhance individuals' ability to cope effectively with problems encountered daily.[12] Early research applying this model to clinical populations focused on PST as a treatment for adults with major depressive disorder.[13] Subsequently, this approach has been successfully applied to a wide range of psychological disorders, medical problems, and clinical populations.[11] In addition, PST has been effective across different modes of implementation (e.g., individual, group, telephone, Internet) and has been applied as a means of enhancing patients' adherence to other medical or psychosocial interventions.[14]

SOCIAL PROBLEM-SOLVING

According to this approach, the type of problem-solving processes invoked in real-life contexts, due to the significant emotional overlay involved, are somewhat different from those primarily involved in solving intellectual or logic problems.[15,16] As such, it is referred to as *social problem-solving* (SPS). SPS is defined as the process by which people attempt to identify, discover, or create adaptive means of coping with a wide range of stressful problems, both acute and chronic, encountered during the course of daily living. Moreover, it reflects the process whereby people direct their coping efforts at altering the problematic nature of a given situation, their reactions to such problems, or both. Rather than representing a singular type of coping behavior or activity, SPS represents the multidimensional process of identifying and implementing various coping responses to adequately address or match the unique features of a given situation.[17]

Social problem-solving comprises two general, but partially independent, components: (1) problem orientation (PO) and (2) problem-solving style.[18] PO represents the set of cognitive-affective schemas regarding people's generalized beliefs, attitudes, and emotional reactions concerning real-life problems, as well as their ability to successfully cope with such difficulties. Originally thought of as being two ends of the same continuum,[19] recent research has continued to characterize the two forms of POs as impacting health outcomes independent of positive and negative PO.[17]

A *positive PO* involves the tendency for individuals to (1) perceive problems as challenges rather than major threats to one's well-being; (2) be optimistic in believing that problems are solvable; (3) have a strong sense of self-efficacy regarding their ability to handle difficult problems; (4) believe that successful problem-solving usually involves time and effort; and (5) view negative emotions as important sources of information necessary for effective problem-solving to occur (e.g., where one's negative emotions "signal that a problem exists").

A *negative PO* refers to the tendency of individuals to (1) view problems as major threats to one's well-being; (2) generally perceive problems as being too difficult or unsolvable; (3) maintain doubts about their ability to cope with problems successfully; and (4) become particularly distressed when faced with problems or when experiencing negative emotions.

The second major dimension, *problem-solving style*, refers to the core cognitive behavioral activities that people engage in when attempting to solve stressful problems. Three different styles have been identified: rational problem-solving, avoidant problem-solving, and impulsive-careless problem-solving.[18,20] *Rational problem-solving* is the constructive approach that involves the systematic application of the following set of specific skills: (1) *problem definition and formulation*, clarifying the nature of a problem, delineating a realistic set of problem-solving goals and objectives, and identifying obstacles to reaching such goals; (2) *generation of alternatives*, brainstorming a range of possible solution strategies geared to overcome the identified obstacles; (3) *decision-making*, predicting the likely consequences of the various alternatives, conducting a cost-benefit analysis based on these identified outcomes, and developing a solution plan that is geared to achieve the problem-solving goal; and (4) *solution implementation and verification*, carrying out the solution plan, monitoring and evaluating the consequences of such a plan, and determining whether one's problem-solving efforts have been successful or need continuing.

In addition to a rational problem-solving style, two other styles have been identified, both of which, in contrast, are generally dysfunctional or ineffective in nature.[18] An *impulsive/careless style* is the problem-solving approach whereby individuals tend to engage in impulsive, hurried, and careless attempts at problem resolution. *Avoidant problem-solving* is a maladaptive problem-solving style characterized by procrastination, passivity, and over-dependence on others to provide solutions. People who typically engage in these styles tend to worsen existing problems and create new ones.

RELEVANCE OF PST FOR PSYCHOSOCIAL ONCOLOGY

The conceptual relevance of PST for persons with cancer and their caregivers is embedded in a general problem-solving model of stress, whereby the experience of cancer is conceptualized as both a major negative life event and the cause of a series of stressful daily problems.[21] Both sources of stress are further hypothesized to increase the likelihood that a cancer patient, as well as the identified caregiver, can experience significant psychological distress, such as depression and anxiety. However, one's problem-solving ability is conceptualized as an important moderator of these relationships, whereby effective problem-solving ability should reduce the probability of experiencing distress, even when confronted by cancer-related difficulties.

The core assumptions of the general model have been supported by research findings regarding multiple populations.[11] Relevant to psychosocial oncology, in our study with recently diagnosed cancer patients, individuals characterized by less effective problem-solving also reported higher levels of anxiety and depressive symptomatology, as well as greater numbers of cancer-related problems.[22] In a further study, it was found that under *similarly high levels of cancer-related stress,* those patients who were characterized as *ineffective* problem-solvers reported *higher* levels of depression compared to their cancer patient counterparts who were characterized as *effective* problem-solvers.[23]

Regarding cancer caregivers, among spouses of men diagnosed with prostate cancer, effective problem-solving has been associated with less emotional distress.[24] More specifically, higher levels of avoidance style, impulsive/careless style, and negative PO were associated with greater mood disturbance, whereas the opposite was true with regard to higher levels of rational problem-solving and a positive PO. In addition, McClure et al. found that spouses/partners of adult cancer patients with greater positive orientations were less likely to experience depression.[9]

Given the identified relationships between SPS and emotional distress among cancer patients and their informal caregivers, it appears that teaching these individuals effective SPS skills can lead to lowered emotional distress.[25] We conducted a three-arm randomized clinical trial to evaluate the efficacy of PST in reducing emotional distress among cancer patients.[26] One condition involved 10 hours of individual PST, whereas a second arm involved 10 hours of PST for both the patient and a designated caregiver (e.g., spouse/partner, family member). This second treatment protocol assessed the enhanced effects of formalizing a social support system where the role of the caregiver was conceptualized as a "problem-solving coach." Unfortunately, with specific relevance to the topic of this book, we did not assess the impact of PST on the caregivers themselves, only the patients. The third arm involved a treatment-as-usual control.

Results of this investigation at post-treatment across several self-report ratings, clinician ratings, and ratings by the significant other provide strong supportive evidence of the overall efficacy of PST for decreasing emotional distress and improving the overall quality of life of cancer patients. Specifically, patients in both treatment conditions demonstrated significant improvement compared to individuals in the control condition. At post-treatment, no differences were found between these two conditions. However, at a 6-month follow-up assessment, on approximately half of the variables assessed, patients who received PST along with a significant other continued to improve significantly beyond those individuals receiving PST alone, highlighting the advantage of formally including a collaborator in treatment. These positive effects of PST were not only statistically significant, but also highly clinically significant. Moreover, improvements in problem-solving were found to correlate significantly with decreases in psychological distress and improvements in overall quality of life.

The efficacy of PST to reduce emotional distress and improve coping of cancer patients has been supported by several additional clinical trials (see Nezu and Nezu[27] for a review, plus Hirai et al.[28] and Hopko et al.[29] for more recent examples). It is notable that in a follow-up to their initial study, Hopko and colleagues found that PST led to a continued decrease in depression among a sample of breast cancer patients at 12 months post-treatment and engendered a decrease in suicidal ideation.[30]

PROBLEM-SOLVING FOR CANCER CAREGIVERS

Based on our PST treatment protocols, we also developed the Prepared Family Caregiver Course, which provided information within the following categories to family caregivers of cancer patients: (1) understanding the problem; (2) when to get professional help; (3) what can be done to deal with, as well as prevent, a problem; (4) identifying obstacles when they arise and planning to overcome them; and (5) carrying out and adjusting the plan.[31,32] This course was aimed at helping caregivers develop problem-solving plans across a variety of physical (e.g., fatigue, hair loss, appetite difficulties) and psychosocial (e.g., depression, anxiety) problems that cancer patients commonly experience. We used the acronym *COPE* to highlight various problem-solving operations, where *C* indicates creativity, *O* optimism, *P* planning, and *E* expert information. One open trial that included family caregivers of patients with advanced cancer found that this protocol led to reduced emotional tension, increased confidence, and improved positive problem-solving among the caregivers.[33] Another more recent open trial including caregivers of patients undergoing hematopoietic stem cell transplantation found the COPE protocol to engender significant improvements in caregiver self-efficacy and physical health and significant decreases in emotional distress.[34] In another randomized controlled trial comparing COPE with usual care, COPE also led to significant improvements regarding quality of life for caregivers of patients with advanced cancer, although not for the patients themselves.[35]

Table 10.1 lists clinical trials evaluating the efficacy of problem-solving–based interventions specifically for caregivers of cancer patients. While not a systematic review, perusal of this table suggests that PST is an effective

Table 10.1 CLINICAL TRIALS OF INTERVENTIONS BASED ON PROBLEM-
SOLVING FOR CANCER CAREGIVERS

Authors	Patient Group	Caregiver Group	Conditions	Basic Results
Hawes et al.[36]	Men with prostate cancer	66 spouses/ partners	1. PST 2. Standard care (SC)	PST = SC
McMillan et al.[37]	Hospice patients with advanced cancer	Family caregivers	1. PST (COPE) + hospice care (HC) 2. Emotional support + HC 3. HC alone	PST > both comparison groups re: better caregiver quality of life, reduced caregiver burden
Meyers et al.[35]	Adults with advanced cancer	476 family caregivers	1. PST (COPE) 2. Usual care (UC)	PST > UC
Sahler et al.[38]	Newly diagnosed children with cancer	80 mothers	1. PST 2. SC	PST > SC re: increased SPS and reduced negative affect
Sahler et al.[39]	Newly diagnosed children with cancer	309 mothers (English and Spanish speaking)	1. PST 2. Nondirective support (NDS)	PST = NDS at posttest; however, mothers in PST continued to show significant improvement re: distress, whereas NDS mothers showed no further gains
Sahler et al.[40]	Newly diagnosed children with cancer	430 mothers (English and Spanish speaking)	1. PST 2. UC	PST > UC re: increased problem-solving and decreased negative affectivity; younger, single mothers profited the most from PST

treatment approach to help cancer caregivers better cope with the stress related to the caregiving experience. However, because there are only a handful of such studies, a logical recommendation is a call for additional research in terms of quantity and methodological rigor. Moreover, future studies should be geared toward identifying mechanisms of action, moderators of treatment, long-term effects of PST, and effective treatment implementation approaches.

CLINICAL GUIDELINES

This final section provides a brief overview of problem-solving–based clinical guidelines. Note that the following represents a revised form of PST that we recently developed, emotion-centered problem-solving therapy (EC-PST).[15,16] Based on advances in clinical psychology and affective neuroscience, we revised the earlier treatment protocol to help individuals cope with the emotional aspects of significant stressors rather than rely solely on improving their cognitive problem-solving skills.

A major underlying precept of this model involves four major obstacles that may exist for individuals when attempting to successfully resolve stressful problems encountered in real-life contexts:

1. Ineffective problem-solving strategies
2. "Cognitive/brain overload"
3. Poor motivation or feelings of hopelessness
4. Limited ability to engage in effective emotional regulation.

Emotion-centered problem-solving therapy involves training individuals in four major problem-solving "toolkits" or skill sets that address each of the four general barriers:

1. Planful problem-solving
2. Problem-solving "multitasking"
3. Motivation for action
4. "Stop and slow down"

Next are descriptions of these four toolkits.

Planful Problem-Solving Toolkit: Fostering Effective Problem-Solving

The planful problem-solving toolkit provides training in four general planful problem-solving tasks. The first is *problem definition*, which involves having individuals separate facts from assumptions when describing a problem, delineate a realistic and attainable set of problem-solving goals and objectives, and identify obstacles that prevent one from reaching such goals. This model advocates delineating both *problem-focused goals*, which include objectives that entail changing the nature of the situation so that it no longer represents a problem (e.g., dealing with medical insurance issues), and *emotion-focused goals*, which include objectives that involve moderating one's cognitive-emotional reactions to unchangeable situations (e.g., coping with death anxiety).

The second task, *generating alternatives*, involves brainstorming a range of possible solution strategies geared to overcome the identified obstacles using various brainstorming techniques. *Decision-making*, the third planful problem-solving task, involves predicting the likely consequences of the generated alternatives, conducting a cost-benefit analysis based on these identified outcomes, and developing a solution plan geared to achieve the articulated problem-solving goal(s). The last activity, *solution implementation and verification*, entails having individuals optimally carry out the solution plan, monitor and evaluate the consequences of the plan, and determine whether their problem-solving efforts were successful or need continuing.

Problem-Solving Multitasking Toolkit: Overcoming Brain Overload

The problem-solving multitasking toolkit set of tools is provided to help individuals cope with a ubiquitous human limitation when facing stressful situations: "brain or cognitive overload." Due to limitations in one's ability to manipulate large amounts of information in working memory while attempting to solve complex problems or make effective decisions, especially when stressed, individuals are taught to use three "multitasking enhancement" skills: externalization, visualization, and simplification. These skills are considered foundational to effective problem-solving, similar to basic skills including effective aerobic exercise, such as stretching, breathing, and maintaining a healthy diet.

Externalization involves displaying information "externally" as often as possible. Individuals are taught to write ideas down, draw diagrams, charts, or maps, make lists, and audiotape ideas. In this manner, one's working memory is not overly taxed and the ability to concentrate on other activities, such as creatively thinking of various solutions, is enhanced. The *visualization* tool is presented as using one's "mind's eye" or visual imagery to (1) better clarify the nature of a problem, (2) practice carrying out a solution (imaginal rehearsal), and (3) reduce high levels of negative arousal (i.e., a form of guided imagery whereby one is directed imaginally to go on a peaceful vacation). *Simplification* involves "breaking down" problems to make them more manageable. Here, people are taught to simplify complex problems into more manageable, smaller problems and goals and translate complex, vague, and abstract concepts into more simple, specific, and concrete language.

Enhancing Motivation for Action Toolkit: Overcoming Reduced Motivation and Feelings of Hopelessness

The enhancing motivation for action toolkit specifically addresses potentially relevant PO issues, such as reduced motivation and feelings of hopelessness. The first tool would be used if a person is hesitant to carry out an action plan to solve a problem. People are taught to list consequences that may occur if they do not carry out an action plan. In addition, they are directed to delineate a series of outcomes that are possible if the plan is carried out and somewhat successful in reaching a desired goal. The comparison of these two lists can lead to enhanced motivation to implement one's solution plan. It can also lead to the identification of a deficient or limited action plan that would signal the revision of the plan.

A second tool in this skill set involves using visualization to further enhance motivation and specifically to reduce feelings of hopelessness. The use of visualization here, which is different from that described within the multitasking toolkit, is to help individuals to sensorially experience what it "feels" like to successfully solve a difficult problem; in other words, to "see the light at the end of the tunnel or the crossing ribbon at the finishing line." With this strategy, the clinician's goal is to help people create the experience of success in their "mind's eye," and vicariously experience the potential reinforcement to be gained. They are specifically taught *not* to focus on "how" the problem got solved, rather to focus on the feelings associated with having *already* solved it. The central goal of this strategy is to have individuals create their own positive consequences (in the form of affect, thoughts, physical sensations, and behavior) associated with solving a difficult problem as a major motivational step toward overcoming low motivation and feelings of hopelessness, as well as minimizing the tendency to engage in avoidant problem-solving.

"Stop and Slow Down:" Overcoming Emotional Dysregulation

The stop and slow down toolkit becomes especially important to emphasize in situations where the primary goal of EC-PST involves the decrease of clinically significant emotional distress (e.g., depression, suicidal ideation, generalized anxiety). It is also useful for preventing extant emotional concerns from becoming particularly problematic. Individuals are taught a series of steps to enhance their ability to modulate (as opposed to "eradicate") negative emotional arousal in order to more effectively apply a systematic approach to solving problems (i.e., to be able to optimally use the various planful problem-solving skills). It is also presented to individuals as the overarching "map" to follow when attempting to cope with stressful problems that engender strong emotional reactions and is included as the major treatment strategy for fostering adaptive emotional regulation skills. It is also included in EC-PST as a means of minimizing impulsive/careless attempts at problem-solving and avoidance of the problem.

According to this approach, people are first taught to become "emotionally mindful" by being more aware of, and specifically attentive to, when and how they experience negative emotional arousal. They are taught to notice changes in physical (e.g., headache, fatigue, pain); mood (e.g., sadness, anger, tension); cognitive (e.g., worry, thoughts of negative outcomes); or behavioral (e.g., urge to run away, yelling, crying) indicators. For certain individuals, additional training may be necessary to increase the accuracy by which they attempt to identify and label emotional phenomena. Next, they are taught to "stop" and focus on what is happening to increase awareness of what is engendering this arousal. They are directed to engage in behaviors (e.g., shouting out loud, raising one's hands) that can aid them in "putting on the brakes" in order to better modulate their emotional arousal (i.e., prevent the initial arousal from evoking a more intense form of the emotion together with its "full-blown" concomitant negative thinking, state-dependent negative memories, negative affect, and maladaptive behaviors).

Next, to meaningfully be able to stop, individuals are further taught to "slow down," that is, to decrease the accelerated rate at which one's negative emotionality can occur. Various specific techniques are provided and practiced, offering a choice among a pool of potentially effective "slowing down" tools. These include counting down from 10 to 1, diaphragmatic breathing, guided imagery or visualization, "fake yawning," meditation, exercise, talking to others, and prayer. Individuals are also encouraged to identify and use strategies that have historically been helpful to them.

An overall acronym, *SSTA*, is then taught, where the *T* and *A* pieces refer to "thinking" and "acting," that is, the four planful problem-solving tasks (i.e., defining the problem and setting realistic goals, generating alternative solutions, decision-making, solution implementation and verification). In other words, it is only once individuals are slowed down that they are able to "think and act" in a rational manner to effectively attempt to cope with the stressful problem situation that initially evoked the negative emotional stress reaction.

Guided Practice

A major part of the EC-PST intervention involves providing feedback and additional training to individuals in the four toolkits as they continue to apply the model to current problems they are experiencing. In addition, EC-PST encourages individuals to "forecast" future stressful situations, whether positive or negative, in anticipation of how such tools can be used in the future to minimize potential negative consequences.

CASE EXAMPLE

The following is a brief description of how EC-PST can be applied to a cancer patient-caregiver dyad.

Background

Betty is a 43-year-old, white female who was referred by her oncologist because of symptoms of depression. She was previously diagnosed with stage II breast cancer and is currently beginning chemotherapy. Although her prognosis appears to be positive regarding her physical health, she remains depressed and worried about the future. She has an aunt who underwent a double mastectomy a few years ago, which is constantly on her mind. She admits that she is scared that her husband, Steve, would no longer find her sexually attractive if she undergoes such surgery despite his admonitions that this would not be the case. Betty's oncologist suggested that because Steve appears to be very interested in doing "whatever I can to help," both should seek counseling together. Although Betty was initially against seeking any type of therapy, she was also concerned that her continued depression might be an extra burden on Steve, especially since he acquired new responsibilities at work related to a recent promotion. As such, she decided to pursue EC-PST.

Assessment and Case Formulation

The first two sessions of therapy were aimed at developing an initial case formulation that could help create a treatment plan for both Betty as the cancer patient and Steve as the informal caregiver. This included both quantitative strategies (e.g., self-report questionnaires) and qualitative strategies (e.g., interview questions, use of visualization exercises).

Assessments were conducted individually and together. In addition to confirming elevated levels of clinical depression and anxiety, it appeared that Betty has a strong negative PO regarding the overall cancer experience. Although it was a struggle, Steve fights to maintain a positive orientation, believing that "there is always something that can be done." Further inquiries indicated that Betty's negative orientation further impacts her planful problem-solving abilities, whereby she has difficulties with many aspects of her current life, including basic activities of daily living. However, it appears that prior to her cancer diagnosis, she functioned effectively, having successfully maintained a part-time job as a high school librarian, which she left once the cancer treatment began. An analysis of Steve's problem-solving skills suggests that they are strong and likely the reason for his continued success at work. However, he did reveal that he was concerned that his wife's continued depression may adversely affect her physical health, as she continued to feel fatigued, socially avoidant, and preoccupied with the future. He also noted that it is difficult at times to be a caregiver as he often is confused about how best to be of help.

As a standard part of EC-PST, the case formulation was shared with both Betty and Steve, noting both their strengths and limitations. As part of psychoeducation, it was highlighted that being depressed after a cancer diagnosis is normal, but that sustained mood disturbance can lead to additional negative consequences, such as poor adherence to medical advice and poor overall emotional well-being. In addition, depression can have a negative effect on their relationship, leading to additional stress. It was suggested that any serious medical illness can lead to myriad "smaller problems," which serve as additional stressors. Collectively, this overwhelming sense of stress could increase the likelihood that the depression would not likely change on its own, especially if Betty has any future adverse side effects from the chemotherapy (e.g., increased fatigue, hair loss, nausea). Suggesting that EC-PST involves teaching both partners a series of skills to more effectively cope with such stressors, both "big and small," fostered Betty's motivation to participate in the counseling.

Proposed Initial Treatment Plan

Based on an initial case formulation, a tailored EC-PST protocol for this couple should initially include the following clinical components in the following order:

1. *Emotion regulation training.* Despite her ability to function success-fully prior to having cancer, this new experience represented a major source of stress that greatly impacted Betty's mood and ability to be optimistic. This was compounded by her fear of needing radical breast surgery like her aunt. As such, it would appear more fruitful to initially focus on teaching and helping Betty to apply the stop and slow down tools to provide her with skills to better manage her reactions to both interoceptive and external cues that trigger negative emotions. Steve should be taught these skills as well to (a) serve as a coach to foster his wife's ability to apply such tools (e.g., help her to better identify triggers that exacerbate the depressive symptoms) and (b) use these skills himself to prevent caregiver burden and feeling overwhelmed.

2. *Overcoming feelings of hopelessness.* The toolkit involving the use of vis-ualization to overcome feelings of hopelessness should be provided to Betty alongside emotion regulation training as she frequently lapses into feelings of despair. This would help her to be more hopeful that learning emotion regulation tools can ultimately lead to overcoming depression. In addition, Steve can help devise a relevant pool of visu-alization exercises for Betty to apply and practice.

3. *Planful problem-solving.* A more formal training in these skills should follow the previous approaches with a focus on demonstrating how such an approach can be helpful in overcoming specific problems, such as communicating with other people, dealing with med-ical staff, handling insurance concerns, coping with negative side effects of chemotherapy, and so forth. It is possible that as treat-ment continues, additional problems may occur whereby new goals can be articulated.

4. *Overcoming brain overload.* Training in this set of tools should be closely tied to the emotion regulation training, as when Betty begins to think about her aunt, she becomes overwhelmed, which leads to her becoming more sad, anxious, and flooded with negative memories, rather than attempting to stop and slow down and engage in more adaptive ways of coping.

The EC-PST for this dyad should entail the sequence of clinical components just mentioned with the focus on helping Betty and Steve overcome her depression and prevent his becoming "burned out" as a caregiver. An emphasis on their mutual training should be placed on having Betty practice the various tools both in and between sessions to foster skill acquisition and application, with Steve serving as a coach. It would be important to continuously underscore the notion that serving as a caregiver and simultaneously having a full-time career can also be stressful. As such, both need to use various problem-solving tools to mitigate the negative effects of the myriad daily stressors they encounter as a function of the cancer experience. Even though both Betty and Steve have above-average intellectual abilities, all EC-PST clients receive numerous handouts to enhance learning with the suggestion that such information (which would include various training worksheets) should be kept for future reference. Monitoring change should occur throughout the course of treatment, focusing on both symptom reduction and improvements in the various skill sets that were the focus of treatment. Due to Betty's initial elevated depression, particular attention should be paid to the emergence of suicidal ideation over time. If a sufficient decrease in depression does not occur within a reasonable period of time, the therapist should review the initial case formulation to determine what needs to be revised. We encourage therapists to view themselves as "clinical problem-solvers" applying many of the same planful problem-solving principles described previously and to perceive their goal in this context as "how I can best help this person achieve his or her goals." Prior to terminating EC-PST, an additional focus would be to help this couple predict future stressful circumstances to be better prepared to cope with them.

CONCLUSIONS

Informal caregivers of patients with cancer can experience significant emotional distress, such as depression and anxiety. In essence, the responsibilities and burdens associated with the caregiving experience can be very stressful. Research has indicated that a caregiver's ability to effectively handle stressful experiences can significantly moderate the relationship between stress and distress such that the likelihood of experiencing emotional difficulties related to caregiving is attenuated. Problem-solving therapy (PST) is a psychosocial intervention that teaches a series of skill sets geared to foster people's ability to effectively manage stress. Studies document the efficacy of such an approach in reducing distress among cancer patients, as well as cancer patient caregivers. This chapter provided a description of PST for these populations, as well as the underlying rationale for why it is relevant for these individuals. A brief description of treatment guidelines regarding an updated version of PST, emotion-centered problem-solving therapy (EC-PST) was included in addition to a clinical example that delineated its application with a patient-caregiver dyad.

REFERENCES

1. Ferlay J, Shin HR, Bray F, Forman D, Mathers C, Parkin DM. Estimates of worldwide burden of cancer in 2008: GLOBOCAN 2008. *Int J Cancer*. 2010;127:2893–2917.

2. Edwards B, Clarke V. The psychological impact of a cancer diagnosis on families: the influence of family functioning and patients' illness characteristics on depression and anxiety. *Psychooncology*. 2004;13:562–576.

3. Lewis FM, Fletcher KA, Cochrane BB, et al. Predictors of depressed mood in spouses of women with breast cancer. *J Clin Oncol*. 2008;26:1289–1295.

4. Northouse LL, Katapodi MC, Schafenacker AM, et al. The impact of caregiving on the psychological well-being of family caregivers and cancer patients. *Semin Oncol Nurs*. 2012;28:236–245.

5. Soothill K, Morris SM, Harman JC, et al. Informal carers of cancer patients: what are their unmet psychosocial needs? *Health Soc Care Community*. 2001;9:464–475.

6. Osee BHP, Vernooij-Dassen MJFJ, Schadé E, et al. Problems experienced by the informal caregivers of cancer patients and their needs for support. *Cancer Nurs*. 2006;29:378–388.

7. Hodges LJ, Humphris GM, Macfarlane G. A meta-analytic investigation of the relationship between the psychological distress of cancer patients and their carers. *Soc Sci Med*. 2005;60:1–12.

8. Hagedoorn M, Sanderman R, Bolks HN, et al. Distress in couples coping with cancer: a meta-analysis and critical review of role and gender effects. *Psychol Bull*. 2008;134:1–30.

9. McClure KS, Nezu AM, Nezu, CM. Social problem solving and depression in couples coping with cancer. *Psychooncology*. 2012;21:11–19.

10. Northouse LL, Katapodi M, Song L, et al. Interventions with family caregivers of cancer patients: meta-analysis of randomized trials. *CA Cancer J Clin*. 2010;60:317–339.

11. Nezu AM, Nezu CM, D'Zurilla TJ. *Problem-Solving Therapy: A Treatment Manual*. New York, NY: Springer; 2013.

12. D'Zurilla TJ, Goldfried MR. Problem solving and behavior modification. *J Abnorm Psychol*. 1971;78:107–126.

13. Nezu AM. Efficacy of a social problem-solving therapy approach for unipolar depression. *J Consult Clin Psychol*. 1986;54:196–202.

14. Nezu AM, Nezu CM, Perri MG. Problem solving to promote treatment adherence. In: O'Donohue WT, Levensky ER, eds. *Promoting Treatment Adherence: A Practical Handbook for Health Care Providers*. New York, NY: Sage; 2006:135–148.

15. Nezu AM, Nezu CM, Hays AM. Problem-solving therapies. In: Dobson K, ed. *Handbook of Cognitive-Behavioral Therapies*. 4th ed. New York, NY: Guilford Press; in press.

16. Nezu AM, Nezu CM. Emotion-centered problem-solving therapy. In: Wenzel A, ed. *Handbook of Cognitive Behavioral Therapy*. Washington, DC: American Psychological Association; in press.

17. Nezu AM. Problem solving and behavior therapy revisited. *Behav Ther*. 2004;35:1–33.

18. D'Zurilla TJ, Nezu AM, Maydeu-Olivares A. Social problem solving: theory and assessment. In: Chang EC, D'Zurilla TJ, Sanna LJ, eds. *Social Problem Solving: Theory, Research, and Training*. Washington, DC: American Psychological Association; 2004:11–27.

19. D'Zurilla TJ, Nezu A. Social problem solving in adults. In: Kendall PC, ed. *Advances in Cognitive-Behavioral Research and Therapy*. Vol. 1. New York, NY: Academic Press; 1982:202–274.

20. D'Zurilla TJ, Nezu AM, Maydeu-Olivares A. *Manual for the Social Problem-Solving Inventory—Revised*. North Tonawanda, NY: Multi-Health Systems; 2002.

21. Nezu AM, Nezu CM, Houts PS, Friedman SH, Faddis S. Relevance of problem-solving therapy to psychosocial oncology. In: Bucher JA, ed. *The Application of Problem-Solving Therapy to Psychosocial Oncology*. Binghamton, NY: Haworth Medical Press; 1999:5–26.

22. Nezu CM, Nezu AM, Friedman SH, et al. Cancer and psychological distress: two investigations regarding the role of problem solving. In: Bucher JA, ed. *The Application of Problem-Solving Therapy to Psychosocial Oncology*. Binghamton, NY: Haworth Medical Press; 1999:27–40.

23. Nezu AM, Nezu CM, Faddis S, DelliCarpini LA, Houts PS. Social problem solving as a moderator of cancer-related stress. Paper presentation at: Annual Convention of the Association for Advancement of Behavior Therapy; November 1995; Washington, DC.

24. Malcarne V, Banthia R, Varni JW, Sadler GR , Greenbergs HL, Ko CM. Problem-solving skills and emotional distress in spouses of men with prostate cancer. *J Cancer Educ*. 2009;17(3):150–154.

25. Nezu AM, Nezu CM, Friedman SH, Faddis S, Houts PS. *Helping Cancer Patients Cope: A Problem-Solving Approach*. Washington, DC: American Psychological Association; 1998.

26. Nezu AM, Nezu CM, Felgoise SH, McClure KS, Houts PS. Project Genesis: assessing the efficacy of problem-solving therapy for distressed adult cancer patients. *J Consult Clin Psychol*. 2003;71:1036–1048.

27. Nezu AM, Nezu CM. Psychological distress, depression, and anxiety. In: Feuerstein M, ed. *Handbook of Cancer Survivorship*. New York, NY: Springer; 2007:323–338.

28. Hirai K, Motooka H, Ito N, et al. Problem-solving therapy for psychological distress in Japanese early-stage breast cancer patients. *Jpn J Clin Oncol*. 2012;42(12):1168–1174.

29. Hopko DR, Armento ME, Robertson S, et al. Brief behavioral activation and problem-solving therapy for depressed breast cancer patients: randomized trial. *J Consult Clin Psychol*. 2011;79(6):834.

30. Hopko DR, Funderburk JS, Shorey RC, et al. Behavioral activation and problem-solving therapy for depressed breast cancer patients: preliminary support for decreased suicidal ideation. *Behav Modif*. 2013;37(6):747–767.

31. Bucher JA, Houts PS, Nezu CM, Nezu AM. Improving problem-solving skills of family caregivers through group education. In: Bucher JA, ed. *The Application of Problem-Solving Therapy to Psychosocial Oncology*. Binghamton, NY: Haworth Medical Press; 1999:73–84.

32. Houts PS, Nezu AM, Nezu CM, Bucher JA. The prepared family caregiver: a problem-solving approach to family caregiver education. *Patient Educ Couns*. 1996;27:63–73.

33. Cameron JI, Shin JL, Williams D, Stewart DE. A brief problem-solving intervention for family caregivers to individuals with advanced cancer. *J Psychosom Res*. 2004; 57(2):137–143.

34. Bevans M, Wehrlen L, Castro K, et al. A problem-solving education intervention in caregivers and patients during allogeneic hematopoietic stem cell transplantation. *J Health Psychol.* 2014;19(5):602–617.

35. Meyers FJ, Carducci M, Loscalzo MJ, Linder J, Greasby T, Beckett LA. Effects of a problem-solving intervention (COPE) on quality of life for patients with advanced cancer on clinical trials and their caregivers: simultaneous care educational intervention (SCEI): linking palliation and clinical trials. *J Palliat Med.* 2011;14(4):465–473.

36. Hawes SM, Malcarne VL, Ko CM, et al. Identifying problems faced by spouses and partners of patients with prostate cancer. *Oncol Nurs Forum.* 2006;33(4):807–814.

37. McMillan SC, Small BJ, Weitzner M, et al. Impact of coping skills intervention with family caregivers of hospice patients with cancer. *Cancer.* 2006;106(1):214–222.

38. Sahler OJZ, Varni JW, Fairclough DL, et al. Problem-solving skills training for mothers of children with newly diagnosed cancer: a randomized trial. *J Dev Behav Pediatr.* 2002; 23(2):77–86.

39. Sahler OJZ, Dolgin MJ, Phipps S, et al. Specificity of problem-solving skills training in mothers of children newly diagnosed with cancer: results of a multisite randomized clinical trial. *Jpn J Clin Oncol.* 2013;31(10):1329–1335.

40. Sahler OJZ, Fairclough DL, Phipps S, et al. Using problem-solving skills training to reduce negative affectivity in mothers of children with newly diagnosed cancer: report of a multisite randomized trial. *J Consult Clin Psychol.* 2005;73:272–283.

CHAPTER 11

Family Therapies

TAMMY A. SCHULER, DAVID W. KISSANE,
AND TALIA I. ZAIDER

PURPOSE AND OVERVIEW

When an individual is diagnosed with advanced cancer, the effects are not confined to the patient alone. They are experienced throughout the entire family. *Most caregivers are family members providing informal care,* and it is estimated that informal caregivers provide 70%–80% of care for cancer patients.[1] Thus, family members must simultaneously cope with the emotional turmoil brought on by the illness and its management while adjusting to major upheaval in their usual roles, daily life, and finances. Family caregivers in the cancer setting are most frequently spouses or partners and are predominantly female and middle-aged, though more men are now taking on caregiver roles.[2,3]

An aging society conferring more age-related cancer diagnoses, trends toward higher cancer survival rates, and the transfer of care from the hospital to ambulatory settings and the home have substantially increased the burden of caregiving for cancer patients' families.[1,4] Families receive little preparation before they are required to carry out caregiving roles, and the intricacies of modern cancer care continue to grow in complexity.[5] Families must often provide round-the-clock support to help manage patients' symptoms from cancer and its treatment and possibly conditions that are comorbid to the cancer. This increased responsibility for the family caregiver comes at great cost to the overall functioning of the family, which is greatly affected by the role changes, alterations in family structure, and financial stressors. Consequently, families require a great deal of support from the healthcare team and community, but the degree to which they actually receive support is variable.[6,7]

As families continue to become increasingly involved in patient care, it becomes all the more important to be able to assess the capacity of the family to work effectively as a caregiving system. Although all families struggle with caring for a member with advanced cancer, some families— such as those who functioned poorly to begin with—tend to struggle even more. Poor family functioning has been associated with worse psychosocial outcomes for both patients and their loved ones.[8,9] As such, a vital clinical goal is to identify and support the "at-risk" families with poor functioning in particular.

This chapter illustrates the complex interactions between cancer and the quality of family relationships, delineates the state of the literature on family interventions and screening, describes the family-focused grief therapy (FFGT) model (a prophylactic family-based intervention that begins during palliative care and continues into bereavement for high-risk families), and integrates empirically supported clinical recommendations for interventions to treat families at high risk for worse psychosocial outcomes.[10,11] In addition to research findings, we offer anecdotal commentary from our experiences in working with families coping with cancer. For the most part, we have opted to discuss interventions appropriate for multiple family members rather than dyads. *Given the high proportion of primary caregivers who are family members, the development and study of FFGT included a large number of caregivers at its foundation. We thus believe FFGT is an appropriate treatment for caregivers who are at risk for worse psychosocial outcomes.*

THE IMPACT OF CANCER DIAGNOSIS ON THE FAMILY

For families coping with cancer, the cancer experience may start at diagnosis, but it does not end on completion of treatment. Family members remain a primary source for support and care across remission, recurrence, survivorship, palliative care, and at the time of the patient's death if that occurs.[12] The associated challenges can seem insurmountable and may persist for years. Caregivers routinely report emotional distress and uncertainty and often experience physical health issues of their own, such as insomnia, fatigue, and overall poorer physical health.[13] Despite these difficulties, the majority of interventions are primarily designed to address patient care, which is certainly an important goal. Nonetheless, although there are now more resources available for caregivers than in the past, intervention content for caregivers is still often an incidental occurrence in the context of patient-focused interventions.[5]

Higher family caregiver burden is associated with deleterious consequences for both caregivers and patients. Among 85 dyads of underserved minority patients with advanced solid tumors treated at public hospitals and their family member/non–family member caregivers, caregivers experiencing high levels of emotional distress at a baseline assessment tended to continue to experience high levels of emotional distress across the 20-week follow-up period.[14] In contrast, caregivers experiencing low levels of emotional distress at baseline showed a significant decrease in emotional distress during the 20-week follow-up period. Moreover, specifically being a family member caregiver and caring for a more severely ill patient were significant predictors of whether the caregiver would belong to the high or the low symptom burden group.[14]

In a qualitative study of spouse and partner caregivers' experiences, caregivers interviewed by Trudeau-Hearn et al. (2012) also cited "compounding hardships" and having responsibilities to provide care for multiple individuals as potential contributors to heightened emotional and physical distress.[15] A recent clinical review identified being female, having low educational attainment, living with the patient, more hours spent caregiving, emotional distress, isolation, financial stressors, and lack of choice in being a caregiver as particular risk factors for increased caregiver burden.[16] Although adverse effects on caregivers' mental and physical health can continue beyond the duration of the caregiving role,[7] among those interviewed by Trudeau-Hearn et al., current caregivers reported poorer physical health compared to widowers who reported being in better health after their spouse had passed away.[15] Caregiver burden may even impact patient and caregiver mortality. Higher caregiver burden is known to be related to increased caregiver mortality risk.[13] Moreover, in a randomized controlled trial (RCT) of an early education and support intervention for patients with advanced cancer and their family caregivers, lower survival in patients with a caregiver was significantly related to higher caregiver burden.[17]

It is important to note that the caregivers interviewed by Trudeau-Hearn et al. in 2012 reported having paradoxical feelings regarding their caregiving experience.[15] Despite the growing body of literature on caregiver burden, providing care for a family member is not always a wholly negative experience, and there are positive aspects to caregiving, which also receive attention in the research literature.[7] Although the positive aspects of caregiving are not thought to mediate the stressors experienced, caregivers do report some degree of finding caregiving strengthening their relationship and to be satisfying and rewarding.[18-20]

In preparatory observational work of caregiving families before the development of the FFGT model, using the Brief Symptom Inventory (BSI) and Beck Depression Inventory (BDI) as standardized measures of clinical concern, one-third of partners and one-quarter of adult offspring (average age 28 years; 60% female) carried clinically significant distress.[21] An additional noteworthy finding was that offspring carried significantly higher anger than patients. Using "caseness" norms for the hostility subscale of the BSI, while only 9% of patients and 13% of spouses exhibited hostility caseness, 26% of the adult children were cases of high hostility in the caregiving family. Poor family communication, anticipatory grief, and caregiving burden were predictors of this noteworthy anger among the offspring of these palliative care patients. Although not always directly involved in caregiving tasks, adult offspring of cancer patients are a potentially vulnerable population affected by illness and whose distress may be in need of clinical attention.

BRIEF OVERVIEW OF FAMILY THERAPY RESEARCH

Family therapies treat families as the "unit of care," rather than the caregiver alone. The majority of family therapies in chronic illness focus on cardiovascular disease, cancer, stroke, arthritis, dementia, and psychosis populations.[22-30] Accordingly, the majority of family intervention research includes middle-aged patient populations and their family members,[5,10] with less focus on coping with chronic illness in pediatric and adolescent populations.[31] Although there is some existing literature describing family-based interventions with ill pediatric populations, much of the existing literature on family therapies to decrease burden of caregiving for a child includes families coping with childhood mental health diagnoses and juvenile incarceration.[32,33]

Family therapies utilize a variety of components to treat families coping with chronic illnesses. These therapies generally include those related to support, psychoeducation, problem-solving/skills building, cognitive behavioral/behavior change, coping, complementary and alternative medicine, existential concerns, grief, respite, family relationships, or multiple component therapies/approaches.[22-30,34-39] Intervention formats range from dyads (such as a patient and their caregiver spouse, parent, or child),[29,34,40,41] to individual family units,[24] to multiple family groups.[42]

A 2010 meta-analytic study analyzed data from 52 relevant RCTs (including 8,896 patients) evaluating the effects of family-based interventions for adult patients compared to standard treatment. Results indicated that family involvement was associated with better mental and physical health for the patient, as well as better health for the family members. Effects remained stable across time. Furthermore, the study authors, who categorized the interventions as relationship-focused or psychoeducational, indicated that *data favored relationship-focused family interventions compared with psychoeducational interventions.*[22] A 2011 review of couples-based psychosocial interventions for couples facing cancer identified 14 relevant studies. Among these, eight studies concluded there was overall improvement in emotional distress and coping for patients, and eight studies also reported overall improvement for partners, whereas an additional five showed partial improvement for patients and three demonstrated partial improvements for partners.[43]

Applebaum et al. in 2013 reported that structured, goal-oriented, time-limited, multicomponent interventions seem to have the best feasibility and offer the most benefit for informal caregivers of cancer patients.[37] Meta-analytic reports also touted multicomponent interventions as offering the most benefit for caregivers of dementia patients.[29,44]

FAMILY FUNCTIONING AND THE IMPORTANCE OF EARLY SCREENING

When a well-functioning family receives the diagnosis of advanced cancer, members share caregiving responsibilities and are largely supportive during the cancer experience and bereavement period.[45] A dysfunctional family, however, may inadvertently disrupt these processes.[46] Thus, the healthcare team requires screening methods by which families that may be most "at risk" for poor psychosocial outcomes can be identified.

A classification system, which guides screening, was developed with Australian patients and families.[8,45] To extend this work, we confirmed this procedure with a cohort of 1,809 American palliative care patients.[9,47] This overall line of research determined how to identify two types of well-functioning families (showing high cohesiveness, good support, and ability to resolve conflicts) as well as intermediate-functioning families (30% of families) and two types of dysfunctional families (showing lower cohesiveness, lower expression, and greater conflict; 15%–20% of families during prebereavement, increasing to 30% of families during early bereavement, who were thought to be intermediate

families affected by the stress of bereavement).[8,9] The at-risk intermediate and dysfunctional Australian families reported significantly higher
depressive symptomatology and global psychological morbidity. These
at-risk families also reported poorer social adjustment regardless of
partnered/marital status.[8] These data illustrate the decline in psychosocial functioning from well-functioning, to intermediate, to dysfunctional family types.[8]

*This body of family functioning literature dovetails with the caregiver burden
literature, which, as previously described, indicates that caregivers experiencing
high levels of distress tend to experience poorer psychosocial outcomes across
time.*[12,14] Thus, screening to identify at-risk families, including caregivers
who may experience higher burden, is of utmost importance and should be
a priority for the healthcare team.[16]

FAMILY-FOCUSED GRIEF THERAPY
Background

There is strong evidence that the quality of family relationships affects
the onset or perpetuation of each members' individual distress during
the course of the cancer trajectory.[48] Therefore, using family-focused
interventions is critical.[46] We developed and tested a family-centered psychosocial intervention called *family-focused grief therapy* for families coping
with advanced cancer. The FFGT model utilizes the screening technique
described previously, in the context of the regular healthcare setting, to
identify at-risk families.[8,49] Families identified as at risk are offered FFGT,
an intervention that has a primary aim to prevent or offset poor psychosocial outcomes (such as depressive symptoms and prolonged grief disorder)
through the improvement of communication, cohesiveness, conflict management, and overall family functioning when the ill family member has
passed away.

Families begin FFGT during palliative care and continue into bereavement. The onset of care prior to loss and continuity of care in bereavement are unique features of FFGT and allow families to actively alter the
course of their adaptation to the patient's death. FFGT is a time-limited,
transportable, and manualized intervention, implemented with training
and supervision of master's level therapists for treatment fidelity.[50] FFGT
received empirical support through an RCT with Australian patients and
families.[51] A second RCT examined the dose effectiveness of FFGT (6 vs.
10 therapy sessions or usual care) with American patients and families.
Better outcomes for complicated grief were shown for 10 sessions versus

usual care for "low-communicating" and "high-conflict" families compared with "low-involvement" families. In the usual care arm, 15.5% of bereaved family members developed prolonged grief disorder by 13 months of bereavement compared with 3.3% of those who received 10 sessions.[52]

Assessment Phase

Family-focused grief therapy begins with the engagement phase, which aims to build rapport and gather background information on the story of illness and the family's coping response. The therapists also inquire about dimensions of family functioning and concerns for particular members. A major goal of this phase is to evaluate the family's communication, cohesiveness, and conflict because these three aspects of family functioning direct our classification system and are particularly foundational to familial relations.[53] Also, therapists use genograms for additional insight into strengths, vulnerabilities, relational patterns, and major family events in family history as they relate to the current context. The assessment phase concludes with treatment plan formulation and development of a focused agenda.[46]

Intervention Sessions

Intervention sessions generally occur every 3 to 4 weeks and are regularly held in the inpatient setting or the family's home as the patient's illness progresses. During this phase, therapists review the concerns identified during the engagement phase, underscore family strengths, and continue the discussion of coping and grief. Family communication, cohesiveness, and conflict are addressed at each session, and the therapist prompts families to describe their progress in terms of the major areas of concern identified during the engagement phase.

The work on communication, cohesiveness, and conflict often evolves following the patient's death. Therapists work with the families to help them engage in adaptive communication of feelings. Encouraging this type of shared grief is also helpful in building cohesiveness within the family. In another unique feature of FFGT, therapists frequently attend funerals to foster the therapeutic connection, while paying their respects to the bereaved. Continuation of therapy following bereavement ensures continuity of care for the grieving family and builds on the family's relationship with the therapist's direct experiences with the deceased. The deceased's wishes and motives may direct subsequent sessions. Meaning-making, coming to terms with fresh roles, and continuing relational changes are key foci.[46]

Consolidation and Termination Sessions

As signs of resolution following bereavement emerge, the length of time between sessions is increased, and then therapy termination is prepared for openly. The final FFGT sessions include relapse prevention strategies aimed at maintaining change and the consideration of future approaches to sustain the changes that the family has made. A frequent strategy is to invite the family to anticipate and identify relational patterns that may be problematic in the future and to consider how they might handle these problematic behaviors when they arise.

During this stage of FFGT, it is likely that the family is still coping with the loss of their loved one. The continuity of care by FFGT therapists can prove to be advantageous in terms of reminiscing and achieving family goals.

At therapy termination, the therapist may share personal feelings for the benefit of the family. In our experience, saying good-bye often generates genuine feelings of sadness for the therapist, which are acknowledged and used to reaffirm the impact of the therapist's work with the family. The therapist conveys his or her faith in the ability of the family to maintain the important changes they have made and belief that the family will be able take responsibility for continuing their work together in the future.[46]

CASE EXAMPLE

A 70-year-old mother of five adult children was battling progressive and advanced colorectal cancer. She was aware that her 80-year-old husband of some 49 years, who did his best as her caregiver, would find it hard to keep going without her. Screening of this family had shown reduced communication and some tension within the family. The patient, as matriarch, kept them all together. She was forthright in expressing her sadness at leaving them all, and the family as a whole expressed concern for their father, who had been valiant in taking on instrumental roles in the household. Humor and honesty were identified as protective strengths of the family, while silence and holding back had been their modus operandi in dealing with the cancer thus far. When a family is about to lose its emotional lynchpin, there is some sense of threat regarding what the future will bring.

This family met four times with the therapist across 3 months before the matriarch of the family died. They acknowledged their love and gratitude as they communicated more openly with one another. In bereavement, the father created a shrine for his wife and seemed needy in his grief. His children struggled with how much support to offer, as they now took on a caregiving role for their father. In subsequent months, some tension emerged as the children felt unable to meet all of their father's needs. However, they kept talking together about this predicament and in the process shared their efforts in a balanced and less burdensome manner.

The six sessions of therapy that occurred over the first 12 months of bereavement helped the family adapt to new roles as the caregiving balance changed. They became united in efforts to support and console their father in his grief. The therapy room, with its strong memories of their mother's wish for her husband to be cared for, helped to hold and organize the family in this task. Mutuality, respect, and love prevailed; grief was shared; and the family moved forward by successfully adapting to new roles. A more open communication style proved a strength and a metaphor for the mother's gift to her family.

NEWER AREAS IN FAMILY CAREGIVER RESEARCH

Although most family-based therapies involve in-person meetings with a practitioner, many family-based therapies are now provided via telehealth services and other technologies (such as eHealth and mHealth) for intervention delivery. Alternative formats that decrease travel burden on the family (such as those used during FFGT)[46] can be particularly important when families live in remote locations with few services or when the patient is very ill, as in the case of advanced cancer.[25] Existing data indicate that such interventions appear to be feasible, acceptable, and effective.

In 2015, Badr et al. reported results from a pilot study of a telephone-based dyadic psychosocial intervention developed for advanced lung cancer patients and their caregivers. Thirty-nine patients within 1 month of treatment initiation and their caregivers participated. Intervention participation, versus usual medical care, was associated with improvements in emotional distress and caregiver burden. Moreover, the study showed low attrition rates, suggesting that the telephone-based format was acceptable to patients and their caregivers.[54]

In a later, separate study, Badr and colleagues reported initial development and evaluation data from a dyadic, web-based intervention designed to improve self-management in oral cancer survivors and to improve quality of life (QOL) for their caregivers. Results indicated that the survivors and caregivers were interested in using an online program, and that providing tailored website content and features based on the person's role as survivor or caregiver was important.[55] Steel et al. (2016) randomized 261 patients with advanced cancer and 179 family caregivers to a web-based collaborative care intervention or enhanced usual care. For patients with clinical levels of symptoms at the baseline assessment, those in the collaborative care intervention showed significant decreases in emotional distress, pain, and fatigue, and improvements in QOL and immune functioning (interleukin [IL] 6, IL-1β, IL-1α, IL-8, and natural killer cell numbers) 6 months later, compared with those in the enhanced usual care arm. Moreover, reductions in caregiver emotional distress was shown 6 months later for caregivers whose loved ones were randomized to the collaborative care intervention.[56]

Another new area of research involves family interventions targeted toward those with increased hereditary susceptibility toward developing cancer. A Portuguese research group held multifamily discussion groups for four families with individuals at risk of developing colorectal cancer and their families. Although the study was small, families reported feeling better able to cope with genetic illness afterward. The authors concluded that it is important for family-based approaches to genetic susceptibility to incorporate the stage the cancer is diagnosed, and that because of the reproductive implications of susceptibility, a wider range of family members (and possibly adolescents) should be involved.[57]

CONCLUSIONS: ADVANCES IN FAMILY THERAPY IN ONCOLOGY

Family-focused grief therapy is an effective family-based intervention that we believe to be an appropriate treatment for caregivers who are at risk for worse psychosocial outcomes. Other effective family-based interventions for caregivers are also currently available. In addition, there are promising shifts on the horizon for family caregiver intervention research. Ferrell and Wittenberg's 2017 meta-analysis and review describing the evolution of family caregiver research indicated that there has been an increase in RCTs involving family caregivers and that study sample sizes have become larger. The authors indicated that these phenomena may be partially attributable to increased funding for research in this area. Indeed, most major cancer organizations and many major science organizations now provide significant attention to the difficulties faced by caregivers. Furthermore, there has been growth in the number of caregiver research and advocacy groups, and technology has made caregiving resources more easily accessible to clinicians and families. It is also encouraging that there has been an increase in the number of studies that target caregivers rather than just the patients.[12] Currently, most interventions are psychoeducational, and couples-based therapies remain the most prolific intervention format.[12,58]

Limitations in Family Therapy in Oncology

As with any line of research, family therapy research confers certain limitations. First, due to the exceedingly complex nature of family therapy, it is frequently difficult to determine what the "active ingredients" that drive change are. Which intervention components and formats are responsible for the greatest improvements?[12,22] In relation, although family interventions (particularly multicomponent) are thought to be beneficial, acceptable, and applicable,[29,44] effect sizes associated with family interventions tend to be modest,[16,22,29] and interventions are not always equally effective for patients and caregivers.[43] Moreover, Ferrell and Wittenberg in 2017 identified a decrease during the past several years in the reporting of treatment fidelity for family caregiver intervention studies.[12]

Second, there is a need for realistic application of these evolving family caregiver intervention models to clinical practice. Involvement in faraway intervention studies can be extremely time consuming and unrealistic for families, who are already coping with a major burden and who may not have access to state-of-the-art facilities. This is where the flexibility and transportability approach utilized by FFGT is especially important.[46] There has been a recent increase in the use of multidisciplinary providers to deliver interventions as well as greater attention to the use of telephone delivery and other technologies that can be used from the home.[12] Nonetheless, important practice questions such as how interventions should be delivered, at what point in the cancer trajectory they should be provided, and intervention duration remain challenging.[43]

Third, most family therapy research participants are white. This is unsurprising, as this sample demographic composition remains the general state of affairs for most research studies in cancer and other areas. Ferrell and Wittenberg in 2017 identified a "noticeable tendency for researchers to exclude caregiver race and ethnicity as a reported caregiver demographic variable" (p. 322).[12] This approach is, of course, incongruous with the literature, which underscores cultural influences on family caregiving and demographic trends.[12,25,59] Though we have written some reports on cultural influence,[60,61] there is a clear need for research testing interventions that are more sensitive to cultural influences and true demographics.[12] Regarding other demographic influences, the majority of family caregiving research in oncology has studied middle-aged adults caring for other adults.[62] While there is a growing body of research,[31] longitudinal work is needed to understand the impact of caring for a child or adolescent/young adult with cancer and a child, adolescent, or young adult caring for another family member with cancer in order to develop optimally effective interventions.[62]

Finally, the relation between receiving family therapy in cancer and changes in caregiver burden as an outcome is not fully clear. It is assumed that a large proportion of family members enrolled in family therapy studies in cancer are caregivers, but the exact proportions may not be known. Caregiver burden is not always used as an outcome in family therapies in cancer, although other important associated outcomes such as emotional distress and QOL are regularly assessed.[16] Even when caregiver burden is assessed, burden may be an outcome that is too broad to be consistently measured and affected by intervention participation.[28] The need for valid measurement of caregiver outcomes in family therapy studies to properly evaluate the effects on caregivers is clear.[16,28]

Closing Words

There is a central role for caregiver education and support to empower the main caregiver to execute relevant tasks competently. Family therapy interventions recognize that these tasks are executed in a broader relational context that can support or constrain the main caregiver's well-being. A distinct and equally important intervention target has therefore been the poorly functioning family, who struggles to provide care for a family member who is ill or perhaps dying. We have focused primarily on the latter approach, with an evidence base demonstrating that much can be done preventively with such families to optimize outcomes that include bereavement. Family-centered care is richly endorsed as part of the mission of hospice care. The FFGT model is one example of how this can be implemented cost effectively while simultaneously targeting those most in need.

ACKNOWLEDGMENTS

We would like to thank the clinical research staff of the FFGT study, the caregivers who make a difference in patients' lives each day, and the FFGT families who volunteered to share with us their personal experiences during caregiving and bereavement.

REFERENCES

1. Lambert SD, Levesque J V., Girgis A. Impact of cancer and chronic conditions on caregivers and family members. In: Koczwara B, ed. *Cancer and Chronic Conditions.* New York, NY: Springer Nature; 2016:159–202.
2. National Alliance for Caregiving (NAC) and American Association of Retired Persons (AARP) Public Policy Institute. *Caregiving in the US.* Washington, DC: Public Policy Institute; 2015.
3. Russell R. The work of elderly men caregivers: from public careers to an unseen world. *Men Masc.* 2007;9(3):298–314. doi:10.1177/1097184X05277712
4. Braun M, Mikulincer M, Rydall A, Walsh A, Rodin G. Hidden morbidity in cancer: spouse caregivers. *J Clin Oncol.* 2007;25(30):4829–4834. doi:10.1200/ JCO.2006.10.0909
5. Northouse LL, Katapodi MC, Song L, Zhang L, Mood DW. Interventions with family caregivers of cancer patients: meta-analysis of randomized trials. *CA Cancer J Clin.* 2010;60(5):317–339. doi:10.3322/caac.20081.
6. Given BA, Given CW, Sherwood PR. Family and caregiver needs over the course of the cancer trajectory. *J Support Oncol.* 2012;10(2):57–64. doi:10.1016/ j.suponc.2011.10.003
7. Weitzner MA, Haley WE, Chen H. The family caregiver of the older cancer patient. *Hematol Oncol Clin North Am.* 2000;14(1):269–281. doi:10.1016/ S0889-8588(05)70288-4
8. Kissane DW, Bloch S, Onghena P, McKenzie DP, Snyder RD, Dowe DL. The Melbourne family grief study, II: psychosocial morbidity and grief in bereaved families. *Am J Psychiatry.* 1996;153(5):659–666. doi:10.1176/ajp.153.5.659
9. Schuler TA, Zaider TI, Li Y, et al. Perceived family functioning predicts baseline psychosocial characteristics in US participants of a family focused grief therapy trial. *J Pain Symptom Manage.* 2017;54(1):126–131. doi:10.1016/ j.jpainsymman.2017.03.016
10. Kissane DW, Parnes F, eds. *Bereavement Care for Families.* New York, NY: Routledge; 2014.
11. Kissane, DW, Bloch S, eds. *Family Focused Grief Therapy: A Model of Family-Centred Care During Palliative Care and Bereavement.* Buckingham, UK: Open University Press; 2002.
12. Ferrell B, Wittenberg E. A review of family caregiving intervention trials in oncology. *CA Cancer J Clin.* 2017;67:318–325. doi:10.3322/caac.21396
13. Sharpe L, Butow P, Smith C, McConnell D, Clarke S. The relationship between available support, unmet needs and caregiver burden in patients with advanced cancer and their carers. *Psychooncology.* 2005;14:102–114. doi:10.1002/pon.825

14. Palos GR, Mendoza TR, Liao KP, et al. Caregiver symptom burden: the risk of caring for an underserved patient with advanced cancer. *Cancer.* Mar 1;117(5):1070–9. doi: 10.1002/cncr.25695. Epub 2010 Oct 19.
15. Trudeau-Hern S, Daneshpour M. Cancer's impact on spousal caregiver health: a qualitative analysis in grounded theory. *Contemporary Family Therapy: An International Journal;* Dec 2012; 34(4):534.
16. Adelman RD, Tmanova LL, Delgado D, Dion S, Lachs MS. Caregiver burden: a clinical review. *JAMA.* 2014. Mar 12;311(10):1052–60. doi: 10.1001/jama.2014.304.
17. Dionne-Odom JN, Hull JG, Martin MY, et al. Associations between advanced cancer patients' survival and family caregiver presence and burden. *Cancer Med.* 2016. May;5(5):853–62. doi: 10.1002/cam4.653. Epub 2016 Feb 10.
18. Salmon JR, Kwak J, Acquaviva KD, Brandt K, Egan KA. Transformative aspects of caregiving at life's end. *J Pain Symptom Manage.* 2005;29(2):121–9. doi:10.1016/j.jpainsymman.2004.12.008
19. *Res Aging.* 2004;26(4):429–453. doi:10.1177/0164027504264493
20. Cohen CA, Colantonio A, Vernich L. Positive aspects of caregiving: rounding out the caregiver experience. *Int J Geriatr Psychiatry.* 2002;17:184–188. doi:10.1002/gps.561
21. Kissane DW, Bloch S, Burns WI, Patrick JD, Wallace CS, McKenzie DP. Perceptions of family functioning and cancer. *Psychooncology.* 1994;3(4):259–269. doi:10.1002/pon.2960030403
22. Hartmann M, Bäzner E, Wild B, Eisler I, Herzog W. Effects of interventions involving the family in the treatment of adult patients with chronic physical diseases: a meta-analysis. *Psychother Psychosom.* 2010;79(3):136–48. doi: 10.1159/000286958. Epub 2010 Feb 20.
23. Drossel C, Fisher JE, Mercer V. A DBT skills training group for family caregivers of persons with dementia. *Behav Ther.* 2011. Mar;42(1):109–19. doi: 10.1016/j.beth.2010.06.001. Epub 2010 Nov 19.
24. Bowman KF, Rose JH, Radziewicz RM, O'Toole EE, Berila RA. Family caregiver engagement in a coping and communication support intervention tailored to advanced cancer patients and families. *Cancer Nurs.* 2009; Jan-Feb; 32:73–81. doi:10.1097/01.NCC.0000343367.98623.83
25. Eisdorfer C, Czaja SJ, Loewenstein DA, et al. The effect of a family therapy and technology-based intervention on caregiver depression. *Gerontologist.* 2003 Aug;43(4):521–31. doi:10.1093/geront/43.4.521
26. Roddy S, Onwumere J, Kuipers E. A pilot investigation of a brief, needs-led caregiver focused intervention in psychosis. *J Fam Ther.* 2015. 4(37):529–545. doi:10.1111/1467-6427.12054
27. Cheng HY, Chair SY, Chau JPC. The effectiveness of psychosocial interventions for stroke family caregivers and stroke survivors: a systematic review and meta-analysis. *Patient Educ Couns.* 2014 Apr;95(1):30–44. doi: 10.1016/j.pec.2014.01.005. Epub 2014 Jan
28. Acton GJ, Kang J. Interventions to reduce the burden of caregiving for an adult with dementia: a meta-analysis. *Res Nurs Heal.* 2001 Oct;24(5):349–60. doi:10.1002/nur.1036
29. Laver K, Milte R, Dyer S, Crotty M. A systematic review and meta-analysis comparing carer focused and dyadic multicomponent interventions for carers of people with dementia. *J Aging Health.* 2017 Dec;29(8):1308–1349. doi: 10.1177/0898264316660414. Epub 2016 Jul 25.

30. Losada A, Márquez-González M, Romero-Moreno R, et al. Cognitive–behavioral therapy (CBT) versus acceptance and commitment therapy (ACT) for dementia family caregivers with significant depressive symptoms: results of a randomized clinical trial. *J Consult Clin Psychol.* 2015 Aug;83(4):760–72. doi: 10.1037/ccp0000028. Epub 2015 Jun 15.

31. Kazak AE, Simms S, Barakat L, et al. Surviving Cancer Competently Intervention Program (SCCIP): a cognitive-behavioral and family therapy intervention for adolescent survivors of childhood cancer and their families. *Fam Process.* 1999 Summer;38(2):175–91.

32. Foley K, McNeil CB, Norman M, Wallace NM. Effectiveness of group format parent-child interaction therapy compared to treatment as usual in a community outreach organization. *Child Fam Behav Ther.* 2016 38(4):279–298. doi:10.1080/07317107.2016.1238688

33. Keiley MK. Multiple-family group intervention for incarcerated adolescents and their families: a pilot project. *J Marital Fam Ther.* 2007 Jan;33(1):106–24. doi:10.1111/j.1752-0606.2007.00009.x

34. Northouse LL, Mood DW, Schafenacker A, et al. Randomized clinical trial of a brief and extensive dyadic intervention for advanced cancer patients and their family caregivers. *Psychooncology.* 2013;22:555–563. doi:10.1002/pon.3036

35. McMillan SC, Small BJ, Weitzner M, et al. Impact of coping skills intervention with family caregivers of hospice patients with cancer. *Cancer.* 2006;106(1):214–222. doi:10.1002/cncr.21567

36. Chawla N. A multiple-behavior lifestyle intervention for cancer patients and their families delivered in a community-based oncological and hematologic treatment clinic. *J Fam Psychother.* 2011;22(1):74–81. doi:10.1080/08975353.2011.551101

37. Applebaum AJ, Breitbart W. Care for the cancer caregiver: a systematic review. *Palliat Support Care.* 2013 Jun;11(3):231–52. doi: 10.1017/S1478951512000594. Epub 2012 Oct 10.

38. Guldina MB, Vedsted P, Jensen AB, Olesena F, Zachariae R. Bereavement care in general practice: a cluster randomized clinical trial. *Fam Pract.* 2013;30:134–141. doi:10.1093/fampra/cms053

39. Demark-Wahnefried W, Jones LW, Snyder DC, et al. Daughters and Mothers Against Breast Cancer (DAMES): main outcomes of a randomized controlled trial of weight loss in overweight mothers with breast cancer and their overweight daughters. *Cancer.* 2014;120:2522–2534. doi:10.1002/cncr.28761

40. Shields CG, Rousseau SJ. A pilot study of an intervention for breast cancer survivors and their spouses. *Fam Process.* 2004;43(1):95–107. doi:10.1111/j.1545-5300.2004.04301008.x

41. Manne S, Mee L, Bartell A, Sands S, Kashy DA. A randomized clinical trial of a parent-focused social-cognitive processing intervention for caregivers of children undergoing hematopoetic stem cell transplantation. *J Consult Clin Psychol.* 2016;84:389–401. doi:10.1037/ccp0000087

42. Ostroff J, Ross S, Steinglass P, Ronis-Tobin V, Singh B. Interest in and barriers to participation in multiple family groups among head and neck cancer survivors and their primary family caregivers. *Fam Process.* 2004;43:195–208. doi:10.1111/j.1545-5300.2004.04302005.x

43. Baik OM, Adams KB. Improving the well-being of couples facing cancer: a review of couples-based psychosocial interventions. *J Marital Fam Ther.* 2011 Apr;37(2):250–66. doi: 10.1111/j.1752-0606.2010.00217.x.

44. Abrahams R, Liu KPY, Bissett M, et al. Effectiveness of interventions for co-residing family caregivers of people with dementia: systematic review and meta-analysis. *Aust Occup Ther J.* 2018 Jun;65(3):208–224. doi: 10.1111/1440-1630.12464. Epub 2018 Mar 12.

45. Kissane DW, Bloch S, Dowe DL, et al. The Melbourne family grief study, I: perceptions of family functioning in bereavement. *Am J Psychiatry.* 1996;153(5):650–658. doi:10.1016/0924-9338(96)88882-1

46. Masterson MP, Schuler TA, Kissane DW. Family focused grief therapy: a versatile intervention in palliative care and bereavement. *Bereave Care.* 2013;32(3):117–123. doi:10.1080/02682621.2013.854544

47. Schuler, TA, Zaider, TI, Li Y, et al. Typology of perceived family functioning in an American sample of patients with advanced cancer. *J Pain Symptom Manage.* 2014;48:281–288.

48. Kissane DW, Bloch S, Dowe DL, et al. The Melbourne family grief study, I: perceptions of family functioning in bereavement. *Am J Psychiatry.* 1996;153(5):650–658. doi:10.1016/0924-9338(96)88882-1

49. Kissane D. Family focused grief therapy. *Bereave Care.* 2003;22(1):6–8. doi:10.1080/02682620308657563

50. Chan EKH, O'Neill I, McKenzie M, Love A, Kissane DW. What works for therapists conducting family meetings: treatment integrity in family-focused grief therapy during palliative care and bereavement. *J Pain Symptom Manage.* 2004. Jun;27(6):502–12. doi:10.1016/j.jpainsymman.2003.10.008

51. Kissane DW, McKenzie M, Bloch S, Moskowitz C, McKenzie DP, O'Neill I. Family focused grief therapy: a randomized, controlled trial in palliative care and bereavement. *Am J Psychiatry.* 2006;163(7):1208–1218. doi:10.1176/appi.ajp.163.7.1208

52. Kissane DW, Zaider TI, Li Y, Hichenberg S, Schuler TA, Lederberg M. Dose-effectiveness RCT of preventive family therapy in advanced cancer: benefits for the bereaved. *J Clin Oncol.* 2016;34:1921–1927.

53. Edwards B, Clarke V. The validity of the family relationships index as a screening tool for psychological risk in families of cancer patients. *Psychooncology.* 2005;14(7):546–554. doi:10.1002/pon.876

54. Badr H, Smith CB, Goldstein NE, Gomez JE, Redd WH. Dyadic psychosocial intervention for advanced lung cancer patients and their family caregivers: results of a randomized pilot trial. *Cancer.* 2015;121:150–158. doi:10.1002/cncr.29009

55. Badr H, Lipnick D, Diefenbach MA, et al. Development and usability testing of a web-based self-management intervention for oral cancer survivors and their family caregivers. *Eur J Cancer Care (Engl).* 2016;25:806–821. doi:10.1111/ecc.12396

56. Steel JL, Geller DA, Kim KH, et al. Web-based collaborative care intervention to manage cancer-related symptoms in the palliative care setting. *Cancer.* 2016;122:1270–1282. doi:10.1002/cncr.29906

57. Mendes Á, Chiquelho R, Santos TA, Sousa L. Supporting families in genetic counselling services: a psychoeducational multifamily discussion group for at-risk colorectal cancer families. *J Fam Ther.* 2015;37(3):343–360. doi:10.1111/1467-6427.12016

58. Regan TW, Lambert SD, Girgis A, Kelly B, Kayser K, Turner J. Do couple-based interventions make a difference for couples affected by cancer? A systematic review. *BMC Cancer.* 2012;12:279. doi:10.1186/1471-2407-12-279

59. Marshall CA, Weihs KL, Larkey LK, et al. Like a Mexican wedding: psychosocial intervention needs of predominately Hispanic low-income female co-survivors of cancer. *J Fam Nurs.* 2011;17:380–402. doi:10.1177/1074840711416119

60. Del Gaudio F, Hichenberg S, Eisenberg M, Kerr E, Zaider TI, Kissane DW. Latino values in the context of palliative care: illustrative cases from the family focused grief therapy trial. *Am J Hosp Palliat Med.* 2013;30(3):271–278. doi:10.1177/1049909112448926

61. Mondia S, Hichenberg S, Kerr E, Eisenberg M, Kissane DW. The impact of Asian American value systems on palliative care: illustrative cases from the family-focused grief therapy trial. *Am J Hosp Palliat Med.* 2012;29(6):443–448. doi:10.1177/1049909111426281

62. Faulkner RA, Davey M. Children and adolescents of cancer patients: the impact of cancer on the family. *American Journal of Family Therapy,* 2002;30(1):63–72. doi:10.1080/019261802753455651

Addressing the Needs of Cancer Caregivers

Adaptations of Empirically Supported Treatments

CHAPTER 12

Cognitive Behavioral Therapy for Insomnia for Caregivers

KELLY M. SHAFFER, PATRICIA CARTER,
SHEILA N. GARLAND,
AND ALLISON J. APPLEBAUM

Insomnia is among the most common, distressing, and impairing psychophysiological outcomes experienced by cancer caregivers.[1] Insomnia is defined as a persistent difficulty initiating or maintaining sleep and a subjective report of nonrestorative sleep, despite adequate opportunity for sleep, resulting in significant daytime impairment or distress.[2] Between 40% and 76% of family caregivers for a person with cancer report clinically significant symptoms of insomnia,[3-5] although rates up to 95% have been documented among caregivers of patients with advanced cancer.[6,7] Such rates are higher than the roughly one-third prevalence rate among the general US population[8] and those among caregivers for patients with other chronic medical illnesses like Alzheimer's disease[9] or Parkinson's disease.[10] Caregivers also frequently report worse sleep disturbance than even their loved ones with cancer.[3,11,12] Importantly, once a chronic pattern has been established, the moderate-to-severe symptoms of insomnia tend not to remit naturally.[5] Indeed, studies of bereaved caregivers highlight that severe insomnia symptoms present before the death of the patient, when left untreated, persist up to 5 years later.[13,14] As such, early assessment and intervention targeting insomnia among caregivers is important to attenuate the long-term impact of sleep disturbance on caregivers' well-being.

RISK FACTORS FOR INSOMNIA

General risk factors for insomnia that have been consistently associated with insomnia are older age, female sex, unemployment, lower socioeconomic status, and rotating shift work.[15] Some studies suggest that married individuals have lower levels of insomnia than those who are single, divorced, or separated.[16] Insomnia also has complex, reciprocal relations with psychiatric and medical conditions. Depression and anxiety disorders are particularly bidirectionally related to sleep problems,[6,17–19] and treatment for insomnia has been shown to meaningfully improve these psychiatric symptoms.[20–22] Symptoms and treatments for medical conditions, including chronic pain disorders, cancer, and cardiovascular diseases, also commonly increase insomnia symptoms.[15] Common pharmacologic drug classes associated with insomnia include antidepressants, beta blockers, corticosteroids, decongestants, and stimulants.[23]

In addition to these common general insomnia risk factors, caregivers also face the challenge of providing care to a loved one. Family caregivers are predominately women[24] (insomnia risk factor) and often report increased symptoms of anxiety and depression (insomnia risk factors).[11,24] They often have multiple roles (e.g., wife, mother, employee) and take on the additional role of clinical case manager to assist the person with cancer. Understandably, a majority of cancer caregivers have high caregiving burden, with many feeling as though they are "on call" 24 hours per day,[25] naturally causing disruption to their typical schedules and roles. The added stress and reduced time for self-care appear to increase the risk of adopting coping behaviors that are in direct conflict with obtaining a good night's sleep. Specifically, caregivers report an increased use of caffeine and naps to manage fatigue[4] and alcohol and tobacco use to relax,[26] as well as decreases in amount of exercise[26,27] and stress management activities.[27]

CONSEQUENCES OF INSOMNIA

Insomnia among cancer caregivers has been associated with aggravated psychological and physical health problems, including increased psychological distress,[5] depression,[17] poor quality of life (QOL),[7] and decreased immune functioning.[28] Lack of adequate restorative sleep is also hypothesized to play a role in prolonged grief disorder due to the significant energy frequently required to process grief through the bereavement process.[14] These cross-sectional findings align with longitudinal research among the general population, in which sleep disturbance has been found to play an important role in the onset and maintenance of depression[18] and anxiety disorders.[19,29] Moreover, insomnia is prospectively associated with development of cardiovascular disease,[30] obesity,[31,32] diabetes,[31] and all-cause mortality.[33] As such, addressing cancer caregivers' sleep disturbance is critical to mitigating the notable mental and physical health disparities documented in this population.

Caregivers' sleep disturbance can also be interdependent with their loved ones' sleep disturbance during cancer treatment. A study of women with breast cancer and their bed partners demonstrated, by using actigraphy, an objective measure that infers sleep based on the presence or absence of movement during the night, that both partners' sleep deteriorated across the course of adjuvant chemotherapy.[34] Bed partners' habits and mental health are associated with one's own sleep disturbance.[35,36] Conversely, bed partners can also exert a positive effect on one's sleep, such as promoting consistent social routines and behavioral activation during the day.[37] Given that 39% of caregivers live with the individual with cancer and 16% are spouses,[24] interventions efficacious in improving caregivers' sleep may also produce meaningful, indirect benefits to persons with cancer.

THEORETICAL MODELS OF INSOMNIA

The first behavioral theory of insomnia to gain wide acceptance was the 3P model, later modified to the 4P model to accommodate classical conditioning factors,[38,39] and it is particularly helpful for conceptualizing and explaining the rationale for key components of insomnia treatment (Figure 12.1). This model highlights unique *predisposing, precipitating*, and *perpetuating* factors that, when combined, make certain individuals more likely to experience insomnia, and explain how acute episodes of insomnia eventually become chronic via classical (*Pavlovian*) conditioning. The 4P model begins as a diathesis-stress model and explains the interaction between vulnerability and expression of insomnia whereby a predisposition to insomnia may exist but requires a sufficiently stressful precipitant, or combination of precipitants, before it may be expressed.

Predisposing factors comprise biological features (e.g., older age, female sex) and psychological traits (e.g., tendency to worry) that increase one's vulnerability to insomnia.[40] Precipitating factors are single or multiple occurrences of a sufficiently stressful trigger.[41] In the case of caregivers, this may be the partner's initial diagnosis of cancer, increased responsibilities for nighttime care provision, or a nocturnal accident/injury. Perpetuating factors refer to the behaviors that contribute to the

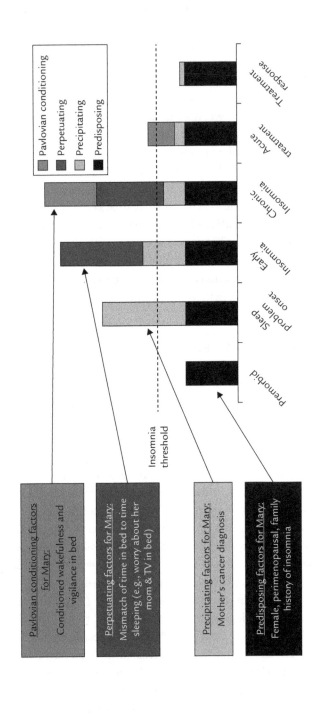

Figure 12.1: Behavioral (4P) model of insomnia.
Figure adapted with permission from Perlis M, Ellis J, Kloss J, Riemann D. Etiology of insomnia. In: Kryger MH, Roth T, Dement WC, eds. *The Principles and Practice of Sleep Medicine.* (Buysse D, section ed.). 6th ed. Philadelphia, PA: 2016:850–865.

persistence or maintenance of insomnia. These are usually activities that an individual engages in to attempt to manage their insomnia, such as going to bed earlier, "trying" harder to sleep, worrying about the effects of poor sleep on next-day functioning, daytime napping, and engaging in activities other than sleep while in bed. When sleep-related stimuli (i.e., the bed, bedroom) are repeatedly paired with insomnia-related wakefulness, a classically conditioned cognitive and somatic arousal response is produced. Thus, the 4P model provides a strong explanation for how acute insomnia can develop into chronic insomnia via these perpetuating and "Pavlovian" factors, even as stress of the initial trigger fades.[38]

Recent adaptations and extensions of the 4P model have further increased the understanding of specific neurological, cognitive, and physiological aspects of insomnia. The *cognitive model* of insomnia suggests that individuals with insomnia have excessive worry and rumination about getting enough sleep and the impact of poor sleep on health and functioning.[42] This model emphasizes targeting cognitive maintaining factors (e.g., attentional bias to fatigue) and eliminating the use of safety behaviors (e.g., caffeine) in the successful treatment of insomnia.[43] The *neurocognitive model* extends these models by suggesting that classical conditioning of sleep-related stimuli with insomnia-related wakefulness can also lead to exaggerated levels of cortical hyperarousal during sleep, which interferes with the ability to initiate or maintain sleep.[44] Indeed, heightened frontal and temporal cortical arousal, associated with stress-induced worry and rumination, has been demonstrated in patients with insomnia.[45] In contrast, the *psychobiological inhibition model* suggests that difficulty with sleep initiation and maintenance is caused by the failure to inhibit wakefulness,[46] as opposed to the conditioned hyperarousal.[44] This model suggests that when a person experiences difficulty sleeping, their attention shifts toward the process of sleep, something that is typically an automatic and passive event. Individuals then exert more active effort to sleep, which further impairs the inhibition of wakefulness. These models demonstrate the complexity of insomnia and the multifaceted contributing factors that may present differently across each caregiver.

COGNITIVE BEHAVIORAL THERAPY FOR INSOMNIA

The recognition that individuals with insomnia exhibit cognitive, physiological, and cortical hyperarousal; demonstrate particular cognitive patterns and attentional biases; strongly endorse problematic sleep-related beliefs; and engage in maladaptive sleep-related behaviors has led to the development of cognitive behavioral therapy for insomnia (CBT-I), a treatment designed to address these interrelated components. Treatment targets the factors perpetuating insomnia by combining behavioral techniques of stimulus control (i.e., developing a strong association between the bed and sleep), sleep restriction (i.e., matching time in bed to current sleep ability to increase homeostatic sleep pressure and facilitate deeper and more restorative sleep), and relaxation strategies (i.e., reduction of cognitive and physiological hyperarousal) with sleep hygiene education and cognitive restructuring of maladaptive beliefs about sleep.[8,47,48] Several reviews and meta-analyses of studies have concluded that CBT-I is a highly effective treatment among the general population[49,50] and patients with cancer.[51,52] Specifically, CBT-I reduces sleep onset latency (SOL), increases sleep efficiency (SE), and increases slow-wave sleep more than hypnotic medications.[53,54] Given the strong evidence base for CBT-I and the relative preference for nonpharmacological treatment among most individuals,[55,56] CBT-I is recommended as a first-line treatment for insomnia.[8]

Traditionally, CBT-I requires four to eight weekly face-to-face meetings with the clinical provider; standard content and session delivery is described in greater detail in Table 12.1. During the intake session, the clinical history is obtained, and the patient is instructed in the use of sleep diaries. No intervention is provided during the first week as it is used to collect the baseline sleep-wake data that will guide treatment for the remainder of therapy. The primary interventions (stimulus control and sleep restriction) are deployed over the course of the next one to two sessions. Once these treatments are delivered, the patient enters into a phase of treatment where total sleep time is upwardly titrated over the course of the next visits. Providers may also use these sessions to discuss sleep hygiene, cognitive techniques, and relaxation strategies as applicable. Treatment concludes with a session reviewing the patient's improvements across treatment and psychoeducation regarding relapse prevention.

KEY POINTS OF ADAPTATION FOR CBT-I WITH CAREGIVERS

Cognitive behavioral therapy for insomnia is also well suited to address etiological factors unique to caregivers' sleep disturbance. However, given the known practical barriers caregivers face in accessing psychosocial treatment and in maintaining adequate opportunity for sleep, CBT-I is ideally tailored and sensitive to caregivers' unique needs. Such areas of adaptation are outlined along with standard CBT-I techniques in Table 12.1. Indeed,

Table 12.1 COGNITIVE BEHAVIORAL THERAPY FOR INSOMNIA: TREATMENT TECHNIQUES AND SUGGESTED ADAPTATIONS FOR CAREGIVERS

Standard Content	Adaptations for Caregivers
Assessment[8,63,64]	
Beginning of Treatment (e.g., Session 1)	
Sleep complaint	*Effect of cancer on role and routine*
• Difficulty falling asleep, staying asleep, or waking early	• Describe a typical day and night
• Poor quality/unrefreshing sleep	• Describe care responsibilities and tasks
• Onset, duration, course of difficulty	
Sleep schedule	
• Times to go to bed/wake-up	
• Factors promoting/inhibiting asleep	
• Number, duration of typical awakenings and associated behaviors	
Comorbid sleep disorders	
• Sleep apnea (e.g., STOPBANG measure [Snoring, Tired, Observed gasping, high blood Pressure, Body mass index, Age over 50, Neck size large, Gender is male])	
• Restless leg syndrome	
Daytime activity, functioning, and impairment	
• Napping frequency, timing, duration	
• Work, healthy lifestyle (e.g., alcohol, exercise), travel factors	
• Daytime impairment and distress	
Safety concerns	
• Assess whether the caregiver has ever fallen asleep at times when it would be dangerous	
• Set a plan to monitor and prevent adverse effects of daytime fatigue	
Sleep diary	
• Demonstrate how to complete and emphasize the importance of recording	
Psychoeducation[48]	
Beginning of treatment (e.g., Session 2)	
Review sleep diary (every session)	*Normalize caregivers' concerns and conflicts regarding self-care*
• Use sleep diary to calculate the average sleep onset latency (SOL), wake after sleep onset (WASO), total sleep time (TST), time in bed (TIB), sleep efficiency (SE = [TST/TIB]*100), and early morning awakening (EMA) over the past week	• Caregivers often experience conflict engaging in self-care activities and tend to prioritize patient needs before meeting their own[65,66]
	• Legitimize and commend caregivers' attention to their own health needs

(continued)

Table 12.1 CONTINUED

Standard Content	Adaptations for Caregivers
Model of insomnia	*Manage expectations for treatment outcome*
• Describe 4P model using the caregiver's own factors	• Treatment success can include improved perceived sleep quality without increased sleep quantity
Content of CBT-I	
• Provide overview of techniques employed in CBT-I, including sleep restriction and stimulus control, and how these treat insomnia by targeting perpetuating factors	• Even small increases in sleep may lead to meaningful improvements in caregivers' daily lives
• Set expectations about short-term increase in fatigue from sleep restriction	

Sleep Restriction[42,67]

Early to midtreatment (e.g., Sessions 2–4)

Reiterate psychoeducation regarding technique	*Flexibility*
• Matches the presenting caregivers' time spent in bed to their current sleep ability	• Develop sleep restriction plan to be feasibly enacted given caregivers' care responsibilities and schedules
• Primary mechanism of change to improve sleep via reducing perpetuating factors and conditioned arousal	• Consider sleep compression,[68] a more flexible and gradual variant of sleep restriction, if caregivers are not amenable to sleep restriction procedures
• May produce short-term daytime drowsiness to build sleep pressure	
Set sleep "prescription"	
• Obtain data from approximately 2 weeks of sleep diaries	
• Calculate TST and TIB	
• Collaboratively identify ideal wake time	
• Subtract sleep ability from ideal wake time to set bedtime	
- Optional: provide 15–30 minutes additional time to sleep window to accommodate average SOL/WASO	
• Never set sleep window to less than 4.5 hours, regardless of sleep ability[40]	
Titrate "prescription" according to 7-day average SE from sleep diaries	
• If SE ≤ 85%: Reduce sleep window by 15–30 minutes	
• If 85% < SE ≤ 90%: Maintain sleep window	
• If SE > 90%: Increase sleep window by 15–30 minutes	
• Continue in this manner until a sleep window is reached that facilitates the caregivers' personal sleep need, ideally 7–8 hours	

Table 12.1 CONTINUED

Standard Content	Adaptations for Caregivers

Stimulus Control
Early to midtreatment (e.g., Sessions 2–4)

Establish that the bed is for sleep and sex only • Eliminate other sleep-incompatible behaviors in bed (e.g., watching TV, worrying) • If the caregiver estimates they have been in bed awake for 20 minutes, instruct him/her to leave bed and engage in a relaxing activity outside the bedroom until drowsy or for a defined period of time (e.g., 30 minutes) before returning to bed	*Use creative, flexible solutions where caregivers are restricted in their ability to adhere (e.g., sleeping on their loved one's couch during caregiving)*

Sleep Hygiene
Mid- to late treatment (e.g., Session 4)

Keep a regular schedule for bedtime, wake time, meals, and daytime activity	
Avoid stimulating activities (e.g., caffeine, screen time, exercise) close to bedtime	
Maintain a healthy lifestyle (e.g., healthy diet and regular exercise)	
Maintain a comfortable sleep environment (e.g., cool temperature, dark, quiet)	

Cognitive Restructuring
Mid- to late treatment (e.g., Session 5)

Assess and address maladaptive beliefs about sleep • "Myth busting" regarding necessity of 7 hours of sleep per night, etc. • Decatastrophize thoughts about the consequences of a night of disrupted sleep	*Assess and address maladaptive beliefs about sleep disturbance on caregivers' ability to care for their loved one*

Relapse Prevention
End of treatment (e.g., Session 6)

Normalize minor sleep disturbances to reinforce adaptive thoughts about sleep *Reiterate improvements demonstrated in sleep diaries from use of CBT-I techniques* *Discuss lapse vs. relapse* • Lapse: a few days of poor quality or disrupted sleep; caregiver should consider what changes may have preceded disruptions (e.g., increased stress, lapse in sleep hygiene) and problem-solve accordingly	*As appropriate, normalize impending changes in distress and sleep patterns according to the cancer trajectory (e.g., through bereavement, transition off treatment) and use "coping ahead" to plan adaptive coping strategies for such changes*

(continued)

Table 12.1 CONTINUED

Standard Content	Adaptations for Caregivers
• Relapse: two or more weeks with a few days of poor quality or disrupted sleep, suggesting a possible return of insomnia; caregiver should reinstitute sleep diaries, institute sleep restriction procedures based on their sleep ability and opportunity, review therapy notes, and/or contact a clinical provider to assist in reapplying CBT-I techniques	

---

the Caregiver Sleep Intervention (CASI) study[22] has demonstrated efficacy of such a tailored CBT-I approach to improve caregivers' perceived
sleep quality and depressive symptoms even as they provided active care
to a loved one with cancer. The program was found to be well received by
caregivers overall, who reported appreciating its accommodation of their
"energy and time constraints" (p. 101) and flexible scheduling of time and
location.

As with all interventions for family caregivers, CBT-I should be delivered
flexibly and with an emphasis on problem-solving and autonomy support.
Assessment will reveal actual barriers that caregivers face in terms of scheduling weekly appointments and following rigid sleep schedules typical of
CBT-I. As with the CASI study[22] and many other caregiver interventions,[57]
hectic schedules must be honored with flexible scheduling times, locations,
and modes of treatment delivery. Although weekly in-person sessions
are typical, practitioners working with caregivers must be prepared to re-
schedule appointments, offer a variety of appointment times, and offer sessions by phone or other telehealth modalities (where allowable). In addition,
Internet-based CBT-I programs have demonstrated strong, sustained effects
on multiple sleep parameters[58,59] and comorbid psychiatric symptoms[20,21]
among both the general population[58,60] and people with cancer.[61]

Infusing problem-solving into sessions can help emphasize the spirit of
flexibility and collaboration by encouraging practitioners and caregivers to
think creatively about ways to fit sessions into their schedules and behavioral changes into their routines. Problem-solving is an effective treatment
component included in many caregiver interventions.[57,62] Problem-solving
is also critical to securing caregivers' willingness to engage in sleep restriction or compression. Based on careful assessment of any nighttime
care task or fears related to fatigue impairing caregiving responsibilities,

problem-solving to accommodate these tasks and ameliorate concerns related to short-term daytime sleepiness from sleep restriction is necessary to ensure caregivers' ability to fully participate in this important treatment component.

Caregivers are experts in their own family structures and needs, yet gentle questioning of rules governing their roles can illuminate opportunities for changes that may improve their QOL. Moreover, as caregivers will be asked to modify, reduce, or eliminate compensatory strategies such as napping, identifying other pleasant and refreshing activities to replace these behaviors will be useful. Implementing regular relaxation exercises may be particularly beneficial for caregivers, given their frequently high levels of stress.

CASE EXAMPLE

We demonstrate use of these techniques with the case example of Mary, a single 56-year-old woman who lived with her 82-year-old mother, for whom she was providing care following a diagnosis of metastatic colon cancer approximately 4 months prior. In Session 1, we focused on assessment in order to build rapport and to formulate an impression of the precipitating and perpetuating factors related to Mary's insomnia. Prior to her mother's diagnosis, Mary reported that she had "no problem" falling asleep and typically slept 8 hours per night. Since her mother's diagnosis, she reported taking approximately 45 minutes to fall asleep, during which time she would frequently worry about her mother's health and their finances. She also reported waking several times throughout the night to listen for, or attend to, her mother. When Mary awoke during the night, she described often looking at the clock, calculating how much sleep she might get and worrying about the effects of insufficient sleep on her functioning the next day. When Mary found it particularly difficult to fall back to sleep, she would watch TV in bed. Mary's sleep diaries showed that she maintained approximately a 7-hour sleep opportunity window, but she only slept about 5 hours per night.

Mary described a typical day as getting up at 6 AM and assisting her mother to the bathroom and dressing, before preparing their breakfast. When her sister, who lived locally, took her mother to appointments, she reported typically napping on the couch for a few hours. Mary worked from 12 pm to 4 pm, having reduced her hours to allow her more time with her mother. She spent evenings cleaning the home and preparing for the following day, often losing track of time and rushing to be in bed by 11 pm, only to lay awake with her mind spinning from the busyness of the day.

We spent the majority of Session 2 providing psychoeducation about the 4P model of insomnia. We described how Mary's own behavioral (e.g., napping, watching TV in bed); cognitive (e.g., worry about consequences of lack of sleep); and caregiving-related (e.g., waking to listen for and assist her mother) factors perpetuated her insomnia (Figure 12.1). This psychoeducation was used to support the rationale for sleep restriction. We collaboratively set a sleep window of 5.5 hours, using Mary's sleep diary data from the past 2 weeks to demonstrate the "mismatch" in her sleep ability (5 hours) versus sleep opportunity (7 hours).

In Session 3, we primarily addressed stimulus control, reviewing the rationale for limiting time and sleep-incompatible behaviors (e.g., worrying, watching TV) in bed. Mary described feeling apprehensive about limiting her worry time, expressing concern that she might forget an important task without this time mulling over the day ahead. In response, she agreed to set a 30-minute worry time in the evenings to be completed at her desk, as well as keep a notepad on her bedside table to write down any thoughts that came to her at night.

In Session 4, we used cognitive techniques and problem-solving to address Mary's difficulty in adhering to the sleep restriction "prescription." Mary struggled with worry that she would sleep through her mother calling for her in the night. Using the downward arrow cognitive technique, Mary described a belief that if she slept through the night, she would miss her mother calling for help to get to the bathroom, and her mother would fall and hurt herself on attempting to go independently. Examining the evidence supporting and contradicting this thought demonstrated that her mother had only needed assistance in the evening three times in the past month, and each time Mary had woken up to her mother's call. Following the steps for problem-solving, Mary agreed to discuss a backup plan with her mother. Together, they decided her mother would use the home phone to speed-dial Mary's cell phone in the event Mary did not respond to her verbal call. With these measures in place, Mary was more comfortable with and adherent to sleep restriction.

By Session 5, Mary's sleep diaries demonstrated a reduction in her SOL and fewer awakenings. When she did wake during the night, she replaced TV with relaxation techniques. However, it remained difficult for her to increase her window of sleep opportunity given the extent of her caregiving, home, and work responsibilities. We took inventory of her various role responsibilities and evaluated whether there were any tasks that could be done less frequently or delegated. One notable finding was that preparing meals took Mary approximately 2 hours per evening. In discussing advantages and disadvantages of possible solutions, Mary reported feeling guilty thinking about not preparing healthy meals nightly for her mother, who had cooked for her family through her childhood. On further discussion and use of cognitive restructuring techniques, Mary acknowledged that her mother would want her to take care of herself and that her sister had offered to cook two nights per week. Accepting her sister's help and cooking ahead over the weekend allowed Mary to move her bedtime earlier and even add in an evening walk.

In Session 6, we continued to discuss and troubleshoot adherence to sleep restriction and stimulus control procedures and reviewed general sleep hygiene education. Given Mary's good application and comprehension of sleep restriction and stimulus control, we collaboratively agreed to 1 week off treatment before the following appointment, allowing a trial for Mary to independently use the CBT-I skills. At the following session (i.e., Session 7 during Week 8 of treatment), Mary's sleep diaries showed an increase in her sleep time to an average of 6 hours per night and SE of 85%. Moreover, she reported less daytime fatigue and worry about sleep, as well as greater ability to concentrate and an overall feeling of well-being. We reviewed relapse prevention strategies, drawing on Mary's established knowledge of the 4P model of insomnia and CBT-I techniques of sleep restriction and stimulus control. Given her treatment gains and consistent use of CBT-I skills, we agreed to terminate treatment.

CONCLUSIONS AND FUTURE DIRECTIONS

Insomnia and associated sleep problems are prevalent among cancer caregivers, are associated with significant psychosocial and physiological consequences, and do not remit naturally. CBT-I tailored to be flexibly, yet rigorously, delivered in a manner that respects caregivers' unique scheduling needs, accommodates their care responsibilities, and addresses their caregiving-related maladaptive thoughts about sleep can help alleviate caregivers' sleep disturbance. As an established first-line treatment for insomnia, CBT-I provides the optimal basis for such a tailored intervention to address the unique experience of insomnia among cancer caregivers. Empirical study is necessary to establish the efficacy and effectiveness of CBT-I delivered in person to cancer caregivers, as is determination of optimal points in the caregiving trajectory (e.g., at diagnosis, transition to survivorship) when CBT-I will be most efficacious and acceptable. Additionally, further evaluation of the efficacy of CBT-I delivered via telehealth modalities is necessary to determine the appropriateness and impact of this treatment for caregivers who are unable to access care in person as a result of temporal and financial demands of traveling to and from treatment centers for care. The establishment and dissemination of empirically supported interventions for insomnia among cancer caregivers has the potential to improve their QOL, enhance care provided by caregivers, lead to improved bereavement outcomes, and attenuate the notable mental and physical health disparities present in this vulnerable population.

REFERENCES

1. Skalla KA, Smith E, Li Z, Gates C. Multidimensional needs of caregivers for patients with cancer. *Clin J Oncol Nurs.* 2013;17(5):500–506.
2. American Psychiatric Association. *Diagnostic and Statistical Manual of Mental Disorders.* 5th ed. Washington, DC: American Psychiatric Association; 2013.
3. Carney S, Koetters T, Cho M, et al. Differences in sleep disturbance parameters between oncology outpatients and their family caregivers. *J Clin Oncol.* 2011;29(8):1001–1006.
4. Lee K-C, Yiin J-J, Lu S-H, Chao Y-F. The burden of caregiving and sleep disturbance among family caregivers of advanced cancer patients. *Cancer Nurs.* 2015;38(4):E10–E18.
5. Morris BA, Thorndike FP, Ritterband LM, Glozier N, Dunn J, Chambers SK. Sleep disturbance in cancer patients and caregivers who contact telephone-based help services. *Support Care Cancer.* 2015;23(4):1113–1120.
6. Carter PA, Chang BL. Sleep and depression in cancer caregivers. *Cancer Nurs.* 2000;23(6):410–415.
7. Carter PA, Acton GJ. Personality and coping: predictors of depression and sleep problems among caregivers of individuals who have cancer. *J Gerontol Nurs.* 2006;32(2):45.
8. Schutte-Rodin S, Broch L, Buysse D, Dorsey C, Sateia M. Clinical guideline for the evaluation and management of chronic insomnia in adults. *J Clin Sleep Med.* 2008;4(5):487–504.
9. Lou Q, Liu S, Huo YR, Liu M, Liu S, Ji Y. Comprehensive analysis of patient and caregiver predictors for caregiver burden, anxiety and depression in Alzheimer's disease. *J Clin Nurs.* 2015;24(17–18):2668–2678.
10. Happe S, Berger K, Investigators FS. The association between caregiver burden and sleep disturbances in partners of patients with Parkinson's disease. *Age Ageing.* 2002;31(5):349–354.
11. Goren A, Gilloteau I, Lees M, daCosta DiBonaventura M. Quantifying the burden of informal caregiving for patients with cancer in Europe. *Support Care Cancer.* 2014;22(6):1637–1646.

12. Langford DJ, Lee K, Miaskowski C. Sleep disturbance interventions in oncology patients and family caregivers: a comprehensive review and meta-analysis. *Sleep Med Rev.* 2012;16(5):397–414.
13. Carlsson ME, Nilsson IM. Bereaved spouses' adjustment after the patients' death in palliative care. *Palliat Support Care.* 2007;5(04):397–404.
14. Carter PA. Bereaved caregivers' descriptions of sleep: impact on daily life and the bereavement process. Paper presented at: Oncology Nursing Society Congress. Oncology Nursing Forum. Jul 2005:32(4):741.
15. Lichstein KL, Taylor DJ, McCrae CS, Petrov ME. Insomnia: epidemiology and risk factors. In: Kryger M, Roth T, Dement W, eds. *Principles and Practice of Sleep Medicine.* 6th ed. Philadelphia, PA: Elsevier; 2017:761–768.
16. Troxel WM, Buysse DJ, Matthews KA, et al. Marital/cohabitation status and history in relation to sleep in midlife women. *Sleep.* 2010;33(7):973–981.
17. Carter PA. Family caregivers' sleep loss and depression over time. *Cancer Nurs.* 2003;26(4):253–259.
18. Bouwmans ME, Conradi HJ, Bos EH, Oldehinkel AJ, de Jonge P. Bidirectionality between sleep symptoms and core depressive symptoms and their long-term course in major depression. *Psychosom Med.* 2017;79(3):336–344.
19. Alvaro PK, Roberts RM, Harris JK. A systematic review assessing bidirectionality between sleep disturbances, anxiety, and depression. *Sleep.* 2013;36(7):1059–1068.
20. Christensen H, Batterham PJ, Gosling JA, et al. Effectiveness of an online insomnia program (SHUTi) for prevention of depressive episodes (the GoodNight Study): a randomised controlled trial. *Lancet Psychiatry.* 2016;3(4):333–341.
21. Thorndike FP, Ritterband LM, Gonder-Frederick LA, Lord HR, Ingersoll KS, Morin CM. A randomized controlled trial of an Internet intervention for adults with insomnia: effects on comorbid psychological and fatigue symptoms. *J Clin Psychol.* 2013;69(10):1078–1093.
22. Carter PA. A brief behavioral sleep intervention for family caregivers of persons with cancer. *Cancer Nurs.* 2006;29(2):95–103.
23. Schweitzer P, Randazzo A. Drugs that disturb sleep and wakefulness. In: Kryger M, Roth T, Dement W, eds. *Principles and Practice of Sleep Medicine.* 6th ed. Philadelphia, PA: Elsevier; 2017:480–498.
24. National Alliance for Caregiving. *Cancer Caregiving in the US: An Intense, Episodic, and Challenging Care Experience.* 2016. https://www.google.com/url?sa=t&rct=j&q=&esrc=s&source=web&cd=1&ved=2ahUKEwizj6KAzKbdAhWkVN8KHThYBCcQFjAAegQIARAC&url=https%3A%2F%2Fwww.caregiving.org%2Fwp-content%2F2Fuploads%2F2016%2F06%2FCancerCaregivingReport_FINAL_June-17-2016.pdf&usg=AOvVaw2R_VG2XyHASkLxne_TJDC-
25. Kim Y, Spillers RL. Quality of life of family caregivers at 2 years after a relative's cancer diagnosis. *Psychooncology.* 2010;19(4):431–440.
26. Chassin L, Macy JT, Seo D-C, Presson CC, Sherman SJ. The association between membership in the sandwich generation and health behaviors: a longitudinal study. *J Appl Dev Psychol.* 2010;31(1):38–46.
27. Acton GJ. Health-promoting self-care in family caregivers. *West J Nurs Res.* 2002;24(1):73–86.
28. Damjanovic AK, Yang Y, Glaser R, et al. Accelerated telomere erosion is associated with a declining immune function of caregivers of Alzheimer's disease patients. *J Immunol.* 2007;179(6):4249–4254.

29. Neckelmann D, Mykletun A, Dahl AA. Chronic insomnia as a risk factor for developing anxiety and depression. *Sleep.* 2007;30(7):873–880.

30. Phillips B, Mannino DM. Do insomnia complaints cause hypertension or cardiovascular disease? *J Clin Sleep Med.* 2007;3(5):489.

31. Buxton OM, Marcelli E. Short and long sleep are positively associated with obesity, diabetes, hypertension, and cardiovascular disease among adults in the United States. *Soc Sci Med.* 2010;71(5):1027–1036.

32. Wu Y, Zhai L, Zhang D. Sleep duration and obesity among adults: a meta-analysis of prospective studies. *Sleep Med.* 2014;15(12):1456–1462.

33. Cappuccio FP, D'Elia L, Strazzullo P, Miller MA. Sleep duration and all-cause mortality: a systematic review and meta-analysis of prospective studies. *Sleep.* 2010;33(5):585–592.

34. Kotronoulas G, Wengström Y, Kearney N. Alterations and interdependence in self-reported sleep-wake parameters of patient-caregiver dyads during adjuvant chemotherapy for breast cancer. Paper presented at: OncologyNursing Forum; May 2016; San Antonio, TX.

35. Revenson TA, Marín-Chollom AM, Rundle AG, Wisnivesky J, Neugut AI. Hey Mr. Sandman: dyadic effects of anxiety, depressive symptoms and sleep among married couples. *J Behav Med.* 2016;39(2):225–232.

36. Troxel WM, Robles TF, Hall M, Buysse DJ. Marital quality and the marital bed: examining the covariation between relationship quality and sleep. *Sleep Med Rev.* 2007;11(5):389–404.

37. Carney CE, Edinger JD, Meyer B, Lindman L, Istre T. Daily activities and sleep quality in college students. *Chronobiol Int.* 2006;23(3):623–637.

38. Perlis M, Shaw P, Cano G, Espie C. Models of insomnia. In: Kryger MH, Roth T, Dement WC, eds. *Principles and Practice of Sleep Medicine.* 5th ed. St. Louis, MO: Elsevier; 2011:850–865.

39. Perlis M, Ellis JG, Kloss J, Riemann D. Etiology of insomnia. In: Kryger MH, Roth T, Dement WC, eds. *Principles and Practice of Sleep Medicine.* 6th ed. Philadelphia, PA: Elsevier & Saunders; 2016:850–865.

40. Spielman AJ, Caruso LS, Glovinsky PB. A behavioral perspective on insomnia treatment. *Psychiatric Clinics of North America.* 1987;10(4):541–553.

41. Drake CL, Roth T. Predisposition in the evolution of insomnia: evidence, potential mechanisms, and future directions. *Sleep Med Clin.* 2006;1(3):333–349.

42. Harvey AG. A cognitive model of insomnia. *Behav Res Ther.* 2002;40(8):869–893.

43. Harvey AG, Tang NK, Browning L. Cognitive approaches to insomnia. *Clin Psychol Rev.* 2005;25(5):593–611.

44. Perlis M, Giles D, Mendelson W, Bootzin R, Wyatt J. Psychophysiological insomnia: the behavioural model and a neurocognitive perspective. *J Sleep Res.* 1997;6(3):179–188.

45. Riemann D, Spiegelhalder K, Feige B, et al. The hyperarousal model of insomnia: a review of the concept and its evidence. *Sleep Med Rev.* 2010;14(1):19–31.

46. Espie CA, Broomfield NM, MacMahon KM, Macphee LM, Taylor LM. The attention–intention–effort pathway in the development of psychophysiologic insomnia: a theoretical review. *Sleep Med Rev.* 2006;10(4):215–245.

47. Morin CM, Barlow DH. *Insomnia: Psychological Assessment and Management.* Vol. 104. New York, NY: Guilford Press; 1993.

48. Perlis ML, Jungquist C, Smith MT, Posner D. *Cognitive Behavioral Treatment Of Insomnia: A Session-by-Session Guide.* Vol. 1. New York, NY: Springer Science & Business Media; 2006.

49. Okajima I, Komada Y, Inoue Y. A meta-analysis on the treatment effectiveness of cognitive behavioral therapy for primary insomnia. *Sleep Biol Rhythms.* 2011;9(1):24–34.

50. Trauer JM, Qian MY, Doyle JS, Rajaratnam SM, Cunnington D. Cognitive behavioral therapy for chronic insomnia: a systematic review and meta-analysis. *Ann Intern Med.* 2015;163(3):191–204.

51. Garland SN, Johnson JA, Savard J, et al. Sleeping well with cancer: a systematic review of cognitive behavioral therapy for insomnia in cancer patients. *Neuropsychiatr Dis Treat.* 2014;10.

52. Johnson JA, Rash JA, Campbell TS, et al. A systematic review and meta-analysis of randomized controlled trials of cognitive behavior therapy for insomnia (CBT-I) in cancer survivors. *Sleep Med Rev.* 2016;27:20–28.

53. Jacobs GD, Pace-Schott EF, Stickgold R, Otto MW. Cognitive behavior therapy and pharmacotherapy for insomnia: a randomized controlled trial and direct comparison. *Arch Intern Med.* 2004;164(17):1888–1896.

54. Sivertsen B, Omvik S, Pallesen S, et al. Cognitive behavioral therapy versus zopiclone for treatment of chronic primary insomnia in older adults: a randomized controlled trial. *JAMA.* 2006;295(24):2851–2858.

55. Morin CM, Gaulier B, Barry T, Kowatch RA. Patients' acceptance of psychological and pharmacological therapies for insomnia. *Sleep.* 1992;15(4):302–305.

56. Vincent N, Lionberg C. Treatment preference and patient satisfaction in chronic insomnia. *Sleep.* 2001;24(4):411–417.

57. Applebaum AJ, Breitbart W. Care for the cancer caregiver: a systematic review. *Palliat Support Care.* 2013;11(03):231–252.

58. Ritterband LM, Thorndike FP, Gonder-Frederick LA, et al. Efficacy of an Internet-based behavioral intervention for adults with insomnia. *Arch Gen Psychiatry.* 2009;66(7):692–698.

59. Ritterband LM, Thorndike FP, Ingersoll KS, et al. Effect of a web-based cognitive behavior therapy for insomnia intervention with 1-year follow-up: a randomized clinical trial. *JAMA Psychiatry.* 2017;74(1):68–75.

60. Koffel E, Kuhn E, Petsoulis N, et al. A randomized controlled pilot study of CBT-I Coach: feasibility, acceptability, and potential impact of a mobile phone application for patients in cognitive behavioral therapy for insomnia. *Health Informatics J.* 2018;24(1):3–13.

61. Ritterband LM, Bailey ET, Thorndike FP, Lord HR, Farrell-Carnahan L, Baum LD. Initial evaluation of an Internet intervention to improve the sleep of cancer survivors with insomnia. *Psychooncology.* 2012;21(7):695–705.

62. O'Toole MS, Zachariae R, Renna ME, Mennin DS, Applebaum A. Cognitive behavioral therapies for informal caregivers of patients with cancer and cancer survivors: a systematic review and meta-analysis. *Psychooncology.* 2017;26(4):428–437.

63. Howell D, Oliver TK, Keller-Olaman S, et al. A Pan-Canadian practice guideline: prevention, screening, assessment, and treatment of sleep disturbances in adults with cancer. *Support Care Cancer.* 2013;21(10):2695–2706.

64. Morin CM, Benca R. Chronic insomnia. *Lancet.* 2012;379(9821):1129–1141.

65. Ramirez A, Addington-Hall J, Richards M. ABC of palliative care. The carers. *BMJ.* 1998;316(7126):208–211.

66. Shaw J, Harrison J, Young J, et al. Coping with newly diagnosed upper gastrointestinal cancer: a longitudinal qualitative study of family caregivers' role perception and supportive care needs. *Support Care Cancer.* 2013;21(3):749–756.

67. Miller CB, Espie CA, Epstein DR, et al. The evidence base of sleep restriction therapy for treating insomnia disorder. *Sleep Med Rev*. 2014;18(5):415–424.

68. Kyle SD, Aquino MRJ, Miller CB, et al. Towards standardisation and improved understanding of sleep restriction therapy for insomnia disorder: a systematic examination of CBT-I trial content. *Sleep Med Rev*. 2015;23:83–88.

CHAPTER 13

Emotion Regulation Therapy for Cancer Caregivers

Targeting Mechanisms of Distress

ALIZA A. PANJWANI, MIA S. O'TOOLE,
ALLISON J. APPLEBAUM, DAVID M. FRESCO,
AND DOUGLAS S. MENNIN

Conservative estimates indicate that 4 million people serve as informal caregivers for cancer patients annually. Caregivers, often family members or friends, experience elevated levels of psychological distress that are comparable to, or greater than, the stress experienced by cancer patients.[1,2] They report a range of emotions, such as sadness, fear, anxiety, anger, and hopelessness.[3,4] Without adequate support, cancer caregivers are at risk for debilitating levels of anxiety and depressive symptoms.[5] These symptoms partly arise from uncertainty experienced in the caregiving role, including uncertainty about care demands and patient prognosis and well-being.

It is natural for caregivers to focus on distressing illness-related events and continually think of ways to change or resolve the situation. While self-referential in nature and engaged with the aim of avoiding and diminishing the experience of negative emotions, this type of mental processing is known as *perseverative negative thinking* (PNT) and includes worry, rumination, and self-criticism. PNT compounds the burden of stress by keeping new counterfactual information from being processed and maintaining negative emotional states, including physiological, behavioral, and psychological stress responses.[6,7] The inability to disengage from PNT exacerbates anxiety and depressive symptoms,[8,9] predicts aberrant functioning in autonomic and endocrine indices,[10] and increases engagement in unhealthy behaviors.[11]

EMOTION REGULATION THERAPY

The chronic and multidimensional uncertainty (e.g., regarding a patient's prognosis) associated with caregiving, combined with the increased engagement of PNT often observed in caregivers,[12,13] can manifest as a clinical presentation closely resembling individuals with generalized anxiety disorder (GAD). Indeed, GAD is among the most common initial diagnoses given to cancer caregivers.[14] Although cognitive behavior therapies (CBTs) demonstrate robust efficacy for treating individuals with anxiety and depression,[15,16] meta-analytic findings demonstrate negligible effects of CBTs among cancer caregivers across physical and psychological symptoms (Hedge's g = 0.09).[7] In traditional cognitive treatment models, an important clinical objective is to teach individuals to observe and challenge inaccuracies in their maladaptive cognitions to reduce emotional struggles. However, as cancer caregivers' negative thoughts often have validity (e.g., "My loved one may die, and I will be alone"),[17] this treatment principle may be less appropriate.

Emotion regulation therapy (ERT) may therefore be particularly suited for treating caregivers, as it was developed to target PNT among individuals with comorbid anxiety and depression. Incorporating principles from CBT and experiential therapy with findings from affective science, ERT is an integrated, mechanism-focused intervention.[6,18] The emotion dysregulation model underlying ERT posits that PNT dysfunction in anxiety and depression can be best understood by: (1) motivational mechanisms, reflecting the functional and directional properties of an emotional response tendency; (2) regulatory mechanisms, reflecting the alteration of emotional response trajectories utilizing less (i.e., attentional) and more (i.e., metacognitive) cognitively elaborative systems; and (3) contextual learning consequences, reflecting the promotion of broad and flexible behavioral repertoires.[18] Distress in those with anxiety and depression is characterized by heightened emotional experiences coupled with negative PNT, which functions as a compensatory strategy to manage the experience of strongly felt emotional and somatic experiences. The overarching goal of ERT is to counteract distress and PNT in pursuit of gratifying, goal-directed actions by: (1) increasing awareness of motivational conflicts; (2) developing regulatory capacities; and (3) adaptively engaging life circumstances whether associated with threat/danger or pleasure/reward.

Emotion regulation therapy has established preliminary efficacy for anxiety and depression through an initial open trial (OT) (N = 20; M_{age} = 32.25, SD = 10.96)[19] and randomized controlled trial (RCT) (N = 63; M_{age} = 38.30, SD = 14.46) of adults diagnosed with GAD with and without co-occurring major depression (examining ERT-linked symptom changes in comparison to a minimal attentional control condition).[20] ERT was well tolerated in both trials, as evidenced by low attrition rates. Gains were maintained at 9 months in clinician-assessed and self-report measures of GAD severity, worry, rumination, trait anxiety, depression symptoms, and quality of life (QOL); within-subject effect sizes exceeded conventions for large effects (Hedge's g = 0.7 to 3.4).[19] RCT patients who received immediate ERT, as compared to a modified attention control condition, demonstrated significantly greater reductions in these indices (Hedge's g = 0.70 to 1.8).[20]

Similarly, a more recent OT using a slightly abbreviated format of ERT and comprising a diverse and disadvantaged sample of young adults (N = 32; M_{age} = 22.25, SD = 2.48) with a primary diagnosis of any anxiety or mood disorder, including GAD, and scoring above threshold on PNT measures, revealed strong ameliorative changes from pre- to post-treatment in worry, rumination, generalized anxiety, anhedonic depression, clinician-rated severity of GAD and major depressive disorder, social disability, and QOL. These gains were also maintained at the 9-month follow-up.[21]

The efficacy of ERT in treating distressed individuals with anxiety and depression led the authors to surmise that this targeted approach may have positive effects on caregivers' ability to successfully navigate painful and conflicting emotional states endemic to caregiving. Though the majority of caregivers do not endorse a formal diagnosis, persistent PNT may exacerbate psychological distress.[13,22] ERT provides clinicians with a framework to address caregiver-specific challenges. Accordingly, the ERT model and its mechanistic components are herein reviewed with examples from caregiver contexts.

MOTIVATIONAL MECHANISMS

Underlying our emotional experiences are two motivational systems: (1) the security system, which involves seeking safety and avoiding threatening stimuli; and (2) the reward system, which involves engaging reward and minimizing loss. In particular, the security system instigates avoidance of threats and safety-seeking behaviors, while the reward system mobilizes behavioral approach and minimization of loss.[23] A motivational "pull" reflects the discrepancy between an individual's current experience versus their desired level of safety or reward. Emotions are integrally tied to motivational systems, serving as cues for when something important needs our attention or requires actions consistent with values and subjective goals. Emotional cues associated with these motivational systems can individually or simultaneously "pull" individuals to act in the direction of security or reward. For instance, a caregiver's pull for safety may be strong: desperately wanting information but concurrently experiencing uncertainty when waiting to learn about chemotherapy side effects on a loved one's health. Likewise, the pull for reward may be strong when longing to spend time with family and friends but prevented from doing so by the patient's health demands. Normative functional responding consists of responding flexibly to situations that evoke conflicts between security and reward systems. Conversely, motivational dysfunction involves motivational imbalance by responding with either heightened focus toward safety and control, resulting in avoidance and escape,[24] or increased focus toward loss and lack of reward, resulting in withdrawal and numbing.

Caregivers often experience mood and sleep disturbances and reduced QOL[3] but report feeling conflicted about self-care.[25] They may desire a reprieve from caregiving but feel guilty about taking time for themselves. Self-care, which may be informed by the reward system and higher order values, often becomes difficult to enact as caregivers are oriented toward threats surrounding the patient[26] and withdraw from previously reinforcing activities, such as hobbies or social interactions. Caregivers may anticipate losing their loved one, while simultaneously wanting to cultivate positive experiences with him or her in the present.[27] Importantly, emotionally navigating such moments becomes difficult when caregivers are hypervigilant and focused on potential loss/threat.

REGULATORY MECHANISMS

Cancer caregivers experience powerful emotions like sadness, fear, and anxiety. When experiencing high emotional intensity, individuals may fail to enhance or diminish emotional experiences in a way that would be suitable for the situation at hand. Emotion regulation strategies refer to any means of changing the emotional tone or trajectory of a situation and vary regarding the degree of cognitive elaboration or linguistic processing needed to engage the strategy.[28] At a less elaborative level, caregivers may respond with maladaptive regulatory strategies such as *attentional rigidity*, which refers to fixating on or avoiding evocative emotional stimuli. For example, a caregiver experiencing intense anxiety may fail to notice a feeling, albeit less intense, of gratitude for social support received from family members.

Previous research corroborates the presence of more verbally elaborative, maladaptive, regulatory strategies among caregivers. These can include PNT, such as worry, rumination, guilt, self-criticism, and self-blame, as well as poor behavioral responding, including withdrawal and substance use.[4,29-31] Although these responses appear superficially different, functionally they are utilized for similar purposes: (1) to gain feelings of control in largely uncontrollable situations; (2) to dampen intensity of emotional experiences or arousal; (3) to escape emotional experiences or arousal; and (4) to find temporary relief. In the long term, these responses can be exhausting and resource depleting and, paradoxically, maintain the emotional states they were intended to diminish or avoid.

Adaptive regulatory responses involve processing emotion and motivational information earlier in the emotion generation process (i.e., closer to when they arise), ideally first through less elaborative and cognitively effortful strategies and, if necessary, utilizing more elaborative, cognitively effortful strategies. Less elaborative strategies reflect *attentional flexibility*, including *orienting* and *allowing*. Orienting denotes the ability to shift, maintain, or broaden focus from one stimulus to another depending on contextual demands.[32] Allowing refers to capacity to sustain attention on emotionally laden information and maintain it in working memory.[6]

Metacognitive regulation skills, such as decentering and reappraisal, are relatively more elaborative. *Decentering* helps individuals gain perspective in time (e.g., thinking of inner experiences as temporary) and space (e.g., thinking of inner experiences as physical objects distinct from oneself) from emotionally salient information.[33,34] *Cognitive reappraisal* helps individuals ascribe a different meaning to a situation to alter its emotional impact.[35] Although these strategies involve greater cognitive effort, they can be deployed when less elaborative strategies are insufficient in promoting adaptive responses. Optimal emotion regulation may begin with engaging less elaborative strategies and becoming increasingly elaborative as needed. Through practicing healthier regulatory strategies, processing the full spectrum of emotions and information contained within, caregivers gain emotional clarity and engage in adaptive responding. In ERT, these advances are fostered through skill-building and are considered crucial to improving the ability to take goal-directed actions under duress.[36]

CONTEXTUAL LEARNING

Utilizing maladaptive emotion regulation strategies can result in inflexible behavioral responses, which often prevent individuals from meeting the demands of stressors such as caregiving. Attentional rigidity obfuscates access to information that bears relevance to the situation.[37] Individuals may fixate on aspects of their emotional experience or ignore cues that prevent optimal behavioral responses.[38] Elaborative regulatory deficits, such as rumination and worry, also result in narrowed coping repertoires. Rumination diminishes the likelihood of new or reward-based learning,[36] steers attention away from goal-directed behavioral responses,[39] and increases emotional reactivity.[40] Worry encourages avoidance of emotional processing, sustains negative affect, and results in overconditioning to threat.[41,42]

In response to immediate emotional cues (e.g., fear about spouse's upcoming oncologist visit) signaling a security motivation, a caregiver may worry about their loved one dying and how to break the news to extended family. For example, a caregiver may ruminate over the decision to move away from their hometown and the loss of familial support during their loved one's illness.[41] These responses may result in sustained, rather than diminished, feelings of anxiety as well as avoidance of accompanying the patient to the appointment altogether. The caregiver may miss opportunities to support the patient and, instead, be mired in their own PNT. As cancer caregiving is frequently a long-term stressor, reactive responses habitualize through negative reinforcement. The overall effect of the use of maladaptive strategies can lead to reduced access and achievement of reward-based goals.[6]

Knowing and providing contextually adaptive behavioral responses are key to optimal functioning. Behavioral flexibility is dependent on the ability to increase awareness of environmental cues and contingencies, gain emotional clarity, and take goal-directed action.[43] Broadening attention to also notice positive emotions, for example, can extend our thoughts and actions, build novel ways of responding, and generate learning that habituates over time. In the first scenario, rather than exclusively focusing on security motivations and, consequently, avoiding accompanying the loved one to his or her appointment, the caregiver may also observe emotions such as affection or pride in being able to help their loved one, which may lead to different behavioral responses (e.g., going for ice cream after the appointment) that generate new learning despite fears of potential loss.

ADAPTING ERT FOR CANCER CAREGIVERS

Emotion regulation therapy required adaptation for cancer caregivers (ERT-C) to be delivered in a feasible, acceptable manner that was maximally attentive to the cancer caregiving context. The content and format of the original ERT manual was adapted by experts/practitioners of ERT and the treatment of caregivers. The sessions were consolidated to 8 from 16 (O'Toole, Mennin, Fresco, & Applebaum, unpublished manual, 2015), within the range of treatments in psychooncology[44] and the context of caregiving.[7] As many caregivers experience distress but do not meet criteria for psychological disorders, a shorter treatment package was deemed appropriate.

The eight 60-minute sessions were planned to be delivered weekly, within a 16-week period, to allow for flexibility and unanticipated events that occur in caregivers' lives. The manual, which included caregiver-specific examples, was reviewed by six caregivers, who then completed in-depth, semistructured interviews and provided feedback on intervention structure, appropriateness, and feasibility.[45] The manual was adjusted accordingly (O'Toole et al., unpublished manual, 2015).

Treatment Protocol
Motivational Awareness Training

To cultivate emotional and motivational clarity, ERT initially focuses on building motivational awareness, or efficient detection of cues that indicate onset of motivational pull(s). Starting with psychoeducation in Session 1 to develop an understanding of emotions and underlying motivations, caregivers are given a rationale about the benefits of becoming accurate observers of their emotions. They are presented with the "orchestra" metaphor, in which each instrument in an orchestra signifies an individual emotion, contributing to the overall composition or symphony, which represents the motivational pull(s). When motivational pulls are balanced, individual sounds of the instruments are discernible. However, during the experience of caring for a loved one with cancer, the security pull may be strong. Within the context of the orchestra, an overrepresentation of threat may be viewed as one or two instruments drowning out others. For instance, the therapist may ask if the caregiver can liken their anxiety to the incessant beat of the drum drowning out other instrumental sounds (i.e., emotions) present.

In Session 2, caregivers are coached to identify reactive responses to their emotions, including PNT (e.g., worry, rumination) and behavioral dysregulation (e.g., smoking, drinking) and become better self-monitors, with the goal of generating more conscious, deliberate actions as troubling situations arise. They are taught that less effort is needed when emotions are "handled" earlier in the unfolding of emotional response rather than later. To illustrate this temporal model of emotion dysregulation, the therapist presents the "snowball" metaphor. Caregivers are asked to imagine a pristine snowball—white, pure, and fluffy—much like our initial emotions (e.g., sadness, fear, love). The unfolding of our emotional response is akin to the snowball rolling down the hill, collecting debris along the way. Once it reaches the bottom of the hill, it no longer resembles a white, fluffy snowball, but instead a solid, icy mass covered with leaves, twigs, and dirt. The reactions to our initial emotions, reactions that distressed caregivers often have, are reflected in the transformation of the initially white fluffy snowball into a dirty, cloudy, hardened snowball (e.g., self-criticism, rumination, worry, avoidance).

Drawing from the snowball metaphor, caregivers are asked to practice self-monitoring between sessions with the Catch Yourself Reacting (CYR) exercise and accompanying form, which helps identify antecedents of strong or difficult emotions, the emotions themselves, and reactive responses. The therapist and caregiver then identify a CYR event that felt especially challenging, reviewing it in-session to offer opportunities for practicing emotion regulation skills. The goal of the CYR is to derive a *counteraction,* or alternative action, for the transpired event. The therapist can also conduct a Do-Over, a cognitive rehearsal task that allows for shaping and refining self-monitoring and cue-detection skills for difficult CYRs (O'Toole et al., unpublished, 2015).

Regulatory Skills Training

The first four sessions help caregivers cultivate increasingly elaborative and adaptive emotion regulation strategies, ranging from mindful attention to metacognitive skills. In Sessions 1 and 2, caregivers learn the attention regulation skills of *orienting* and *allowing,* respectively. Orienting denotes the ability to focus and broaden attention, while allowing refers to the ability to sustain attention even when the attention is focused on difficult emotional exteroceptive and interoceptive stimuli. Sessions 3 and 4 include the metacognitive regulation skills of *decentering* and *reappraisal,* respectively. Decentering encourages individuals to "deindividuate" from feelings, thoughts, and corresponding motivations as well as notice that emotions in a given moment are not synonymous with their essential self. Cognitive reappraisal references the ability to change one's evaluation of an event to alter its emotional significance. The skills are designed to help caregivers gain "clarity for action," that is, help determine the functional utility of emotions and corresponding motivational value in guiding behavior.

Derived from mindfulness-based stress reduction[46] and mindfulness-based cognitive therapy,[47] each mindfulness skill is first introduced and conducted in session. To promote outside practice, audio recordings of each skill are provided. Caregivers are taught Mindful Body Breathing, which focuses attention on bodily sensations and builds breathing awareness, to encourage orienting or anchoring in the present moment. To promote allowing, caregivers practice Mindfulness of Emotions, which involves maintaining contact with difficult feeling states, cognitions, and bodily sensations. The goal of allowing is to, over time, learn to sustain attention on "cloudy," diffuse emotional states until caregivers connect to the primary or initial emotions that reflect underlying security or reward motivations.

To facilitate decentering from objects of the mind (e.g., memories, images, feelings, thoughts), caregivers are invited to internalize a living, breathing tree in the Tree Meditation. Distance is created in time (i.e., "this too shall pass") and space (i.e., placing objects of the mind on branches of the tree) so that while the feelings, thoughts, and sensations are observable and their motivational information apparent, caregivers have created a healthy working distance from their internal milieu and, resultantly, gained clarity on their emotional experience. Reappraisal skills are practiced with the Meditation on Courageous and Compassionate Reframing by adopting self-compassionate and courageous reframes. Caregivers are asked to picture individuals (real or imagined) who remind them of their strengths and promote their capacity to cope through compassion, acceptance, and kindness. These skills are meant to be practiced "offline" via recordings outside of session, while also building corresponding on-the-spot practices in collaboration with the therapist. On-the-spot practices refer to briefer versions of each mindfulness skill and are meant for deployment when confronted with an emotionally distressing moment.

Case Example 13.1

Lara was a 40-year-old married woman with two young children, living in a small apartment. Before becoming a full-time caregiver for her father,

Will, who has stage IV colorectal cancer, Lara and her husband led a busy, active life between managing their household, building their careers, and raising 5- and 7-year olds. Lara's siblings lived across the country and Will was widowed, leaving the sole responsibility of caregiving to Lara and her young family. To afford Will privacy, rest, and quiet, Lara and her husband slept in their living room while Will slept in their bedroom. Lara always had a close father-daughter relationship with Will. Employed as an accountant, Lara took a temporary leave of absence to care for him and had just returned to work part-time a week before her first session of ERT-C.

Over the next two sessions with the aid of CYR exercises, Lara built her self-monitoring skills and learned about orienting (Mindful Body Breathing) and allowing (Mindfulness of Emotions). She started to identify her "top-of-the-hill" emotions regarding events that transpired during the week and began to distinguish between "pulls" for security and reward (and its absence in loss). For example, she observed significant fear and anxiety around Will's upcoming scan, noticing that her pull for security was high— the incessant beat of the "anxiety" drum hard to ignore. Lara anticipated his death and also shared "immense" feelings of sadness and grief when she saw him sleeping, "tuckered out" after just an hour of activity. In other words, her pull for reward was low, leaving her with little desire to engage in fulfilling activities. She also began recognizing when her "snowball rolled down the hill" in CYRs, noting reactive responses like worry and avoidance. Though practicing allowing was challenging, it helped Lara acknowledge that she was responding to her emotions with reactivity.

By Sessions 3 and 4, she had been introduced to decentering (Tree Meditation) and cognitive reappraisal (Meditation of Courage and Compassion) skills. Decentering was particularly helpful when emotions felt intense and larger than life. In a CYR exercise during Session 4, she discussed a difficult moment at work in which job-related duties combined with caregiving responsibilities felt daunting. She rated her pulls for security and reward at an 8 and 2, respectively. Lara felt anxious and nervous, knowing that there would not be much respite at home after her busy workday. Rather than giving herself permission to feel these understandable emotions, she was experientially avoidant. When asked what happened next, Lara said she had to excuse herself from her cubicle. The therapist gently queried about what she was experiencing internally at that moment. "I am not the one with the illness. I shouldn't be feeling sorry for myself," Lara exclaimed in session and proceeded to cry.

This moment created an opportunity for a Do-Over and a full on-the-spot skills response, including orienting, allowing, decentering, and cognitive reappraisal. The therapist asked Lara to close her eyes and imagine herself back in her work cubicle. Guided through on-the-spot orienting, Lara spent several minutes noticing her breath and the different bodily sensations she was experiencing. For on-the-spot allowing, the therapist asked Lara to identify and allow the different emotions she was feeling. Lara shared and sat with what she was experiencing, including her anxiety and tight sensations in her chest. She began to speak after a moment of silence. The therapist gently interrupted, reminding Lara to stay with the difficult feelings and say aloud, "I am giving myself permission to feel whatever I am feeling." Allowing gave Lara time to stay in contact with her emotions and validate them, rather than rushing to self-criticism or guilt.

The therapist transitioned to on-the-spot decentering. As they had practiced in previous sessions, the therapist invited Lara to become the dignified tree, her spine the solid tree trunk rooted in the earth, imagining the different emotions, reactive responses, and motivations as different branches of the tree. She placed each of the objects of her mind at a healthy distance, where she could see them and the information they carry, but not be overwhelmed by them. For on-the-spot reappraisal, the therapist asked Lara to picture the face of her closest friend, kind and encouraging, on one of the tree's branches and pull this image closer to the tree trunk. This friend would say matter of factly and with a knowing smile, "Lara, just think about all the things you do in a given day rather than what you don't do, and that in itself will be telling!" Lara began to smile a little. After a few moments, the therapist asked Lara about a counteraction she would have taken reflecting on that CYR "moment" now. Lara responded with, "Rather than rushing home, I would have taken a 10-minute walk around a nearby, beautiful park, feeling the last bit of the day's sun on my face before heading home."

Experiential Exposure to Promote New Learning

Sessions 5 through 7 consist of developing a *proactive* stance toward meaningful/rewarding activities and broadening one's behavioral repertoire to encourage new learning, despite perceived threat. The experiential exposure work involves three components: delineation of values, imaginal exposure, and conflicting voices task. Caregivers are asked to delineate their values, priorities, and principles. The therapist works with caregivers to identify values that remain meaningful, but with which they are not living consistently (e.g., relationships, work, self-care).[48] As self-care is challenging for most caregivers, the therapist may utilize the "oxygen mask" metaphor: When flying on an airplane, the safety instructions are to put on "your" oxygen mask first before helping others. The rule is in place because if the individual in question runs out of oxygen, the ability to help others is dramatically reduced. The same may be said of caregiving, particularly when caring for a loved one living with a chronic illness such as cancer.

The question then asked is: What step(s), even if small, can be taken in service of this value *today*? Through the *imaginal exposure* (or "Do It") task, caregivers envision taking the values-consistent action and, in doing so, are exposed to perceived fears, disappointments, and reactive responses that serve as internal obstacles. These internal struggles include motivational conflicts (e.g., security motivations blocking reward efforts) and reactive responding (e.g., self-criticism toward one's emotional responses) and are addressed through an experiential dialogue task, known as the *conflicting voices task* (CVT).[49]

In the CVT, caregivers engage two parts of themselves in dialogue: (1) the part strongly motivated to retain control, safety, and protection from perceived threat; and (2) the part strongly motivated to seek reward or gratification that comes from living consistently with cherished values. When security and reward are able to hear and acknowledge the needs of the other (e.g., a softening of the "security voice" in response to reward's needs and validation of security's concerns by the "reward voice"), a commitment to taking the proaction (valued action) is made. In addition to in vivo exposures, caregivers are encouraged to conduct exposure practices between sessions to consolidate gains and prepare for the final session.

In this way, exposure work can decrease negative emotional responding that is activated when motivational conflicts are perceived, engender new perspectives or meaning of perceived obstacles, and engage more adaptive emotion regulation skills that encourage values-based proactions. ERT-C targets life decisions in the caregiving context that are influenced by "top-down" (values-informed) and "bottom-up" (motivationally informed) systems.

Case Example 13.2

At this juncture of ERT, in Sessions 5 through 7, Lara was invited to reflect on the values that were important to her but with which she was not living consistently. The therapist and Lara discussed wanting to spend quality time with her family rather than rushing through to-do lists and appointments. A proaction incorporating an activity she enjoyed with quality "family time" was cooking a family dinner, something she found relaxing but had put on the "back burner" for some time now as it did not feel like an "efficient" use of time. For Lara, in many ways, this proaction was one in service of the values of self-care and enriching relationships with loved ones.

In the imaginal exposure task, Lara was asked to picture herself engaging in this action, step by step, while the therapist pulled for her emotions, sensations, and thoughts. Initially, Lara seemed excited about this prospect, noting that she would start with a grocery list, but by the time she got to "unloading groceries from boxes," she described anxiety and irritation. She said aloud, "What am I doing? I'd have to then get rid of these boxes and break them down for recycling. I hate doing that chore. . . . It will take up unnecessary time." At this point, with the voice of reward (i.e., the part of Lara wanting and seeing value in taking the action) and security (i.e., the part of Lara questioning the action by focusing on obstacles such as time pressure) present, the therapist transitioned into the CVT. Lara was invited to visualize the security voice holding her back from following through with her proaction. With the therapist's guidance, she described the security system as a "ram with red horns" hovering over her. The therapist asked Lara to articulate the security voice's (i.e., the ram's) concerns. The security voice, Lara noted, is saying, in an anxious and demanding manner, "Why are you creating more work, making it worse for yourself?" and "You know, it is not possible to do this in your tiny apartment anymore—too many people and too much mess."

Lara then visualized the reward system, the system that wanted her to "approach" and take this proaction as "Tinkerbell, from Peter Pan, a glowing orb floating in front of her." At first, the reward voice (Tinkerbell) sounded frustrated at the blocked proaction, telling the security voice (the ram) to "go listen to a cheesy music playlist and calm down." The therapist gently asked of what the security voice might be afraid. Lara eventually articulated that the security voice did not want her feeling overwhelmed by this proaction. The voice wanted to prevent more hard work for her, to protect her; Lara was having this realization for the first time. At this point, the tone of the reward voice shifted, becoming more helpful and offering ways to allay security's concerns. "We can take this one at a time. We will enlist [husband's] help. After all, he will want to contribute to making this dinner and appreciate it." The reward voice added, "This is about family, us connecting and laughing outside of the cancer."

In response, the security voice acknowledged that it can "ease off self-preservation mode." Lara can ask her husband to help make this dinner. Moreover, the worst-case scenario may not happen, and rather than feeling overwhelmed, there is a chance that Lara will feel warm, satisfied, and happy about engaging in the proaction. When the therapist checked in about where the security and reward voice were in relation to one another,

Lara replied, "I am envisioning the ram and Tinkerbell at the dinner table with the family, no longer so intensely at odds with each other." Lara proceeded to take the proaction in the weeks following this session.

Consolidation of Gains and Termination

The eighth and final session involves review, consolidation of gains, goal-setting, and termination. The therapist and caregiver reflect on progress, highlighting the caregiver's willingness to be her own "agent of change" as well as gains in motivational awareness and regulatory skills. The future is considered, wherein time is devoted to the idea of a continued commitment to living a values-informed life, taking even larger proactive steps. This discussion emphasizes how "ups and downs" are inevitable and expected. In reviewing the mindful regulation skills as tools for moments in which intense emotions (e.g., fear, anxiety, sadness) arise, the message that these skills comprise the caregiver's own ERT-C toolbox is underscored. The goal is to prevent an overreliance on the security system and resulting PNTs and behavioral dysregulation once therapy has ended and, instead, foster the caregiver's independence and self-efficacy. Gaining clarity over security and reward impetuses and promoting balance in these systems can help caregivers face long-term challenges while pursuing a values-informed life.

CURRENT AND FUTURE APPLICATIONS OF ERT-C

An OT comprising 24 caregivers to evaluate the acceptability and initial efficacy of ERT-C was recently completed. ERT-C was well tolerated by 22 treatment completers. Caregivers demonstrated reduced depression and anxiety symptoms, PNT, and emotion regulation deficits with moderate-to-large effect sizes (Hedge's g = 0.36 to 0.92), as indicated by self-report measures and feedback from exit interviews. Although caregiver burden was not reduced, caregivers expressed greater ability to confront caregiving-related challenges in exit interviews.[50] Given the documented difficulties in treating caregivers,[7] these results are promising. Currently, a RCT with a wait-list control group is in its final stage, and another one is planned. The latter will compare ERT-C to supportive psychotherapy and examine PNT as well as its psychoneuroimmunologic correlates. These trials provide encouraging preliminary efficacy of ERT-C while exploring potential moderators (e.g., caregiver characteristics) and mediators (e.g., emotion regulation skills). Although further research on caregiver contexts is needed, ERT-C provides a novel, promising approach for the treatment of psychological distress among cancer caregivers, demonstrating strong ameliorative effects where other traditional models have been largely unsuccessful.

REFERENCES

1. Chambers SK, Girgis A, Occhipinti S, et al. Psychological distress and unmet supportive care needs in cancer patients and carers who contact cancer helplines. *Eur J Cancer Care (Engl)*. 2012;21(2):213–223. doi:10.1111/j.1365-2354.2011.01288.x
2. Couper JW, Bloch S, Love A, Duchesne G, Macvean M, Kissane DW. The psychosocial impact of prostate cancer on patients and their partners. *Med J Aust*. 2006;185(8):428–432.
3. Northouse L, Williams A-L, Given B, McCorkle R. Psychosocial care for family caregivers of patients with cancer. *J Clin Oncol*. 2012;30(11):1227–1234. doi:10.1200/JCO.2011.39.5798
4. Stenberg U, Ruland CM, Miaskowski C. Review of the literature on the effects of caring for a patient with cancer. *Psychooncology*. 2010;19(10):1013–1025. doi:10.1002/pon.1670
5. Girgis A, Lambert S, Johnson C, Waller A, Currow D. Physical, psychosocial, relationship, and economic burden of caring for people with cancer: a review. *J Oncol Pract*. 2013;9(4):197–202. doi:10.1200/JOP.2012.000690
6. Fresco DM, Mennin DS, Heimberg RG, Ritter M. Emotion regulation therapy for generalized anxiety disorder. *Cogn Behav Pract*. 2013;20(3):282–300. doi:10.1016/j.cbpra.2013.02.001
7. O'Toole MS, Zachariae R, Renna ME, Mennin DS, Applebaum A. Cognitive behavioral therapies for informal caregivers of patients with cancer and cancer survivors: a systematic review and meta-analysis. *Psychooncology*. 2017;26(4):428–437. doi:10.1002/pon.4144
8. Verkuil B, Brosschot JF, Putman P, Thayer JF. Interacting effects of worry and anxiety on attentional disengagement from threat. *Behav Res Ther*. 2009;47(2):146–152. doi:10.1016/j.brat.2008.11.003
9. Koster EHW, De Lissnyder E, Derakshan N, De Raedt R. Understanding depressive rumination from a cognitive science perspective: the impaired disengagement hypothesis. *Clin Psychol Rev*. 2011;31(1):138–145. doi:10.1016/j.cpr.2010.08.005
10. Ottaviani C, Thayer JF, Verkuil B, et al. Physiological concomitants of perseverative cognition: a systematic review and meta-analysis. *Psychol Bull*. 2016;142(3):231–259. doi:10.1037/bul0000036
11. Clancy F, Prestwich A, Caperon L, O'Connor DB. Perseverative cognition and health behaviors: a systematic review and meta-analysis. *Front Hum Neurosci*. 2016;10(534). doi:10.3389/fnhum.2016.00534
12. Gaugler JE, Eppinger A, King J, Sandberg T, Regine WF. Coping and its effects on cancer caregiving. *Support Care Cancer*. 2013;21(2):385–395. doi:10.1007/s00520-012-1525-5
13. Steiner JL, Wagner CD, Bigatti SM, Storniolo AM. Depressive rumination mediates cognitive processes and depressive symptoms in breast cancer patients and their spouses. *Fam Syst Health*. 2014;32(4):378–388. doi:10.1037/fsh0000066

14. Longacre ML, Applebaum AJ, Buzaglo JS, et al. Reducing informal caregiver burden in cancer: evidence-based programs in practice. *Transl Behav Med.* 2018;8(2):145–155. doi:10.1093/tbm/ibx028

15. Hofmann SG, Wu JQ, Boettcher H. Effect of cognitive-behavioral therapy for anxiety disorders on quality of life: a meta-analysis. *J Consult Clin Psychol.* 2014;82(3):375–391. doi:10.1037/a0035491

16. Hans E, Hiller W. Effectiveness of and dropout from outpatient cognitive behavioral therapy for adult unipolar depression: a meta-analysis of nonrandomized effectiveness studies. *J Consult Clin Psychol.* 2013;81(1):75–88. doi:10.1037/a0031080

17. Levin TT, Applebaum AJ. Acute cancer cognitive therapy. *Cogn Behav Pract.* 2014;21(4):404–415. doi:10.1016/j.cbpra.2014.03.003

18. Renna ME, Quintero JM, Fresco DM, Mennin DS. Emotion regulation therapy: a mechanism-targeted treatment for disorders of distress. *Front Psychol.* 2017;8:98. doi:10.3389/fpsyg.2017.00098

19. Mennin DS, Fresco DM, Ritter M, Heimberg RG. An open trial of emotion regulation therapy for generalized anxiety disorder and cooccurring depression. *Depress Anxiety.* 2015;32(8):614–623. doi:10.1002/da.22377

20. Mennin DS, Fresco DM, O'Toole MS, Heimberg RG. A randomized controlled trial of emotion regulation therapy for generalized anxiety disorder with and without co-occurring depression. *J Consult Clin Psychol.* 2018;86(3):268–281. doi:10.1037/ccp0000289

21. Renna ME, Quintero JM, Soffer A, et al. A pilot study of emotion regulation therapy for generalized anxiety and depression: findings from a diverse sample of young adults. *Behav Ther.* 2018;49(3):403–418. doi:10.1016/j.beth.2017.09.001

22. Penner LA, Guevarra DA, Harper FW, et al. Self-distancing buffers high trait anxious pediatric cancer caregivers against short- and longer-term distress. *Clin Psychol Sci.* 2016;4(4):629–640. doi:10.1177/2167702615602864

23. Mennin DS, Fresco DM. Emotion regulation as an integrative framework for understanding and treating psychopathology. In: Sloan DM, Kring AM, eds. *Emotion Regulation and Psychopathology: A Transdiagnostic Approach to Etiology and Treatment.* New York, NY: Guilford Press; 2009:356–379.

24. Cassidy J, Lichtenstein-Phelps J, Sibrava NJ, Thomas CL, Borkovec TD. Generalized anxiety disorder: connections with self-reported attachment. *Behav Ther.* 2009;40(1):23–38. doi:10.1016/j.beth.2007.12.004

25. Kelly J, Diane K-W, Pamela SH, et al. The care of my child with cancer: parents' perceptions of caregiving demands. *J Pediatr Oncol Nurs.* 2002;19(6):218–228. doi:10.1177/104345420201900606

26. Borneman T, Chu DZ, Wagman L, et al. Concerns of family caregivers of patients with cancer facing palliative surgery for advanced malignancies. *Oncol Nurs Forum.* 2003;30(6):997–1005. doi:10.1188/03.onf.997-1005

27. Applebaum AJ, Kryza-Lacombe M, Buthorn J, DeRosa A, Corner G, Diamond EL. Existential distress among caregivers of patients with brain tumors: a review of the literature. *Neurooncol Pract.* 2016;3(4):232–244. doi:10.1093/nop/npv060

28. Baddeley A. Working memory: theories, models, and controversies. *Annu Rev Psychol.* 2012;63(1):1–29. doi:10.1146/annurev-psych-120710-100422

29. Carmack Taylor CL, Badr H, Lee JH, et al. Lung cancer patients and their spouses: psychological and relationship functioning within 1 month of treatment initiation. *Ann Behav Med.* 2008;36(2):129–140. doi:10.1007/s12160-008-9062-7

30. Dalton WT, 3rd, Nelson DV, Brobst JB, Lindsay JE, Friedman LC. Psychosocial variables associated with husbands' adjustment three months following wives' diagnosis of breast cancer. *J Cancer Educ.* 2007;22(4):245–249. doi:10.1080/08858190701638764

31. Fitzell A, Pakenham KI. Application of a stress and coping model to positive and negative adjustment outcomes in colorectal cancer caregiving. *Psychooncology.* 2010;19(11):1171–1178. doi:10.1002/pon.1666

32. Wadlinger HA, Isaacowitz DM. Fixing our focus: training attention to regulate emotion. *Pers Soc Psychol Rev.* 2011;15(1):75–102. doi:10.1177/1088868310365565

33. Bernstein A, Hadash Y, Lichtash Y, Tanay G, Shepherd K, Fresco DM. Decentering and related constructs: a critical review and metacognitive processes model. *Perspect Psychol Sci.* 2015;10(5):599–617. doi:10.1177/1745691615594577

34. Fresco DM, Moore MT, van Dulmen MH, et al. Initial psychometric properties of the experiences questionnaire: validation of a self-report measure of decentering. *Behav Ther.* 2007;38(3):234–246. doi:10.1016/j.beth.2006.08.003

35. Gross JJ, Thompson RA. Emotion regulation: conceptual foundations. In: Gross JJ, ed. *Handbook of emotion regulation.* New York, NY: Guilford Press; 2007:3–24.

36. Mennin DS, Fresco DM. What, me worry and ruminate about DSM-5 and RDoC? The importance of targeting negative self-referential processing. *Clin Psychol.* 2013;20(3):258–267. doi:10.1111/cpsp.12038

37. Schultz D, Izard CE, Ackerman BP, Youngstrom EA. Emotion knowledge in economically disadvantaged children: self-regulatory antecedents and relations to social difficulties and withdrawal. *Dev Psychopathol.* 2001;13(1):53–67.

38. Bogdan R, Pizzagalli DA. Acute stress reduces reward responsiveness: implications for depression. *Biol Psychiatry.* 2006;60(10):1147–1154. doi:10.1016/j.biopsych.2006.03.037

39. Joormann J, Nee DE, Berman MG, Jonides J, Gotlib IH. Interference resolution in major depression. *Cogn Affect Behav Neurosci.* 2010;10(1):21–33. doi:10.3758/CABN.10.1.21

40. Gilbert K, Gruber J. Emotion regulation of goals in bipolar disorder and major depression: a comparison of rumination and mindfulness. *Cognit Ther Res.* 2014;38(4):375–388. doi:10.1007/s10608-014-9602-3

41. Hendriksen E, Williams E, Sporn N, Greer J, DeGrange A, Koopman C. Worried together: a qualitative study of shared anxiety in patients with metastatic non-small cell lung cancer and their family caregivers. *Support Care Cancer.* 2015;23(4):1035–1041. doi:10.1007/s00520-014-2431-9

42. Newman MG, Llera SJ, Erickson TM, Przeworski A, Castonguay LG. Worry and generalized anxiety disorder: a review and theoretical synthesis of evidence on nature, etiology, mechanisms, and treatment. *Annu Rev Clin Psychol.* 2013;9:275–297. doi:10.1146/annurev-clinpsy-050212-185544

43. Bonanno GA, Burton CL. Regulatory flexibility: an individual differences perspective on coping and emotion regulation. *Perspect Psychol Sci.* 2013;8(6):591–612. doi:10.1177/1745691613504116

44. Applebaum AJ, Breitbart W. Care for the cancer caregiver: a systematic review. *Palliat Support Care.* 2013;11(3):231–252. doi:10.1017/s1478951512000594

45. Applebaum AJ, Buda KL, O'Toole MS, Hoyt MA, Mennin DS. Adaptation of emotion regulation therapy for cancer caregivers (ERT-C). Poster presentation at:14th Annual Conference of the American Psychosocial Oncology Society; February 2017; Orlando, FL.

46. Kabat-Zinn J. *Full Catastrophe Living: Using the Wisdom of Your Body and Mind to Face Stress, Pain, and Illness*. New York, NY: Delacorte Press; 1990.

47. Segal ZV, Williams JMG, Teasdale JD. *Mindfulness-Based Cognitive Therapy for Depression: A New Approach to Preventing Relapse*. New York, NY: Guilford Press; 2002.

48. Hayes SC, Pistorello J, Levin ME. Acceptance and commitment therapy as a unified model of behavior change. *Couns Psychol*. 2012;40(7):976–1002. doi:10.1177/0011000012460836

49. Greenberg LS. *Emotion-Focused Therapy: Coaching Clients to Work Through Their Feelings*. Washington, DC: American Psychological Association; 2002.

50. Applebaum AJ, Panjwani AA, Buda K, O'Toole MS, Hoyt MA, Garcia A, Fresco DM, Mennin DS. (2018). Emotion regulation therapy for cancer caregivers-an open trial of a mechanism-targeted approach to addressing caregiver distress. *Transl Behav Med.*, Epub ahead of print.

CHAPTER 14

Meaning-Centered Psychotherapy for Cancer Caregivers

ALLISON J. APPLEBAUM

Throughout this textbook, the challenges of providing care to patients with cancer have been highlighted. Caregiver burden is clear and receiving deserved attention from medical communities across the United States and world. The potential benefits of the caregiving role and the opportunity for growth afforded by taking care of a loved one with cancer has received less scientific consideration but is nonetheless an equally important area of focus for our field. This chapter focuses on this potential for growth and an intervention developed specifically to foster an enhanced sense of meaning and purpose in the context of caregiving.

EXISTENTIAL DISTRESS AMONG CANCER CAREGIVERS

A critical, potential driving, element of caregiver burden is existential distress, which has been described as including feelings of hopelessness, demoralization, loss of personal meaning and dignity, feelings of burden toward others, and the desire for death or the decreased will to continue living.[1-3] Cherny and colleagues[4] described existential distress in terms of whether individuals are focused on past (e.g., unfulfilled aspirations and regret), present (e.g., loss of important occupational, social, and familial role functions), and future (e.g., the death of/separation from a loved one) concerns. Included in their description of existential distress are issues related to identity, personal integrity, meaninglessness, hopelessness, death, futility, and religious/spiritual concerns.

Existential distress and suffering experienced by caregivers is common and may lead to increased feelings of guilt and powerlessness.[1] The competing demands of cancer caregiving, other caregiving responsibilities (i.e., childcare), paid employment, and personal life goals have the potential to lead to psychological, spiritual, and existential distress. Our systematic reviews of distress and burden among unique groups of caregivers (e.g., caregivers of patients with brain tumors and those undergoing hematopoietic stem cell transplantations[5,6]) have highlighted existential distress as a key contributor to burden, one that has historically received little attention.

FINDING MEANING IN CAREGIVING

Finding meaning in caregiving has the potential to buffer against caregiver burden. The addition of meaning-based coping[7] to Lazarus and Folkman's original model of stress and coping was based on the reports of caregivers of men with advanced HIV disease,[8] which highlighted their concurrent experience of meaning and suffering in the context of providing care to terminally ill loved ones. They found that caregivers were able to sustain positive morale and develop a sense of resilience during caregiving as a result of finding meaning in this role. Indeed, meaning-based coping has been referenced throughout the health psychology and psychosocial oncology literature as the positive reappraisal and reinterpretation of a stressor.[9] A growing number of studies have documented the experience of benefit finding or post-traumatic growth[10,11] as a result of stressful experiences, and finding meaning has been identified as one mechanism through which positive outcomes can be achieved.[12–22]

According to Frankl, finding meaning is a basic motivational force.[23,24] Meaning-making is rooted in the existential concept of one's ability to find meaning or "make sense" out of suffering. Meaning can be derived in circumstances that leave one feeling powerless, which is often the case with caregiving. Frankl[9,23,25–31] suggested that one may find meaning through the choices one makes (e.g., the attitude caregivers take toward this role), creative endeavors (e.g., how caregivers continue to create their lives while engaging in caregiving responsibilities), and experiences (e.g., gaining a new appreciation for their relationship with the patient). Farran and colleagues applied this framework to the experience of caregivers of patients with dementia[28] and emphasized that the choices caregivers make and the values and responsibilities they assume serve as sources of meaning.

Caregiving is therefore concurrently a potential source of suffering and an opportunity for meaning-making and growth.[29] The ability of caregivers to find meaning in their experience is associated with a host of positive outcomes, including decreased depressive symptoms,[30,31] lower perceived burden and improved self-rated health and adaptive coping,[31-34] increased satisfaction with life and self-knowledge and personal growth.[35] Finding meaning in caregiving has also translated into improved relationships with the patient and feelings of satisfaction, reward, and pride in caregiving.[36] One study examined the relationship between coexisting health problems and quality of life (QOL) among patients with advanced cancer and their caregivers and specifically investigated the mediating and moderating role of meaning-based coping on that relationship.[37] The results indicated that caregiver meaning-based coping mediated relationships between patient comorbidities and caregiver health conditions and patient and caregiver QOL. Meaning-based coping therefore has the potential to mitigate the negative impact of patient illness on caregiver well-being.[37] Finding meaning in caregiving may also have benefits into bereavement, as meaning-making is well documented as a key coping strategy among bereaved caregivers.[38] Indeed, studies have found that families who confront the challenges of cancer and eventual loss can gain a sense of strength;[39] therefore, interventions that target meaning-making before the patient's death have the potential to protect against poor bereavement outcomes.[39,40]

LIMITED INTERVENTIONS FOR EXISTENTIAL DISTRESS AMONG CANCER CAREGIVERS

In a mixed-methods study of the unmet needs and intervention preferences among cancer caregivers,[41] we identified existential distress (including guilt, issues with role changes, sense of identity, and responsibility to the self) as a critical area of concern. Qualitative analysis of 25 caregiver participant responses highlighted a common theme: *An increased sense of meaning would decrease burden.* However, very few caregivers reported naturally engaging in a process of meaning-making. This study included an assessment of both patients and caregivers, and almost unanimously, patients acknowledged the benefits to their caregivers of finding meaning in this role.

Although a number of psychosocial interventions have been developed to target caregiver burden, there is a dearth of interventions that attend to existential distress or meaning-making among caregivers.[42] In our 2013 review of interventions for caregivers,[43] only one specifically targeted existential concerns, although others acknowledged the importance of these issues, including finding meaning through the cancer caregiving experience.[44-48] Since the publication of that review, one additional intervention that attends to caregivers' existential concerns has been reported. Existential behavioral therapy (EBT)[49] was developed to provide support to caregivers of palliative care patients (not limited to cancer) through a manualized, six-session, group psychotherapy intervention that is described as a "third-wave" behavioral therapy[49] integrating traditional cognitive and behavioral therapeutic techniques with existential themes. EBT has been demonstrated to be efficacious in improving anxiety and QOL immediately after completion of the program, as well as depression and QOL one year after completion.[50] Notably, most participants were caregivers of patients with life expectancies of six months or less and included both current and bereaved caregivers of patients with a variety of illnesses. While EBT addresses one element of existential distress, current empirically supported interventions do not adequately attend to the variety of existential concerns among caregivers of patients with cancer. Importantly, the specific context of cancer caregiving varies significantly from the experience of caregivers for patients with other illnesses (e.g., dementias); therefore, interventions developed for this population must account for the unique experience of cancer caregiving.

MEANING-CENTERED PSYCHOTHERAPY

Our group developed Meaning-Centered Psychotherapy (MCP),[51-54] an existential therapeutic model that addresses the existential issues of suffering, guilt, and death. MCP has demonstrated efficacy in improving spiritual well-being and a sense of meaning and in decreasing symptoms of anxiety in patients with advanced cancer. Secondary analyses from a trial of Individual Meaning-Centered Psychotherapy (IMCP)[55,56] indicated that IMCP improved patients' sense of meaning and purpose in life, led to their finding comfort and strength in spiritual beliefs, and led to increases in life productivity. Both individual and group formats of MCP have been developed and tested. Meaning-Centered Group Psychotherapy (MCGP) includes eight 1.5-hour sessions, whereas IMCP involves seven 1-hour sessions. As an established, efficacious intervention, MCP provided a solid foundation for a meaning-making intervention tailored to the unique needs of individuals caring for a loved one with cancer.

MEANING-CENTERED PSYCHOTHERAPY
FOR CANCER CAREGIVERS

The goal of Meaning-Centered Psychotherapy for Cancer Caregivers (MCP-C) is to help caregivers connect—or reconnect—to various sources of meaning in their lives. The four sources of meaning addressed in MCP-C are historical, attitudinal, creative, and experiential. Table 14.1 outlines these sources of meaning and their relevance to the experience of providing care to a patient with cancer.

The *historical* source of meaning refers to meaning that may be derived from the recognition that life is lived in a historical context. This legacy is reflective of the past and is changing and open to new possibilities. In this context, past legacy refers to components of caregivers' upbringing that had a significant impact on who they are, including the cultural, religious, and spiritual values of their family of origin. Particularly important elements of past legacy for caregivers include previous experiences of

Table 14.1 SOURCES OF MEANING AND CAREGIVING

Source	Content
Historical	Legacy given (past), lived (present), and to give (future): Examples include previous experiences of providing or watching others provide care, previous experiences of illness or loss, and family values associated with an ethic of care; taking pride in caregiving; and setting examples for future generations.
Attitudinal	Choosing how one faces limitations associated with caregiving: Reflection on challenges faced before caregiving and previous modes of facing such challenges, such as achievements in the face of adversity and rising above or transcending difficult circumstances. Discussion of choosing new ways to respond to and taking pride in one's attitude. Examples include the choice one makes to provide care, how one faces the limitations that result from caregiving, and choosing to engage fully in the relationship with the patient despite the possibility of its ending.
Creative	Engaging in life and taking responsibility for one's life through creative acts: Examples include courageously engaging fully in the caregiving role and taking responsibility for oneself through improved self-care and discussion of existential and neurotic guilt.
Experiential	Connecting with life through love, beauty, and humor: Examples include feeling and expressing love for the patient via a tight hug or handhold, finding humor in dark moments, and deriving hope for the future from a sense of belonging to something greater than oneself.

providing care or watching others (i.e., parents and grandparents) provide care to friends and family members; past experiences of illness or loss; and religious, spiritual, or familial traditions that promoted commitment to the family. Present legacy refers to the legacy the caregiver is currently living and creating, including engaging in caregiving. Future legacy refers to the impact the caregiver has on others, including how others view him or her in the caregiver role and, importantly, the ways in which this role sets an example for future generations, family members, and friends.

The *attitudinal* source of meaning refers to meaning that may be derived from how one faces limitations and challenges, many of which are endemic to caregiving. Reflecting on how one responds to challenges can be incredibly meaningful, especially because the caregiver role is not generally perceived as a choice. Helping caregivers recognize *how* and *to what extent* they engage in this role may serve as a catalyst for improved self-efficacy. Additionally, highlighting how caregivers choose to face limitations due to caregiving, such as the inability to make advanced plans, interruptions to personal goals and employment, and often a limited amount of time remaining with the patient, can foster the development of new skills, clarified values, and resilience.

The *creative* source of meaning refers to meaning derived from creative acts, including how one creates and takes responsibility for one's life and how one engages in caregiving. Creating one's life requires courage and commitment, as does caring for a loved one who is chronically or terminally ill. An area of creativity that is particularly important for caregivers is responsibility to the self and how one may continue to create one's life fully and attend to one's own needs while providing care to a patient with cancer.

Finally, the *experiential* source of meaning refers to the meaning that may be derived through connecting to the world through our five senses. For example, through a tight handhold or hug, caregivers may feel connected through love for the patient; may be transported from present suffering merely through listening to their favorite music or sharing a laugh at a difficult moment with the patient; or may feel a sense of tranquility through experiencing the beauty of nature, which often serves as a reminder of the continuity of the world and the connectedness of humans and nature.

Meaning-Centered Psychotherapy for Cancer Caregivers may be delivered in group (eight sessions) and individual (seven sessions) formats. The outline for these sessions is presented in Table 14.2. The first two sessions are an introduction to the concept of meaning and meaning-making and a discussion of how being a caregiver has impacted one's identity. The next five (or four in the individual format) sessions are each focused on one of

Table 14.2 INDIVIDUAL MEANING-CENTERED PSYCHOTHERAPY
FOR CANCER CAREGIVERS WEEKLY TOPICS[a]

Session	Session Title	Content
1	Concepts and Sources of Meaning	Introductions; review of concepts and sources of meaning; "Meaningful Moments" experiential exercise; copies of *Man's Search for Meaning*[32] distributed for optional reading.
2	Cancer Caregiving, Identity, and Meaning	Discussion of sense of identity before and after becoming a cancer caregiver; "Who Am I?" experiential exercise; homework reflection on Session 3 experiential exercise.
3	Historical Sources of Meaning (Past, Present, and Future Legacy)	Discussion of life as a legacy that has been given (past), is currently lived (present), and will be given (future); homework reflection on Session 4 experiential exercise and additional suggested assignment to "Share Your Story."
4	Attitudinal Sources of Meaning: Encountering Life's Limitations	Discussion of confronting limitations associated with caregiving; "Encountering Life's Limitations" experiential exercise; introduction to Legacy Project; homework reflection on Session 5 experiential exercise.
5	Creative Sources of Meaning: Engaging Fully in Life	Discussion of creativity, courage, and responsibility; "Creative Sources of Meaning" experiential exercise; homework reflection on Session 6 experiential exercise.
6	Experiential Sources of Meaning: Connecting with Life	Discussion of experiential sources of meaning; "Love, Beauty, and Humor" experiential exercise; homework is planning/completion of Legacy Project for presentation in Session 7.
7	Transitions: Reflections and Hopes for the Future	Review of sources of meaning, reflections on lessons learned; "Hopes for the Future" experiential exercise; good-byes.

[a]When delivered in the group format, the materials for Session 3 are divided between two sessions (Past Legacy for Session 3, and Present and Future Legacy for Session 4).

the four sources of meaning and how caregivers may connect or reconnect with each one of these so that they become resources at various points in the caregiving trajectory. The final session is an opportunity for caregivers to reflect on goals for the future, which may include preparation for their loved one's death and the creation of a new life in the future. Each session includes didactic portions and experiential exercises, the latter of which form the backbone of MCP-C. Through exploring their responses to the experiential exercise questions, MCP-C therapists assist caregivers in understanding the relevance and importance of sustaining, reconnecting with, and creating meaning in their lives and caregiving through the sources of meaning previously described.

CASE EXAMPLE

Mr. X is the 64-year-old husband and primary caregiver of his wife, a 60-year-old retired high school teacher who was diagnosed with advanced endometrial cancer with metastases to the brain nine months before he engaged in MCP-C. He and his wife have two adult daughters who live outside of the New York metropolitan area, where the couple resides. Mr. X had previously worked full-time in real estate, but reduced his hours when his wife was diagnosed and recently took an unpaid leave from work to attend to her growing needs. By the first session of MCP-C, Mrs. X was experiencing several neurocognitive changes associated with brain metastases, including seizures, dizziness, and balance and visual disturbances, as well as occasional speech difficulties and incontinence. As such, she was no longer able to independently complete all activities of daily living, and neither Mr. X nor her physicians believed it was safe for her to spend much time on her own. Mr. X described his wife as someone who, for their 28 years of marriage, was self-sufficient and independent, took care of him, and was even-tempered. Recently, she had become verbally aggressive, irritable and forgetful, and had a significant and growing number of needs. Mr. X had no notable psychiatric history and had never before received professional psychological services. At the time that he enrolled in MCP-C, he was experiencing chronic worry about his wife and his future, which interfered with his sleep and ability to concentrate and was associated with somatic symptoms such as nausea and muscle tension. He also reported at times feeling hopeless about the future, fearful of living life without his wife, and abandoned by his daughters for not being present and helping to care for their mother.

Historical Sources of Meaning

Mr. X identified as a first-generation American, having been raised in a small family of Jewish immigrants from Russia. These key elements of his past legacy had a significant impact on his sense of identity and values. As a young man, he worked in his parents' dry cleaning store, a business they started when they arrived in the United States. He was taught at an early age to have an unquestionable devotion to family. The identification of this element of his past legacy helped Mr. X to clarify why, in part, having his daughters live far away and not involved with helping him to care for his wife was so upsetting. He also described watching his mother take care of his father through his progressive deterioration due to Alzheimer's disease and reported holding an old-fashioned belief in the responsibility of women to provide care, which also contributed to feelings of frustration with and resentment toward his daughters.

Through a discussion of current and future legacy, Mr. X became open to the possibility that the legacy he was currently creating and the one he would give to others in the future could be accomplished in a manner different from that of earlier generations. Specifically, Mr. X recognized that his past legacy had significantly impacted the value he placed on unquestionable support for family and his desire to have his daughters more involved but, concurrently, that he could set a new example for future generations of a more flexible approach to traditional gender roles of care.

Attitudinal Sources of Meaning

Mr. X felt strongly that he had no choice in becoming a caregiver. His daughters did not live locally, and both his and his wife's parents were deceased, although his wife's sister and brother-in-law lived nearby. Nonetheless, he reported finding it difficult to ask friends and extended family for help or to agree to receive help when it was offered to him. Instead, he tended to take on all of the responsibilities of caregiving, in part because he believed that as a "real man" he should be able to handle the challenges he faced on his own.

Through an exploration of the ways in which Mr. X responded to limitations and losses in the past, such as his parents' deaths and a layoff from a previous job, it became clear that he had a history of coping through isolating himself and hiding his emotions. He never allowed himself to cry, and when sad or scared, he would remember his father saying to him as a young child to "keep a stiff upper lip," which he did. He also reported being a problem-solver. For example, when he was laid off from a job due to budget cuts, he immediately put himself on the job market, networked, and used all of his professional and personal resources to learn about new opportunities.

The discussion of attitude allowed for the possibility of a more flexible view of caregiving to emerge. In many ways, Mr. X had chosen the extent to which he was engaging in this role and repeatedly refused offers of assistance from family members and friends. Although he was proud of his current ability to do everything for his wife, he recognized his role in making his current situation more challenging and the possibility that he could respond to caregiving differently. For example, he acknowledged that he could choose to allow more extended family to be involved in caring for his wife and that, through problem-solving, he could activate additional support networks, such as professional support through the help of social workers, in-home skilled nursing aides, and his sister-in-law and her family.

He also recognized the benefit he could derive from beginning to speak openly about his feelings. Keeping a stiff upper lip no longer served him or his wife well, particularly because as her disease would progress and her neurocognitive capacity become increasingly compromised, he would have increased responsibility for decision-making. Mr. X had kept his concerns of his wife's death to himself for fear of upsetting her and in so doing had isolated them both from one another. Through the discussion of attitude, Mr. X realized that although speaking about his fears openly with his wife would be painful, it would allow for increased connectedness between them, more shared responsibility in decision-making while it was possible, and it would facilitate improved communication with her physicians moving forward. Indeed, whereas his previous approach of concealing emotions had left him chronically worried and contributed to insomnia and gastrointestinal distress, the conversation about choosing one's attitude underscored new ways in which Mr. X could respond to his current limitations, which would have a more positive impact on his mental and physical health.

Creative Sources of Meaning

The session on creativity focused on several themes with which Mr. X had struggled long before his wife's diagnosis. First, he described feeling that he had not fulfilled his dreams or used his life to its fullest. As a young adult, he had aspirations to travel and cultivate his musical talents, but the need to work from a young age to contribute financially to his family prevented him from doing so. He and his wife married in their early 20s, and as soon as their first child arrived, the demands of working full-time and being an active husband and father led to his "shoving those dreams away." Through an exploration of creativity, Mr. X identified the importance of these dreams and his current capacity to create his life, despite his current challenges. Mr. X acknowledged that, despite the pain associated with his wife's eventual death, he would have a future that was open to new possibilities for growth and renewal, one that he could shape in a manner that would meet his own needs. He also realized that despite the limitations of caregiving, he did not need to wait until his wife's passing to re-engage in his life and could, for example, practice the guitar while spending time with his wife. *Mr. X began to embrace the possibility of concurrently feeling intense pain and sadness as well as hope.*

A second important theme that emerged was Mr. X's acknowledgment of the courage it had taken him to continue to engage fully in his marital relationship since his wife's diagnosis. He described his 28-year marriage as "solid" and "loving." He reported that his wife rarely verbalized her emotions, the couple said "I love you" to one another on only special occasions, and their manner of solving or resolving arguments in the past was to "let things go" with time. Despite this, there was always a feeling of love and connectedness between them, which became particularly important when their daughters moved away. Since his wife's diagnosis, Mr. X felt an urgency to discuss important issues, such as her wishes for end-of-life care. He also reported conflict regarding his desire to engage more than ever emotionally with her and fear of doing so when their time together was becoming more limited and the inevitability of her death a reality. This session highlighted the courage Mr. X possessed in acknowledging his desires to be more open and helped him recognize that this improved emotional engagement would likely prevent future feelings of guilt and regret after his wife's death.

Finally, the session on creativity highlighted Mr. X's difficulty in taking responsibility for his own needs. He struggled to identify what specifically his own needs were and asking others for help. This was particularly clear at the time of Session 5, after a year of Mr. X's intense caregiving, repeated rejection of others' help, and increasing burden. Discussion with the MCP-C therapist helped Mr. X recognize that he would be unable to continue to provide the level of care his wife required if he continued to neglect his basic needs for sleep and exercise and engaging in activities that could bring brief moments of pleasure. He was also reminded that, over time, as his wife's needs would increase, he would be required to involve others in her care. Additionally, Mr. X recognized that his tendency to take full responsibility for his wife's care was, in part, a means of coping with the uncertainty of her illness and their future, similar to how he had coped with challenges and limitations in the past.

Experiential Sources of Meaning

The session on experiential sources of meaning highlighted this source of meaning as one that Mr. X had engaged at various times throughout his life and one that had the potential to become an even more significant resource for him at the present time, when the demands of caregiving were great. Mr. X reported that in the past, he had found peace and contentment through playing the guitar and through participating in religious services. Since his childhood, he had experienced a sense of connectedness to something much greater than himself through prayer, along with a sense of awe, hope, and peace. Similarly, through music, he would often find the hours "flying by" and would get lost in the present moment. When asked about more recent experiences of connectedness through love, beauty, and humor, Mr. X shared that before her illness, he and his wife attended sporting events together, during which they would get "lost in the moment," cheering for their favorite teams and becoming energized by the crowds. This discussion led Mr. X to think more flexibly about how to continue to engage in these types of activities, despite his wife's limitations, such as through watching sports games together on television. Also highlighted was the sense of peace Mr. X felt at night when he slept holding his wife's hand, something he had done almost every night of their marriage. Despite his wife's limitations, in those moments Mr. X felt cared for, deeply loved, safe, and connected. He recognized that this connectedness was something that he could experience despite the difficult circumstances.

DISCUSSION

Meaning-Centered Psychotherapy for Cancer Caregivers is a novel therapeutic approach intended to address the existential concerns commonly experienced by caregivers of patients with cancer. Based on an empirically supported intervention that has demonstrated efficacy in improving the QOL of patients with advanced cancer, breast cancer survivors, and bereaved parents,[52,53,57,58] MCP-C is the first targeted psychotherapy to address the existential needs of caregivers of patients with cancer.

Although psychiatric diagnoses, such as anxiety and depression, are not discussed directly in the course of MCP-C, such symptoms are conceptualized in the context of caregivers becoming disconnected from various sources of meaning in their lives. Helping caregivers derive a new understanding of, or reconnection with, various sources of meaning has the potential to mitigate depressive and anxious symptomatology often associated with caregiver burden. Through MCP-C, caregivers come to understand the benefits of connecting with meaning in their lives and how these sources of meaning may serve as resources, buffer common symptoms of burden, and diminish despair, especially as loved ones transition to end-of-life care.

MCP-C FOR WEB-BASED DELIVERY

In addition to MCP-C delivered individually and in groups in person, we recently adapted MCP-C for delivery over the Internet to attend to the documented barriers to engaging caregivers in in-person support.[59] The resultant intervention, the Care for the Cancer Caregiver Workshop (CCC Workshop), consists of a series of five self-administered webcasts, each of which includes didactic components, video clips of therapeutic interactions of MCP-C therapists and (trained actors portraying) caregivers demonstrating the MCP-C principles, and a message board where participants may post responses to the experiential exercise questions that form the backbone of MCP-C. The feasibility, acceptability, and preliminary effects of the CCC Workshop were evaluated among 80 caregivers recruited across the United States.[60] Participants completed assessments of meaning and purpose, caregiver burden, depression and anxiety, social support, benefit finding, and spiritual well-being before (T1) and after completion (T2) of the workshop and at 3-months following workshop completion (T3). Moderate effect sizes emerged for meaning in caregiving (0.21 and 0.61 for the CCC arm at T2 and T3, respectively, vs. only 0.04 and 0.09 for the wait-list arm) and depressive symptomatology (at T2, the standardized effect size for the change in the CCC arm was -0.38, compared to -0.17 for the wait-list arm). In mixed-effects modeling, significant improvement in benefit finding emerged (β for interaction = 5.01, p = .03), all in favor of the CCC Workshop. Such effect sizes in this small sample are promising, and as this is the first trial of any Meaning-Centered Psychotherapy self-administered over the Internet, the emergence of these trends underscores the potency of MCP principles and techniques and the potential impact of MCP-C to improve the QOL of caregivers across a variety of delivery modalities.

CONCLUSIONS AND FUTURE DIRECTIONS

Our hope is that through the development and dissemination of MCP-C, an intervention developed specifically to address the existential distress experienced by cancer caregivers, the unique needs of this underserved and highly vulnerable group can be better met by the psychooncology and palliative care communities. Trials are currently under way to examine the impact of MCP-C on distress among unique groups of caregivers, such as caregivers of patients with brain tumors, who often experience significant personality and neurocognitive changes and a rapid disease course. Future studies will also examine whether shorter versions of MCP-C may be more feasible and acceptable to caregivers of patients at the end-of-life.

REFERENCES

1. Chochinov, H.M., L.J. Krisjanson, T.F. Hack, T. Hassard, S. Mcclement, and M. Harlos. Dignity in the terminally ill: revisited. *Journal of Palliative Medicine*, 2006. 9(3): pp. 666–672.
2. Henery, N. Constructions of spirituality in contemporary nursing theory. *Journal of Advanced Nursing*, 2003. 42(6): pp. 550–557.
3. Henoch, I., and E. Danielson. Existential concerns among patients with cancer and interventions to meet them: an integrative literature review. *Psycho-Oncology*, 2009. 18(3): pp. 225–236.
4. Cherny, N.I., N. Coyle, and K.M. Foley. Suffering in the advanced cancer patient: a definition and taxonomy. *Journal of Palliative Care*, 1994. 10(2): pp. 57–70.
5. Applebaum, A.J., M. Kryza-Lacomb, J. Buthorn, A. DeRosa, G. Corner, and E. Diamond. Existential distress among caregivers of patients with brain tumors: a review of the literature. *Neuro-Oncology Practice*, 2016. 3(4): pp. 232–244.
6. Applebaum, A., M. Bevans, T. Son, et al. A scoping review of caregiver burden during allogeneic HSCT: lessons learned and future directions. *Bone Marrow Transplantation*, 2016. 51(11): pp. 1416–1422.
7. Folkman, S., M.A. Chesney, and A. Christopher-Richards. Stress and coping in caregiving partners of men with AIDS. *Psychiatric Clinics of North America*, 1994. 17(1): pp. 35–53.
8. Lazarus, R., and Folkman S. *Stress, Appraisal and Coping*. New York, NY: Springer-Verlag; 1984.
9. Wenzel, L., K. Glanz, and C. Lerman. Stress, coping, and health behavior. *Health Behavior and Health Education*, 2002. 3: pp. 210–239.
10. Hudson, P.L., K. Hayman-White, S. Aranda, and L.J. Kristjanson. Predicting family caregiver psychosocial functioning in palliative care. *Journal of Palliative Care*, 2006. 22(3): pp. 133.
11. Pinquart, M., and S. Sörensen. Differences between caregivers and noncaregivers in psychological health and physical health: a meta-analysis. *Psychology and Aging*, 2003. 18(2): p. 250.
12. Manne, S., J. Ostroff, G. Winkel, L. Goldstein, K. Fox, and G. Grana. Posttraumatic growth after breast cancer: patient, partner, and couple perspectives. *Psychosomatic Medicine*, 2004. 66(3): pp. 442–454.
13. Ayres, L. Narratives of family caregiving: the process of making meaning. *Research in Nursing & Health*, 2000. 23(6): pp. 424–434.

14. Bauer-Wu, S., and C.J. Farran. Meaning in life and psycho-spiritual functioning: a comparison of breast cancer survivors and healthy women. *Journal of Holistic Nursing*, 2005. 23(2): pp. 172–190.

15. Tedeschi, R.G., and L.G. Calhoun, Expert companions: posttraumatic growth in clinical practice. In: R.G. Tedeschi and L.G. Calhoun, eds. *Handbook of Posttraumatic Growth: Research and Practice*. Mahwah, NJ: Erlbaum; 2006: pp. 291–310.

16. Farran, C.J., E. Keane-Hagerty, S. Salloway, S. Kupferer, and C.S. Wilken. Finding meaning: an alternative paradigm for Alzheimer's disease family caregivers. *The Gerontologist*, 1991. 31(4): pp. 483–489.

17. Pargament, K.I., and G.G. Ano. Spiritual resources and struggles in coping with medical illness. *Southern Medical Journal*, 2006. 99(10): pp. 1161–1163.

18. Park, C.L., and S. Folkman. Stability and change in psychosocial resources during caregiving and bereavement in partners of men with AIDS. *Journal of Personality*, 1997. 65(2): pp. 421–447.

19. Pearlin, L.I., J.T. Mullan, S.J. Semple, and M.M. Skaff. Caregiving and the stress process: an overview of concepts and their measures. *The Gerontologist*, 1990. 30(5): pp. 583–594.

20. Rhoades, D.R., and K.F. McFarland. Caregiver meaning: a study of caregivers of individuals with mental illness. *Health & Social Work*, 1999. 24(4): pp. 291–298.

21. Zhang, J., and D.T. Lee. Meaning in stroke family caregiving: a literature review. *Geriatric Nursing*, 2016. 38(1): pp. 48–56.

22. Thornton, A.A., and M.A. Perez. Posttraumatic growth in prostate cancer survivors and their partners. *Psycho-Oncology*, 2006. 15(4): pp. 285–296.

23. Frankl, V.E. Existential analysis and dimensional ontology. In V.E. Frankl, Psychotherapy and Existentialism. New York, NY: Simon & Schuster: 1967: pp. 133–142.

24. Frankl, V.E. Critique of pure encounter: how humanistic is "humanistic psychology"? In *The Unheard Cry for Meaning: Psychotherapy and Humanism*. New York, NY: Simon & Schuster: 1978: pp. 64–78.

25. Frankl, V.E. Man's search for meaning: an introduction to logotherapy. *American Journal of Orthopsychiatry*, 1963. 33(2): p. 390.

26. Frankl, V. Meaninglessness: a challenge to psychotherapy. *American Journal of Psychoanalysis*, 1972. 32(1): pp. 85–89.

27. Frankl, V.E. *The Unheard Cry for Meaning: Psychotherapy and Humanism*. New York, NY: Simon and Schuster; 2011.

28. Farran, C.J., B.H. Miller, J.E. Kaufman, E. Donner, and L. Fogg. Finding meaning through caregiving: development of an instrument for family caregivers of persons with Alzheimer's disease. *Journal of Clinical Psychology*, 1999. 55(9): pp. 1107–1125.

29. Salmon, J.R., J. Kwak, K.D. Acquaviva, K. Brandt, and K.A. Egan. Transformative aspects of caregiving at life's end. *Journal of Pain and Symptom Management*, 2005. 29(2): pp. 121–129.

30. Haley, W.E., L.A. LaMonde, B. Han, A.M. Burton, and R. Schonwetter. Predictors of depression and life satisfaction among spousal caregivers in hospice: application of a stress process model. *Journal of Palliative Medicine*, 2003. 6(2): pp. 215–224.

31. Cohen, C.A., A. Colantonio, and L. Vernich, Positive aspects of caregiving: rounding out the caregiver experience. *International Journal of Geriatric Psychiatry*, 2002. 17(2): pp. 184–188.

32. Frankl, V. *Man's Search for Meaning*. New York, NY: Washington Square Press; 1963.

33. Kim, Y., F. Baker, and R.L. Spillers. Cancer caregivers' quality of life: effects of gender, relationship, and appraisal. *Journal of Pain and Symptom Management*, 2007. 34(3): pp. 294–304.

34. Kramer, B.J. Gain in the caregiving experience: where are we? What next? *The Gerontologist*, 1997. 37(2): pp. 218–232.

35. Thombre, A., A.C. Sherman, and S. Simonton. Religious coping and posttraumatic growth among family caregivers of cancer patients in India. *Journal of Psychosocial Oncology*, 2010. 28(2): pp. 173–188.

36. Hudson, P. Positive aspects and challenges associated with caring for a dying relative at home. *International Journal of Palliative Nursing*, 2004. 10(2): pp. 58–65.

37. Ellis, K.R., M.R. Janevic, T. Kershaw, C.H. Caldwell, N.K. Janz, and L. Northouse. Meaning-based coping, chronic conditions and quality of life in advanced cancer & caregiving. *Psycho-Oncology*, 2017. 26(9): pp. 1316–1323.

38. Asai, M., M. Fujimori, N. Akizuki, M. Inagaki, Y. Matsui, and Y. Uchitomi. Psychological states and coping strategies after bereavement among the spouses of cancer patients: a qualitative study. *Psycho-Oncology*, 2010. 19(1): pp. 38–45.

39. Kim, Y., C.S. Carver, R. Schulz, A. Lucette, and R.S. Cannady. Finding benefit in bereavement among family cancer caregivers. *Journal of Palliative Medicine*, 2013. 16(9): pp. 1040–1047.

40. Brandstätter, M., M. Kögler, U. Baumann, et al. Experience of meaning in life in bereaved informal caregivers of palliative care patients. *Supportive Care in Cancer*, 2014. 22(5): pp. 1391–1399.

41. Applebaum, A.J., C.J. Farran, A.M. Marziliano, A.R. Pasternak, and W. Breitbart. Preliminary study of themes of meaning and psychosocial service use among informal cancer caregivers. *Palliative & Supportive Care*, 2014. 12(2): pp. 139–148.

42. Applebaum, A.J., and W. Breitbart. Care for the cancer caregiver: a systematic review. *Palliative & Supportive Care*, 2013. 11(3): pp. 231–252.

43. Duggleby, W., K. Wright, A. Williams, L. Degner, A. Cammer, and L. Holtslander. Developing a living with hope program for caregivers of family members with advanced cancer. *Journal of Palliative Care*, 2007. 23(1): pp. 24–31.

44. Toseland, R.W., P. McCallion, T. Gerber, C. Dawson, S. Gieryic, V. and Guilamo-Ramos. Use of health and human services by community-residing people with dementia. *Social Work*, 1999. 44(6): pp. 535–548.

45. Kozachik, S.L., C.W. Given, B.A. Given, et al. Improving depressive symptoms among caregivers of patients with cancer: results of a randomized clinical trial. *Oncology Nursing Forum*, 2001. 28(7): pp. 1149–1157.

46. McLean, L.M., J.M. Jones, A.C. Rydall, et al. A couples intervention for patients facing advanced cancer and their spouse caregivers: outcomes of a pilot study. *Psycho-Oncology*, 2008. 17(11): pp. 1152–1156.

47. Northouse, L., T. Kershaw, D. Mood, and A. Schafenacker. Effects of a family intervention on the quality of life of women with recurrent breast cancer and their family caregivers. *Psycho-Oncology*, 2005. 14(6): pp. 478–491.

48. Scott, J.L., W.K. Halford, and B.G. Ward. United we stand? The effects of a couple-coping intervention on adjustment to early stage breast or gynecological cancer. *Journal of Consulting and Clinical Psychology*, 2004. 72(6): pp. 1122.

49. Hayes, S.C. Acceptance and commitment therapy, relational frame theory, and the third wave of behavioral and cognitive therapies. *Behavior Therapy*, 2004. 35(4): pp. 639–665.

50. Fegg, M.J., M. Brandstätter, M. Kögler, et al. Existential behavioural therapy for informal caregivers of palliative patients: a randomised controlled trial. *Psycho-Oncology*, 2013. 22(9): pp. 2079–2086.

51. Breitbart, W., B. Rosenfeld, C. Gibson, et al. Meaning-centered group psychotherapy for patients with advanced cancer: a pilot randomized controlled trial. *Psycho-Oncology*, 2010. 19(1): pp. 21–28.

52. Breitbart, W., S. Poppito, B. Rosenfeld, et al. Pilot randomized controlled trial of individual meaning-centered psychotherapy for patients with advanced cancer. *Journal of Clinical Oncology*, 2012. 30(12): pp. 1304–1309.

53. Lichtenthal, W.G., and W. Breitbart. The central role of meaning in adjustment to the loss of a child to cancer: implications for the development of meaning-centered grief therapy. *Current Opinion in Supportive and Palliative Care*, 2015. 9(1): pp. 46.

54. Breitbart, W., H. Pessin, B. Rosenfeld, et al. Individual meaning-centered psychotherapy for the treatment of psychological and existential distress: a randomized controlled trial in patients with advanced cancer. *Cancer*, 2018. 124(15): pp. 3231–3239.

55. Lichtenthal, W., S. Poppito, and M. Olden. Facets of meaning: differential effects of meaning-centered psychotherapy among advanced cancer patients. Poster presented at: the Association for Death Education and Counseling 30th Annual Conference; Montreal, QC, Canada; 2008.

56. Lichtenthal, W., S. Poppito, and M. Olden. Effects of meaning-centered psychotherapy on facets of meaning among advanced cancer patients: a closer look at the FACIT-Sp. Poster presented at: the 30th Annual Meeting of the Society of Behavioral Medicine; Montreal, QC, Canada; 2009.

57. Lichtenthal, W., C. Sweeney, and K. Roberts. Meaning-centered grief therapy: theory, practice, and promise. Oral presentation accepted for: the Association for Death Education and Counseling 37th Annual Conference; San Antonio; 2015.

58. Lichtenthal, W., M. Tuman, G. Corner, et al. Development of a meaning-centered group for breast cancer survivors: focus group findings and preliminary effects. *Psycho-Oncology*, 2014. 23: pp. 130–131.

59. Applebaum, A. Adaptation of meaning-centered psychotherapy for cancer caregivers (MCP-C) for web-based delivery. *Psycho-Oncology*, 2016. 25: pp. 102.

60. Applebaum, A., K.L. Buda, E. Schofield, et al. Exploring the cancer caregiver's journey through web-based meaning-centered psychotherapy. *Psycho-Oncology*, 2018. 27(3): pp. 847–856.

Delivery of Support to Caregivers in the Community

CHAPTER 15

The Cancer Support Community

A Person-Centered Model of Evidence-Based

Cancer Caregiver Support

JOANNE S. BUZAGLO, ALEXANDRA K. ZALETA,
MARGARET L. LONGACRE, AND MITCH GOLANT

INTRODUCTION

Cancer caregiving is increasingly understood as an intensive, burdensome, and emotionally draining experience.[1-4] Many cancer caregivers are spouses, adult children, or other family members or friends. Indeed, at least one estimate suggests that, in 2015, approximately 2.8 million individuals, or 7% of all caregivers in the United States, provided care due to a primary diagnosis of cancer, and this is likely an underestimate as many provide cancer care secondary to another condition.[3]

Cancer caregivers engage in diverse and demanding roles as they assist patients with physical, emotional, and financial strains of a diagnosis and treatment(s). They commonly perform medical or nursing-related tasks, for which they may be inadequately prepared or trained, and are often part of a patient's healthcare team as they advocate and communicate with, or on behalf of, the patient.[1,3] Depending on the patient's medical condition, caregiving activities span a range of day-to-day and long-term tasks, including travel to doctors' appointments; help deciding among treatment options; management of finances; assistance with eating and tasks of daily living, including personal hygiene; administration of medication, and pro-vision of emotional support to the person with cancer.

The demands of caregiving are associated with physical, emotional, and practical consequences for caregivers. A majority of informal caregivers describe caregiving as moderately to highly stressful, and many caregivers also experience poor mental health outcomes.[2,3,5-8] Such responses among informal caregivers are associated with adverse outcomes for caregivers and patients alike, including decreased caregiver health,[2] poorer care quality,[9] and depressed patient mood.[10] Despite knowing these demands and deficits, caregivers are often inadequately identified and supported. Clinicians rarely ask caregivers whether they need information to care for the patient or themselves (54% and 29%, respectively).[3] These findings are troubling given that having unmet needs is a strong predictor of poorer mental health outcomes for caregivers.[11]

Currently, cancer caregivers are underserved due to a variety of factors, including a lack of information disseminated to practitioners about how to support caregivers, institutions being underresourced to support caregivers given the reimbursement structures and care delivery models common to US healthcare, and a limited availability of community and Internet-based resources. Because the US healthcare system is not currently set up to address the needs of cancer caregivers, community-based organizations can provide a model for how to address unmet needs, as well as provide solutions and services most needed by caregivers.

THE CANCER SUPPORT COMMUNITY'S HISTORY AND MISSION

With this backdrop, the Cancer Support Community's (CSC's) mission is to ensure that all people impacted by cancer are empowered by knowledge, strengthened by action, and sustained by community. Since its inception in 1982 (as the Wellness Community), the CSC has been at the forefront of putting the patient and caregiver experience at the center of all cancer care. In 2009, the Wellness Community and Gilda's Club merged to become the CSC. The combined organization, with more than 50 years of collective experience, provides professional social and emotional support for people impacted by cancer; it works through a network of 55 licensed affiliates of community-based facilities, over 100 satellite locations (including those co-located at hospitals), and a vibrant online community (https://www.cancersupportcommunity.org), touching more than 1 million people annually.

Through decades of working with cancer patients, their families, and caregivers, CSC has developed a portfolio of evidence-based programs that address important concerns of these individuals. CSC offers all services free of charge to people ever diagnosed with any type or stage of cancer and for their caregivers or family members, including children, spouses, partners, and siblings. Services include support groups, educational programs, exercise and nutrition classes, children's support programs, and social activities that are provided at community-based affiliates in group or one-on-one format. Moreover, to broaden access, these support services are also available through the CSC Helpline and online.

Importantly, services are provided by trained and certified mental health professionals. CSC is the largest nonprofit employer of psychosocial oncology mental health professionals in the United States, with decades of experience in delivering evidence-based psychosocial support.

As an institution dedicated to serving the emotional and social needs of cancer patients and their families, CSC has developed a theoretical framework to create a road map for supporting caregivers effectively. This framework is the CSC Person-Centered Model of Care (previously known as CSC's Patient Empowerment Model[12]), which describes a series of actions, self-care behaviors, and attitudes that caregivers can take to enhance their ability to support their loved ones and to support their own health and well-being.

CANCER SUPPORT COMMUNITY'S PERSON-CENTERED MODEL OF CARE

When CSC first opened in June 1982, a primary objective of its programs and services—education, support groups, and social events—was to inform people with cancer how to participate with their healthcare team in making treatment decisions and encourage them to do so and how to enhance their quality of life. It was theorized that all of these patient efforts—actions, behaviors, and attitudes—would enhance their quality of life and, perhaps, improve their physical well-being.

Within the first year, we learned that while CSC's programming was helping patients in communicating with their doctors, learning more about their illness, and giving and receiving support, many patients were having difficulties with how cancer affects their relationships with spouses, family, and children.[13] To address these unmet needs, we expanded our support services to include all people affected by cancer, including caregivers and family members.[14,15]

In the mid-1990s, CSC embarked on a series of studies with Stanford University and the University of California, San Francisco (UCSF) to evaluate the effectiveness of our support programming.[16] Our work demonstrated that people attending CSC's professionally led support groups reported benefits including improved relationships with their doctors and healthcare team and enhanced access to cancer-related information and resources. Participants also reported the ability to develop a new attitude toward living with cancer and to make important life changes, whether those changes were reflected in major life decisions, such as a job change, or more subtle changes, such as spending more time with friends and family or exploring a new interest. Participation was also associated with improved outcomes, including decreased depression and anxiety and reduced existential and trauma-like symptoms.[17] Based on these findings, CSC developed a programmatic framework to delineate the person-centered approach embodied by our support services for patients and caregivers (Figure 15.1).[16]

Cancer Support Community's Person-Centered Model of Care guides all of CSC's professionally led programs and provides a theoretical framework for the development and evaluation of innovative programs, instruments, and initiatives.

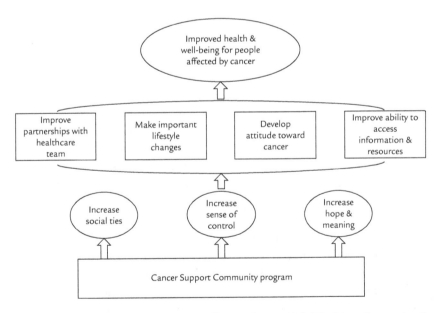

Figure 15.1: Cancer Support Community Person-Centered Model of Care for people affected by cancer.

CSC PERSON-CENTERED RESEARCH INITIATIVES

In 2008, CSC established the Research and Training Institute (RTI) to examine the critical role of social and emotional support by designing studies to help people affected by cancer, giving them the opportunity to share their collective experience to inform new programs, research, and policy. Since that time, the RTI has committed to the development, evaluation, and implementation of person-centered tools and interventions that have been disseminated across its affiliate network, Helpline, online community, and clinical settings. In 2014, the RTI expanded two of its signature research programs to elevate the caregiver voice: the Cancer Experience Registry: Caregivers, an online research initiative; and CancerSupportSource® (CSS)—Caregiver (CSS-CG), a caregiver distress screening and referral program. These initiatives were launched in order to adopt a person-centered approach in identifying and addressing the many issues a caregiver can face.

Cancer Experience Registry: Caregivers

Clinical advances such as new drug therapies and more sophisticated diagnostic tools have extended lives and improved survival rates of many patients across the cancer spectrum. Yet, the complete cancer experience remains less understood by patients, caregivers, and healthcare providers alike. In particular, the emotional and psychosocial effects of cancer are complex and not simply ancillary to the cancer experience. Instead, they have practical implications for how patients and care teams address issues like treatment adherence, complications, and managing side effects.

Since 2013, the Cancer Experience Registry, developed by the CSC's RTI, has provided an opportunity for people impacted by cancer to share perspectives about issues that matter to them and to ensure their experiences are communicated to the broader cancer community, with the goal of making a difference in how people are treated and in the care they receive. The registry is an online research study approved by the Internal Review Board that documents insights from patients across the cancer experience spectrum, illuminates key areas that impact patients' lives, and informs stakeholders looking for data-driven care solutions and broad system change. The findings from the registry assist in quantifying for healthcare providers, advocates, and policymakers the social and emotional gaps in care and treatment to better inform and shape policy and improve quality of life for all those impacted by cancer.

In December 2014, the CSC expanded the registry to include a Caregiver Specialty Registry. This specialty registry documents the experiences of people who are caring for—or have cared for—people affected by cancer. The CSC defines a caregiver as anyone who provides physical, emotional, financial, spiritual, or even logistical support to someone affected by cancer. Many caregiver participants are spouses and loved ones who live with patients; others are nonfamily members. The registry includes standardized, validated questionnaires (e.g., the Patient Reporting Outcomes Measurement Information System, 29-item short form)[18] as well as questions developed by CSC in collaboration with a project advisory council. Guided by a model of community-initiated research collaboration,[12] the Caregiver Advisory Council—made up of healthcare providers, behavioral scientists, patient advocates, industry representatives, and caregivers—supports the efforts of the registry by providing continued support and guidance on outreach, research, and the dissemination of findings. Specifically, the advisors advocated for specific areas of focus, provided review and feedback on the survey questions, and collaborated on dissemination of findings.[19,20]

In order to attract a broad spectrum of caregivers of people impacted by cancer to the registry, the CSC employs a comprehensive recruitment strategy that leverages the robust CSC affiliate network, online community, and national helpline and works with key advocacy organizations to raise awareness of the registry. Outreach is ongoing, with open enrollment to all caregivers and survivors at any point along the care continuum (https://www.cancerexperienceregistry.org).

To date, over 1,000 caregivers have enrolled in the registry from the United States and internationally. Participants are predominately female (82%), white (87%), and educated (55% college degree or higher); they represent individuals from diverse settings (34% urban, 22% rural) and economic backgrounds (22% < $40K annual income; 24% ≥ $100K). Some caregivers find it difficult to identify themselves as such, particularly if they are unpaid family members who live with the patient. The survey asks caregivers whether they meet the registry's definition of caregiving, and 88% believe they do; 74% report that they are currently a caregiver for a person with a cancer diagnosis. Three-quarters (75%) live with the person under their care. A majority of patients receiving care are male (60%); care recipients range in age from 1 to 89 years (average age = 57 years). Fifty-two percent of caregiver respondents are caring for a spouse and 26% for a parent, for an average duration of 5.4 years.

Notably, 68% of caregiver respondents report having no choice in becoming a caregiver. One in five (20%) spend more than 100 hours per week on caregiving. Sixteen percent of caregivers spend between 21 and 40 hours per week on caregiving, 22% spend 11–20 hours, and 22% of caregivers report spending 10 hours or less. Only 17% of respondents report having any formal training as a caregiver; of these, the largest portion (39%) received 1 hour or less of formal training. Forty-seven percent of respondents wish they had more formal training than they received.

Quality of Life, Unmet Needs, and Caregiver Burden. Many caregivers are thrust into their role unexpectedly, with little to prepare them, and feel overwhelmed by the amount of assistance they need to provide to the patient. For example, among a subsample (n = 149) of caregiver respondents in the registry, many desired support across a variety of physical, emotional, and practical aspects of life.[20] Among these respondents, 48% reported substantially worse (>1 standard deviation)[18] levels of anxiety, 31% reported worse levels of depression, and 37% reported substantially worse levels of fatigue as compared to the general US population. Self-care, time management, financial matters, and understanding the patient's disease were identified as areas of elevated need for support. Seventy-two percent wanted more help understanding the patient's medical condition, treatment, and prognosis; 64% wanted more support for themselves; and 62% wanted more support in managing stress. Financial matters were also a significant area of concern: 62% were hoping for at least some support understanding the resources available to them, and 61% wanted help understanding state and local benefits. Greater caregiver burden, lower preparedness for providing care, and less self-perceived knowledge about the patient's cancer were associated with greater unmet caregiver need, after controlling for the number of hours of care provided and level of assistance needed by the patient with activities of daily living (p < .001). These findings underscore the importance of understanding caregivers' unmet needs and highlight important topics to be addressed through education and support services.

Formal Training and Caregiving. Cancer caregivers are often called on to provide instrumental (practical) support, as well as emotional support to the person for whom they provide care. Among a subsample (n = 424) of cancer caregivers enrolled in the registry,[19] approximately one-half (56%) felt prepared to respond to patient emergencies, care for physical needs (52%), and get information from the healthcare system (50%). Only 40% felt prepared to care for the emotional needs of the patient, and 29% were prepared to handle caregiving stress. Among respondents, only 17% reported having received formal caregiver training (typically ≤ 1 hour in duration). Those who underwent formal caregiver training tended to report greater preparedness to provide physical care to the patient (p < .001), but not greater preparedness to provide emotional support (p = .20). These results highlight the need for oncology care systems, including community-based organizations, to develop and test new approaches to training and supporting caregivers in addressing their unmet needs and in providing both physical and emotional support to cancer patients.

CancerSupportSource—Caregiver

It is often difficult for patients and their families to receive necessary supportive services.[21,22] This is problematic in part because addressing distress and psychosocial needs has been associated with a decrease in patient hospitalization frequency and length of stay, number of physician office and emergency room visits, and number of prescriptions received.[23,24] Caregiver distress affects the well-being of the patient and their own quality of life and health outcomes. Thus, caregivers need to be emotionally, physically, and practically equipped in order to care for cancer patients. While screening for distress among patients is recommended to enhance quality of care,[25] there has been an absence of validated measures to identify and address unmet psychosocial needs of caregivers. It is critical to identify caregivers at risk for unmet needs and distress in order to improve quality of life and health outcomes for patients and caregivers. However, within the oncology care system, caregivers are not the identified patient. It is a system-wide challenge to identify caregiver unmet needs and distress and provide targeted resources to improve outcomes.

As a response to this unmet need, CSC developed a novel distress screening tool for cancer caregivers based on CSS, a web-based distress screening and referral tool for people with cancer. CSS has demonstrated robust psychometric properties[26] and is offered in 25- and 15-item forms, including a Spanish language adaptation. CSS allows for easy identification of patients' top concerns and includes subscales that can identify individuals at risk for clinically significant levels of depression and anxiety.[27] Its caregiver adaptation, CSS-CG, is, to our knowledge, the first and only validated cancer caregiver distress screening tool. This tool has been validated through CSC's national, community-based, nonprofit affiliate network offering free psychosocial support for people ever diagnosed with cancer and their families.

The CSS-CG is a flexible tool that has the capacity to be completed at home, in the office, or in clinic. Caregivers are asked to rate their level of concern (0–4) about a series of items related to their emotional well-being, self-care, caregiving role, and patient's well-being. After responding to each concern, caregivers can choose what type of support they would like for that concern (e.g., receive additional information; speak to someone; or no action at this time). For electronic administration, a threshold can be set to trigger these follow-up preferences if a certain level rating is assigned to an individual concern; for example, respondents can be asked if they wish to speak to someone only if an item is rated 2 or higher.

Following completion of CSS-CG, a clinical report and a respondent report are automatically generated. Staff can review caregiver concerns, risk for clinically significant levels of depression or anxiety, and requests for support. Caregivers can immediately receive a report with information (e.g., customized fact sheets with links to educational materials and community resources) they have requested during the survey. This flexible format allows for prioritization of respondents' concerns and desired assistance. The electronic platform allows for secured data management to ensure Health Insurance Portability and Accountability Act (HIPAA) compliance and provides the capacity for integration of reporting into the electronic medical record. Surveys can be automatically scheduled, and results can be accessed through the electronic medical record (EMR) or system's reporting engine.

The initial development of CSS-CG was conducted through CSC's affiliate network, the largest professionally led nonprofit network of cancer support worldwide. In phase I, three focus groups (N = 24 caregivers) were conducted at CSC affiliates to seek caregiver input about how the patient version of CSS could be modified to support their needs. New scale items (e.g., feeling guilty) were developed and scale directions were modified to enhance applicability to caregivers. Subsequently, 10 individual feedback interviews were conducted with caregivers to assess impressions and understanding of the proposed scale items. The initial CSS-CG tool contained 47 items, where respondents rated their level of concern (0 = *Not at all*, 1 = *Slightly*, 2 = *Moderately*, 3 = *Seriously*, 4 = *Very seriously*) with the option to request additional written information or speak to someone about each concern. Items were broadly clustered into three themes: concerns about emotions and self-care (27 items), concerns about caregiving roles and responsibilities (11 items), and concerns about patient well-being (9 items).

The primary validation of CSS-CG was conducted at 10 nationally located CSC affiliate sites, where 246 caregivers were recruited and then completed web-based and paper survey versions of the 47-item tool.[28] Item performance was assessed for (1) strong item discrimination; (2) endorsement for request for assistance among concerned individuals; (3) correlation with validated caregiver and quality-of-life assessment tools; (4) statistical reliability and test-retest stability; (5) contribution to unique variance in overall distress; and (6) scale multidimensionality via exploratory factor analysis. Top concerns included worry about the future, disruptions in home life, patient's pain/discomfort, changes in patient's mood/behavior, and patient's eating and nutrition. Exploratory factor analysis and thematic review suggested that caregiver distress items are distributed across four factors: (1) emotional well-being; (2) self-care; (3) caregiving tasks; and (4) patient well-being.[29] Test-retest stability measured by the Intraclass Correlation Coefficient (ICC) ranged from 0.57 to 91. Statistical criteria and expert review led to the exclusion of 13 items, revision of 12 items, and combination of 3 pairs of items. The revised CSS-CG scale comprises 33 items.

The CSC is conducting a secondary validation study on the revised 33-item CSS-CG scale. Data are currently being collected through the Cancer Experience Registry. The goal of this secondary validation is to ensure a robust, reliable measure that minimizes burden for caregiver respondents. Results from this secondary validation are pending. Additional validation will include examining the utility and psychometric performance of CSS-CG in diverse clinical and care settings. Future goals for implementation include understanding how to best identify caregivers in multiple settings, including primary care, oncology practices, and other potential venues, and how to connect caregivers to resources available within the community.

With respect to CSC's overall research efforts, our next steps are to continue to understand the caregiver experience through the mechanism of the Cancer Experience Registry and CSS-CG to identify gaps in care and opportunities for program development. Findings from the registry directly inform the development of educational and support services at CSC. In addition, CSC is committed to implementing caregiver distress screening, referral, and follow-up across our affiliate network as well as diverse oncology care and other healthcare settings (family and internal medicine) to explore its impact on patient, caregiver, and cost-related outcomes.

CSC PERSON-CENTERED SUPPORT
AND EDUCATION SERVICES

The information that CSC learns from its research initiatives supports a range of evidence-based support and education services available, free of charge. Recognizing the unique experience of caregivers, CSC has developed many programs and services that address the specific challenges of caring for a loved one with cancer. CSC's support and education resources can be accessed by visiting its website (https://www.CancerSupportCommunity. org) and are outlined as follows:

Cancer Support Helpline®. CSC's toll-free *Cancer Support Helpline* (888-793-9355) provides emotional support as well as information and referral to local, regional, and national resources to anyone affected by a cancer diagnosis, including cancer caregivers. The Cancer Support Helpline is staffed by licensed mental health professionals and resource specialists.

Frankly Speaking About Cancer® **(FSAC).** CSC'S landmark cancer education series provides trusted information for cancer patients and their loved ones. Through a variety of delivery mechanisms (publications, online, in-person programs, and radio show), CSC presents information about cancer in a conversational way. To date, CSC has reached hundreds of thousands of people whose lives have been affected by cancer. Our FSAC programs have distributed more than 955,000 FSAC publications, delivered more than 1,980 FSAC workshops and webinars, and hosted nearly 400 radio show episodes. In the past 2 years, FSAC videos have been viewed more than 93,804 times. Many FSAC series have specific videos and chapters of booklets and books for caregivers. Recent offerings from within the FSAC series for caregivers are available at https://www.cancersupportcommunity.org/caregivers and include

- *FSAC: Caregiver* print and PDF booklet
- *FSAC: Support From a Distance* PDF booklet
- Caregiver video testimonials
- Web landing page; compiles all of FSAC: Caregiver resources in one place
- *FSAC: When the Woman You Love Has Breast Cancer*
- *FSAC: De cuidador a cuidador—Compartiendo nuestras experiencias durante el cuidado a mujeres con cáncer de seno*
- eLearning Quick Guide *Ten Tips for Caregivers*
- Webinar—Addressing the Needs of Lung Cancer Caregivers

Services at CSC Affiliates (Including Gilda's Clubs): CSC has affiliate and satellite locations around the country that offer free, comprehensive, personalized, and essential services, including caregiver, patient, or family support and bereavement groups; educational workshops; exercise, art, and nutrition classes; and social activity programs specifically designed for people affected by cancer.

MyLifeLine is an online platform designed to reduce the stress of communication and reduce isolation by building a person-centered community guided by the patient and caregiver. MyLifeLine has transformed the experience of cancer patients over the past decade and joined CSC in 2018 to bring together more than 30,000 patients, survivors, and loved ones in search of connection and community. Patients or a designated caregiver may set up a personalized webpage to share updates on the patient's experience, post support needed, enable friends and family to sign up to drop off a meal and provide a ride to the clinic (https://csc.mylifeline.org).

Grassroots Network. CSC's Cancer Policy Institute provides updates on policy issues that impact the health and well-being of cancer patients and survivors. Anyone impacted by cancer may join the network to make their voice heard by federal and state policymakers at https://www.CancerSupportCommunity.org/join-our-movement.

IMPLICATIONS AND RECOMMENDATIONS

The CSC is committed to serving and supporting the whole patient, including the growing demands placed on caregivers. It is essential to meet patients and families where they are in the cancer trajectory and support them in learning whatever they need to know to enhance their health and well-being. To that end, the CSC has created tools that identify caregivers' greatest needs and direct caregivers to programs designed for them. The development and implementation of these research and programmatic efforts are consistent with several recommendations from the National Academies of Sciences, Engineering, and Medicine,[30] including routine needs assessment for caregivers, training of healthcare and social service providers to provide evidence-based support tailored to caregiver needs as well as referrals to community-based services, and the development, implementation and dissemination of caregiver programs in diverse settings.[30]

The CSC is poised to continue the development and expansion of its research and programmatic initiatives. Future research efforts are needed to develop, test, and evaluate additional innovative programs to meet the needs of caregivers. The first challenge will be to understand how to reach caregivers in diverse settings. In particular, can distress screening be implemented in the oncology practice—where caregivers are not the primary patient? Or, would it be more effective to implement distress screening at family practices where caregivers seek care or at community-based organizations? Are there opportunities to explore integrating the cancer patient and caregiver dyad in a healthcare system, and what would that look like? The second challenge is to understand how and where to link caregivers to evidence-based support and education programs. Implementation research is required in order to identify effective ways to provide targeted and tailored support of caregivers in the community. Given the high burden of demand already placed on caregivers, it will be important to evaluate the effectiveness of innovative technology designed to deliver accessible interventions and to connect caregivers to communities of support. The third challenge is to demonstrate the cost benefits of providing caregiver support. Outcomes include health-related quality of life for the patient and the caregiver, healthcare utilization of the patient and the caregiver, loss of productivity in the workforce, and overall impact on the family. Demonstrating the value of integrating caregiver support into oncology care will help establish payment models that support the vital role of the caregiver.

REFERENCES

1. Kim Y, Schulz R. Family caregivers' strains: comparative analysis of cancer caregiving with dementia, diabetes, and frail elderly caregiving. *J Aging Health*. 2008;20(5):483–503.
2. Bevans M, Sternberg EM. Caregiving burden, stress, and health effects among family caregivers of adult cancer patients. *JAMA*. 2012;307(4):398–403.
3. Hunt GH, Longacre ML, Kent EE, Weber-Raley L. *Cancer Caregiving in the US: An Intense, Episodic, and Challenging Care Experience*. Bethesda, MD: National Alliance for Caregiving, Cancer Support Community and National Cancer Institute; 2016.
4. Stenberg U, Ruland CM, Miaskowski C. Review of the literature on the effects of caring for a patient with cancer. *Psychooncology*. 2010;19(10):1013–1025.
5. Romito F, Goldzweig G, Cormio C, Hagedoorn M, Andersen BL. Informal caregiving for cancer patients. *Cancer*. 2013;119:2160–2169.
6. Northouse LL, Katapodi MC, Song L, Zhang L, Mood DW. Interventions with family caregivers of cancer patients: meta-analysis of randomized trials. *CA Cancer J Clin*. 2010;60(5):317–339.
7. Northouse LL, Katapodi MC, Schafenacker AM, Weiss D. The impact of caregiving on the psychological well-being of family caregivers and cancer patients. *Semin Oncol Nurs*. 2012;28(4):236–245.
8. Kent EE, Longacre ML, Weber-Raley L, Hunt GH. Cancer versus non–cancer caregivers: an analysis of communication needs from the 2015 Caregivers in the U.S. study. J Clin Oncol. 2016;34(26)(suppl):4.
9. Litzelman K, Kent EE, Mollica M, Rowland JH. How does caregiver well-being relate to perceived quality of care in patients with cancer? J Clin Oncol. 2016;34(29):3554–3561.
10. Litzelman K, Yabroff KR. How are spousal depressed mood, distress, and quality of life associated with risk of depressed mood in cancer survivors?

Longitudinal findings from a national sample. *Cancer Epidemiol Biomarkers Prev.* 2015;24(6):969–977.

11. Kim Y, Kashy DA, Spillers RL, Evans TV. Needs assessment of family caregivers of cancer survivors: three cohorts comparison. *Psychooncology.* 2010;19(6):573–582.

12. Golant M, Buzaglo J, Thiboldeaux K. The engaged patient: The Cancer Support Community's Integrative Model of Evidence-Based Psychosocial Programs, Services, and Research. In: Holland JC, Breitbart WS, Butow PN, Jaconsen PB, Loscalzo MJ, McCorkle R, eds. *Psycho-Oncology.* 3rd ed. New York, NY: Oxford University Press; 2015:710–716.

13. Benjamin HH. *From Victim to Victor.* Los Angeles, CA: Tarcher; 1987.

14. Benjamin HH. *The Wellness Community Guide to Fighting for Recovery From Cancer.* Los Angeles, CA: TarcherPerigee; 1995.

15. Golant M. Caregiving: Your role as a strengthened ally. *Coping With Cancer.* March/April Issue 2002;16.

16. Holland JC. *Psycho-oncology.* New York, NY: Oxford University Press; 2015.

17. Giese-Davis J, Brandelli Y, Kronenwetter C, et al. Illustrating the multi-faceted dimensions of group therapy and support for cancer patients. *Healthcare.* 2016;4(3):48.

18. Cella D, Yount S, Rothrock N, et al. The Patient-Reported Outcomes Measurement Information System (PROMIS): progress of an NIH roadmap cooperative group during its first two years. *Med Care.* 2007;45(5)(suppl 1):S3–S11.

19. Zaleta AK, McManus S, Miller MF, Johnson JJ, Buzaglo JS. Preparedness for care and formal training of family cancer caregivers. Paper presented at: American Psychosocial Oncology Society 15th Annual Conference; February 2018; Tucson, AZ.

20. Zaleta AK, Miller MF, Longacre ML, Johnson J, McManus S, Buzaglo JS. Unmet needs, caregiver burden, and quality of life among a community sample of cancer caregivers. Poster presented at: American Psychological Association Annual Convention; August 3–6, 2017; Washington, DC.

21. Cohen GI. ASCO Educational Book, Cancer clinical trials: A primer for participation of community physicians. Alexandria, VA, American Society of Clinical Oncology, 2002:283–289.

22. Edwards BK, Brown ML, Wingo PA, et al. Annual report to the nation on the status of cancer, 1975–2002, featuring population-based trends in cancer treatment. *J Natl Cancer Inst.* 2005;97(19):1407–1427.

23. Sobel DS. The cost-effectiveness of mind-body medicine interventions. *Prog Brain Res.* 2000;122:393–412.

24. Mausbach BT, Yeung P, Bos T, Irwin SA. Healthcare costs of depression in patients diagnosed with cancer. *Psychooncology.* 2018;27(7):1735–1741.

25. Holland JC, Bultz BD. The NCCN guideline for distress management: a case for making distress the sixth vital sign. *J Natl Compr Canc Netw.* 2007;5(1):3–7.

26. Miller MF, Mullins CD, Onukwugha E, Golant M, Buzaglo JS. Discriminatory power of a 25-item distress screening tool: a cross-sectional survey of 251 cancer survivors. *Qual Life Res.* 2014;23(10):2855–2863.

27. Zaleta AK, Miller MF, McManus S, Golant M, Buzaglo JS. Factor structure and validity of CancerSupportSource®: a revised 25-item distress screening tool for cancer survivors. Poster presented at:2018 National Comprehensive Cancer Network 23rd Annual Conference; March 2018; Orlando, FL.

28. Longacre ML, Applebaum AJ, Buzaglo JS, et al. Reducing informal caregiver burden in cancer: evidence-based programs in practice. *Transl Behav Med.* 2018;8(2):145–155.

29. Zaleta AK, Longacre ML, Miller M, et al. Refining a validated distress screening tool for caregivers of cancer patients in a community-based sample. Poster presented at: National Comprehensive Cancer Network 22nd Annual Conference; March 2017; Orlando, FL.

30. National Academies of Sciences Engineering and Medicine. *Families Caring for an Aging America.* Washington, DC: National Academies Press; 2016.

CHAPTER 16

American Cancer Society's Delivery of Support to Caregivers in the Community

RACHEL S. CANNADY AND KATHERINE SHARPE

CAREGIVER STORY

My wife was recently diagnosed with breast cancer and we've been relying on the American Cancer Society's transportation assistance to get to her appointments. If it weren't for this service, I don't know what we would do. When we call to coordinate our ride, we are always impressed by the level of service from the staff who are extremely polite. This transportation program has been just as much a support for me as it has been for my wife. The American Cancer Society has given us much more than just getting us to and from treatment, they have been a valuable resource and we are both so grateful.

—R. O., caregiver

INTRODUCTION

More than 15.5 million Americans with a history of cancer were alive on January 1, 2016, and by January 1, 2026, this number is projected to reach more than 20 million.[1] As they battle this disease, they depend on their family caregivers for support.

Cancer is an issue for the entire family, not just the cancer patient.[2] Rapid advances in care for cancer patients have increased the caregiving responsibilities and needs of families.[3,4] Given the shift from inpatient to outpatient cancer care and shorter hospital stays, reliance on family members or friends has become an essential extension of the healthcare team.

Caregivers are typically responsible for myriad complex tasks, such as gathering cancer- and treatment-related information, arranging medical appointments, driving the patient to and from treatment, monitoring symptoms and treatment side effects, and helping their loved one cope with emotional distress.[5,6] Add to this the conflicting, multiple roles of managing a home and family, as well as employment demands, caregivers often feel overwhelmed with the enormity of responsibilities, which can contribute to high levels of caregiver burden.[7,8]

Throughout the care trajectory, a number of questions may surface that the caregiver does not feel equipped to answer or even have the time to resolve. He or she may feel unprepared for medical tasks required and lack support for proper instruction.[5] He or she may also feel exhausted and burned out from the relentless, around-the-clock requirement of their physical and emotional resources. Often, caregivers lack instrumental or social support as the needs of the patient become paramount. Cancer caregivers need specific information and support programs and services to help them in their role,[4,9] and many are increasingly looking for support outside the cancer centers where their loved ones are receiving support.

The American Cancer Society (ACS) is committed to the support of cancer caregivers. Addressing the needs of caregivers is consistent with the ACS's mission and goals to measurably improve the quality of life (QOL; physical, psychological, social, and spiritual) of all cancer survivors and their caregivers from the time of diagnosis and for the balance of life.

The ACS is uniquely qualified to make a difference in the fight against cancer by continuing its leadership position in supporting high-impact research; improving the QOL for those affected by cancer; preventing and detecting cancer; and reaching more people, including the medically underserved, with the reliable cancer-related information they need. With nearly 5,000 staff members spanning across six regions in the United States and a volunteer base of approximately 2 million people, ACS's existing network of national, state, and local staff and volunteers uniquely positions the organization to improve access to caregiver support services and resources.

This chapter describes how ACS has used its intramurally funded research to inform the development of evidence-based programs and services designed to optimally support caregivers across the cancer trajectory.

Caregiver Research and the American Cancer Society

In the early 2000s, very few studies had been conducted to assess the QOL and adjustment of family caregivers of cancer patients. This limited the ability to better identify cancer caregivers most at risk for having unmet needs or best practices for effective interventions that are tailored, as well as targeted, to the specific groups in need. It is therefore critical to understand the unique challenges these caregivers experience to develop relevant, evidence-based programs to support them.

In 2002, ACS initiated the largest QOL study of caregivers of cancer patients to date: the *National Quality of Life Survey for Caregivers*. This nationwide, longitudinal study followed family caregivers at 2 years,[10] 5 years,[11] and 8 years[12] after their loved one's diagnosis. The study's aims were to (1) identify the prevalence and variability of family caregivers of cancer patients; (2) determine the efficacy of the family's involvement in different dimensions of care tasks; (3) identify the unmet needs of family caregivers; (4) examine the consequences of family care on QOL, which refers to the degree of psychological and physical well-being of patients and family caregivers; and (5) investigate the aforementioned issues across different age and ethnic populations of patients on a trajectory of cancer survivorship. For almost two decades, findings from the study have helped describe what it is like to be a family caregiver during all phases of the disease and has provided necessary information to other researchers, policymakers, and those designing evidence-based programs to help families and caregivers of those diagnosed with cancer.

Among the most notable findings is information from a validation study of a Needs Assessment of Family Caregivers—Cancer measure.[13] Data revealed the top unmet needs of cancer caregivers across the care trajectory (Table 16.1). Caregivers tend to experience the highest level of need in the psychosocial domain of care—needs primarily centered on how to assist their loved one with anxiety, depression, fear, and anger. Throughout the care trajectory, caregivers were more likely to have needs regarding addressing their loved one's emotional distress as well as their own, adjusting to lifestyle changes, getting information about their loved one's cancer, understanding/navigating medical or insurance coverage, and talking to the patient about his or her concerns.

Results from the National Quality of Life Survey for Caregivers have been used to inform caregiver content developed for the ACS website (https://www.cancer.org), have provided empirical support for the creation of a comprehensive resource for caregivers, and have been used to

Table 16.1 CAREGIVER UNMET NEEDS

Top Unmet Needs of Cancer Caregivers	2 Years Postdiagnosis (n = 896)	5 Years Postdiagnosis (n = 608)
Helping your loved one deal with emotional distress	38%	21%
Dealing with your own emotional distress	31%	12%
Dealing with lifestyle changes	27%	11%
Getting information about the cancer your loved one was diagnosed with	27%	10%
Talking to your loved one about concerns	26%	7%
Being satisfied with your relationship with your loved one	25%	10%
Meeting your personal needs	25%	9%
Having enough insurance coverage for your loved one	20%	12%

Source: Kim et al.[13] Reprinted from *Psycho-Oncology*. 2010;19:573–582. This material is reproduced with the permission of John Wiley & Sons, Inc.

help motivate the ACS leadership to pursue a program of support dedicated specifically to those providing care to people with cancer. With the identification and understanding of caregivers' top unmet needs, the ACS is uniquely positioned to build a nationwide platform of standardized support to those who devote countless hours to their loved ones with cancer.

AMERICAN CANCER SOCIETY'S CAREGIVER SUPPORT PROGRAM

Established in 2015, the Caregiver Support Program aims to meet caregivers where they are in the cancer journey. In recent years, the field of caregiving has been burgeoning, especially with the latest reports released from the National Alliance for Caregiving and partners,[4,14] which profile the caregiver experience and provide actionable next steps for health systems and policymakers. Increased attention has been focused on the development of effective caregiver support services aimed at reducing caregiver burden and improving QOL. The focus has also turned to designing relevant and accessible interventions to help caregivers manage their own emotional distress, find meaning in their caregiving experience, and find support in their day-to-day activities; all of these are critical to ensuring the highest QOL for cancer caregivers.

The ACS remains committed to providing integral support to cancer caregivers, and as part of this commitment, targeted information, education, and support have been provided to caregivers to meet their unique and varied needs. The ACS suite of support services for caregivers aims to (1) build confidence in their role as a caregiver; (2) develop caregiving skills in key areas; (3) assist in the management of their own health and wellness (both psychosocial and physical); and (4) design services that are accessible through multiple modalities and channels.

Cancer-specific organizations, like the ACS, primarily tend to provide the majority of support to those diagnosed with cancer while offering peripheral information and support specific to caregivers. With the delegation of the Caregiver Support Program, there is organizational commitment dedicated to the sole focus of those providing care to loved ones with cancer.

A description of resources that follows is organized in two categories: (1) caregiver-focused support (with the caregiver being the intended beneficiary); and (2) caregiver support by proxy (with the patient being the intended beneficiary but peripheral support to the caregiver). Table 16.2 provides a list of URLs for all support sources described.

Table 16.2 AMERICAN CANCER SOCIETY RESOURCES FOR CAREGIVERS

Resource	URL/Contact
ACS website	https://cancer.org
Caregiver page	https://www.cancer.org/caregivers
ACS Caregiver Resource Guide	https://www.cancer.org/caregiverguide
Online bookstore	https://www.cancer.org/bookstore
National Cancer Information Center	(Available 365/24/7) 1-800-227-2345; online chat on https://cancer.org, Monday–Friday 7 am to 6:30 pm CST
Springboard Beyond Cancer: Caregivers	https://survivorship.cancer.gov
Cancer Survivors Network	https://csn.cancer.org
Hope Lodge	https://www.cancer.org/hopelodge
Hotel Partnership	https://www.cancer.org/patientlodging
Road To Recovery	https://www.cancer.org/roadtorecovery
Relay For Life	https://www.cancer.org/relay
Making Strides Against Breast Cancer	https://www.cancer.org/strides

Caregiver-Focused Support

Caregiver Web Page

When a family member or friend is diagnosed with cancer, one of the first things people turn to is the Internet. They search for information about cancer, its treatment and side effects, and how to provide care to their loved one with cancer. Distilling the countless sources of information can feel overwhelming, even for the savviest Internet user. Thus, ACS content staff have been thoughtful about the way information is organized on the website. Prided on comprehensive, trustworthy information, the ACS medical and editorial content teams have developed a wealth of cancer information. With the website redesign and launch in January 2016, the caregiver section provides an easily navigable experience covering topics such as what it means to be a caregiver, managing work-related and financial issues, managing treatment side effects, and taking care of oneself as a caregiver. On https://www.cancer.org/caregivers, one can explore all of the care-related information created for family members and friends of cancer patients.

Caregiver Resource Guide

In spring 2017, ACS released its first caregiver-specific product, the Caregiver Resource Guide. This comprehensive compendium of information is a curation of various content from the ACS website to help organize the care experience and reduce "infoxication." The 120-page guide offers information on each of the following topics:

- *Cancer Caregiving*: Provides information about what caregivers do and how their role is important in the cancer journey; also provides tips for being an effective caregiver
- *Caregiver Self-Care*: Provides information about healthy lifestyle choices with guidelines to support physical activity and nutrition
- *Communication*: Provides tools to better express thoughts and feelings about cancer to the patient as well as the cancer care team
- *Cancer Information*: Provides the basics about what cancer is, how it develops, common cancer myths, how cancer is treated, and how people may change both physically and mentally as a result of having cancer; addresses the financial implications of cancer
- *Cancer Treatment*: Briefly describes surgery, chemotherapy, and radiation and their respective side effects; also provides resources in the event that treatment stops working

- *Patient Nutrition*: Describes how eating the right kinds of foods before, during, and after treatment can help patients feel better and stay stronger
- *Coping*: Describes the most common psychosocial concerns around cancer (i.e., anxiety, fear, and depression) and how caregivers can help patients cope with them
- *Caregiver Resources*: Describes support groups and resources available in multiple online environments offered through the ACS and beyond, as well as in-person support groups offered in various communities nationwide

Aspects of the aforementioned needs assessment from the National Quality of Life Survey for Caregivers helped inform development of the Cancer Resource Guide, with priority given to those areas where needs were most prevalent. Distribution of the guide is made available through health systems across the country by way of ACS patient navigators and other ACS-related cancer liaison staff within hospitals. An online, interactive version is available at https://www.cancer.org/caregiverguide, and the guide in its entirety is also available for download.

Springboard Beyond Cancer: Caregivers

In collaboration with the National Cancer Institute, ACS developed an online tool to help cancer patients with self-management; the tool is designed to enable and empower them to achieve their care goals by instilling confidence in managing their health outcomes. Caregivers are an integral part of making self-management successful. This online platform allows patients and caregivers to identify goals, create a plan, identify potential challenges, monitor their progress, and reassess the plan to allow them to communicate more effectively with the healthcare team.

Detailed information about providing care is organized into six sections: (1) Being a Caregiver; (2) Care for Your Body; (3) Care for Your Mind; (4) Finding Meaning and Peace; (5) After Treatment Ends; and (6) End-of-Life Care and Bereavement. Each section contains directives on building an Action Deck for caregivers to refer to with links to additional information and resources and empowering caregivers to take ownership of the outcomes of their care experience.

Refer to https://survivorship.cancer.gov and click *Get Support* from the navigation ribbon at the top of the page.

The National Cancer Information Center

Like patients, caregivers contact the ACS via telephone, email, and online chat requesting information, service referrals, support programs, and other general service requests. The ACS National Cancer Information Center (NCIC) is open 24 hours a day, 7 days a week, for listening, encouraging, and providing answers. Since 1997, the NCIC has received more than 20 million calls, emails, chats, and social media posts with inquiries about cancer information and resource navigation, clinical trial matching, health insurance assistance, event-related questions, and donation processing. Services are provided in English, Spanish, and more than 200 other languages via a translation service.

Caregivers typically account for nearly 30% of the total service requests received. Cancer information caregivers receive helps empower them to participate in decision-making, communicate with their loved one's healthcare team, and cope with the issues that arise through the cancer journey. When caregivers contact ACS, they have access to patient navigators who are trained to listen to patients and caregivers, guide them along their journey, and connect them to the resources they need, including helping to coordinate the patient's ride to and from treatment appointments and lodging if they need to travel away from home for treatment. The ACS also connects patients and caregivers to local and national resources, including help with managing the appearance-related side effects of treatment, emotional support, and other resources that help them throughout their experience. In addition, oncology and pediatric oncology nurses assist with more medically complex questions that help empower patients and caregivers by providing them with health information for potentially better health outcomes. The NCIC can also assist patients and caregivers with questions about their options and rights if they are about to lose their insurance or already have lost their coverage and share patient stories with the ACS nonprofit, nonpolitical advocacy affiliate, the ACS Cancer Action Network^{SM} (https://www.acscan.org/) to help improve advocacy efforts. Call 1-800-227-2345 to speak to a Cancer Information Specialist or to chat online, go to https://www.cancer.org.

Caregiver Books

The ACS creates and publishes books to help people navigate the cancer experience when it touches their lives or the lives of members of their family. As the world's leading publisher of books on cancer, ACS has won more than 100 awards for content and design excellence since 2006. Highlighted here are three books devoted specifically to caregiving:

American Cancer Society Complete Guide to Family Caregiving: The Essential Guide to Cancer Caregiving at Home; Authors: Julia A. Bucher, Peter S. Houts, Terri Ades; ISBN 9780944235003. Whether a spouse, partner, adult child, friend, or other family member, the caregiver plays a crucial role in a patient's cancer journey. This book is filled with practical information on a wide range of issues that a family caregiver might encounter when caring for a loved one at home. From physical and emotional conditions to dealing with healthcare providers and insurance carriers, caregivers will use this resource in countless ways. Offering thorough, concise checklists, questions to ask the doctor, signs and symptoms to note, and where and when to turn for more help, this book also includes a comprehensive list of specific resources.

Cancer Caregiving A to Z: An At-Home Guide for Patients and Families; Authors: Experts from the American Cancer Society; ISBN 9780944235928. This book is an indispensable quick reference for those who care for loved ones at home. Organized in a straightforward alphabetical format, this book covers more than four dozen critical topics in cancer caregiving, including how to handle problems such as appetite changes, confusion, depression, fatigue, and fevers. The book guides caregivers in how to identify problems early, along with warning signs for when it is time to call the doctor. Whether caring for oneself at home or providing care for a loved one, this useful guide can help improve quality of care and QOL for those with cancer.

How to Help Your Friend With Cancer; Author: Colleen Fullbright; ISBN 9781604432244. Sometimes people may not know what to say or do when a friend has cancer for fear that something might come out wrong. Written by a cancer survivor whose friends made her journey easier, *How to Help Your Friend With Cancer* provides the guidance needed to be the best friend you can be, every step along the way. This book contains more than 100 suggestions, along with practical tips and relatable advice that anyone can use to help a friend get through the cancer experience.

Caregiver Support by Proxy

Caregiver support can also be delivered through programs and services originally targeted to meet patients' needs; thus, they are considered support by proxy.

Hope Lodge and Hotel Partnership

Getting the best care sometimes means cancer patients and their caregivers must travel away from home for outpatient treatment. This can place an extra emotional and financial burden on patients and caregivers during an already challenging time. ACS's lodging programs can help make this difficult situation easier for both cancer patients and their families.

Since 1984, Hope Lodge has provided nearly 5 million free, no-cost nights of lodging in a home-away-from-home environment for adult cancer patients and their caregivers. More than just a roof over their heads, it is a nurturing setting where patients and caregivers can share stories and offer each other emotional support. Guests have access to shared kitchens, laundry rooms, and other common areas. There are currently 32 Hope Lodge locations in 24 states throughout the United States and Puerto Rico, with an additional 6 locations in development (Figure 16.1). To learn more, visit https://www.cancer.org/hopelodge.

The American Cancer Society, in a cooperative effort with hotels across the country, also provides overnight accommodations to cancer patients and caregivers who must travel for outpatient treatment and need assistance with lodging at free or deeply discounted rates. The program is open to cancer patients of all ages and their caregivers, including pediatric patients accompanied by a parent and patients traveling with children. All accommodations are provided based on eligibility requirements and are subject to availability and to restrictions imposed by the participating hotels. Requests for lodging are met on a first-come, first-served basis. To find out more, visit https://www.cancer.org/patientlodging.

In 2017, the ACS lodging program provided more than 520,000 nights of free or reduced-rate lodging to more than 32,000 patients and caregivers, saving them nearly $50 million. Not having to worry about where to stay, or how to pay for lodging, allows patients to focus on getting better and allays financial concerns of caregivers.

Road to Recovery and Transportation Program

One of the biggest roadblocks to cancer treatment can be the lack of transportation. An estimated 3.6 million Americans delay or have difficulty getting needed medical care each year due to the lack of available and affordable transportation to treatment. Caregivers may help, but over the course of several months, they may not always have the time or resources to provide every ride. This is why a successful transportation assistance program can be a tremendous asset.

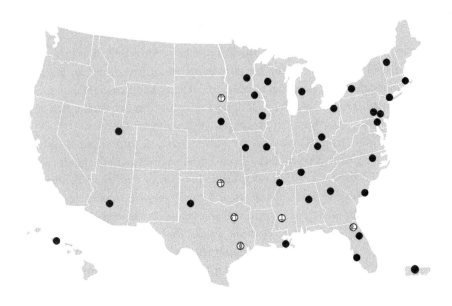

● Existing Locations (32)	
Atlanta, GA	Lubbock, TX
Baltimore, MD	Marshfield, WI
Birmingham, AL	Memphis, TN
Boston, MA	Minneapolis, MN
Burlington, VT	Nashville, TN
Charleston, SC	New Orleans, LA
Cincinnati, OH	New York, NY
Cleveland, OH	Omaha, NE
Gainesville, FL	Philadelphia, PA
Grand Rapids, MI	Phoenix, AZ
Greenville, NC	Rochester, MN
Hershey, PA	Rochester, NY
Honolulu, HI	Salt Lake City, UT
Iowa City, IA	San Juan, PR
Kansas City, MO	St. Louis, MO
Lexington, KY	Tampa, FL
⊕ Planned Locations (6)	
Dallas, TX	Jacksonville, FL
Houston, TX	Oklahoma City, OK
Jackson, MS	Sioux Falls, SD

Figure 16.1: American Cancer Society Hope Lodge locations, existing and planned.

By calling the NCIC, a Cancer Information Specialist will assist patients or caregivers by coordinating a ride with an ACS volunteer driver, coordinating a ride with a local partnering organization to provide transportation, or referring to a network of community organizations that may provide transportation services. In 2017, nearly 350,000 rides were provided to more than 25,000 patients. Since the inception of the transportation program in 2005, over 8 million rides have been provided, serving nearly 475,000 patients. The Road To Recovery program is at the very heart of ACS's work of removing barriers to quality healthcare by providing patients and, at times, their caregivers transportation to treatment and other cancer-related appointments. To learn more about these transportation programs, visit https://www.cancer.org/roadtorecovery or call 1-800-227-2345.

Cancer Survivors Network

The Cancer Survivors Network (CSN), launched in 2000, is the largest online peer support community for cancer patients, survivors, and caregivers. CSN objectives include to (1) encourage mutual support and self-expression; (2) facilitate exchange of experiences and practical information; (3) decrease feelings of isolation; and (4) increase feelings of belonging and community. Users are able to get and give support and practical tips; search, find, and connect with others like them; read and comment on others' stories and blogs; see their photos and other personal expressions; take part in discussion boards and live chats; tell their story, create a blog, and share photos, art, poems, music, and other personal expressions; and send secure messages to other members via a private CSN email.

A study of the CSN community by ACS researchers showed that caregivers are more likely to be recurrent visitors to the site.[15] These data demonstrate the effectiveness of the online, supportive environment for caregivers. Some have considered this platform their "lifeline" in the cancer journey as they connect with others like them. To register and create a profile on CSN, visit https://csn.cancer.org.

Events

American Cancer Society event staff have standardized the way patients, survivors, and caregivers are engaged in participation. Making participants feel welcomed, valued, and cared for goes beyond the date of the event and extends into year-round engagement.

Relay For Life. With nearly 4 million participants worldwide, Relay For Life is ACS's signature fundraiser cancer walk. Relay is staffed and coordinated by volunteers in more than 4,500 communities and 30 countries; these volunteers give of their time and effort because they believe it is time to take action against cancer. At each event, members take turns walking around a track or designated path; the event lasts 6–24 hours, and each team is asked to have a member on the track at all times to signify that cancer never sleeps. Relay's motto is: "Cancer patients don't stop because they're tired, and for one night, neither do we."

Relays around the globe acknowledge the importance of the caregiver role and pay tribute to them with event regalia, including a caregiver sash, a caregiver banner, and a designated caregiver area. They are also recognized through their Caregiver Lap around the track during the opening ceremonies of each event, which is especially meaningful. To learn more about and sign up for Relay For Life, visit https://www.cancer.org/relay.

Making Strides Against Breast Cancer. Every 3- to 5-mile Making Strides Against Breast Cancer walk unites communities to support each other by honoring those touched by the disease and raising awareness and funds to save lives from breast cancer. Thanks to the determination of Making Strides supporters, the ACS funds innovative breast cancer research, promotes education and risk reduction, and provides comprehensive patient support to those who need it most. With more than 200 events across the country, including nearly 1.5 million participants, Making Strides is one of the largest gatherings of lives touch by breast cancer. To learn more about and sign up for a Making Strides Against Breast Cancer, visit https://www.cancer.org/strides.

Patient-Focused Books Related to Caregiving

What to Eat During Cancer Treatment, Second Edition; Authors: Experts from the American Cancer Society, Jeanne Besser, Barbara Grant; ISBN 9781604432565. This cookbook contains more than 130 recipes, including 100 new dishes, to help cancer patients maintain sound nutrition while going through treatment. The book provides practical tips and suggestions to help patients and their caregivers anticipate—and overcome—the major challenges of eating well during treatment. The book's primary focus is on the seven most common eating-related side effects of cancer treatment (nausea, diarrhea, constipation, trouble swallowing, sore mouth, unintentional weight loss, and taste alterations) and the foods that will be acceptable when these side effects occur. Chapters are organized by these side effects, and introductory information for each section is based on evidence-based research and sound clinical experience. The book appeals to both people undergoing treatment and the caregivers who are providing support.

American Cancer Society Complete Guide to Nutrition for Cancer Survivors: Eating Well, Staying Well During and After Cancer; Editors: Barbara Grant, Abby S. Bloch, Kathryn K. Hamilton, Cynthia A. Thomson; ISBN 9780944235782. Eating well is important for everyone, but it is essential for people with cancer. This book offers the latest information about using nutrition to optimal advantage during the cancer journey and beyond. Good nutrition can bolster energy levels, boost the immune system to fight off infection, and minimize the side effects of treatment. Eating well will also contribute to healing and wellness after the stress of cancer therapy. This book not only offers ACS's best advice on cancer-fighting foods, but also shows how eating a balanced, healthy diet and being physically active can provide a solid foundation for a long, healthy life.

What Helped Get Me Through: Cancer Survivors Share Wisdom and Hope; Author: Julie Silver; ISBN 9781604430042. This book, edited by a breast cancer survivor, succinctly relates the experiences, both practical and sensitive, of hundreds of cancer survivors, including celebrities such as Carly Simon and Scott Hamilton, who candidly relate what helped get them through every aspect of their cancer journey. The wisdom and hope offered in this book will be invaluable to newly diagnosed patients and their families, as well as their doctors and caregivers.

CONCLUSIONS

In March 2018, the National Alliance for Caregiving released a report entitled, *From Insight to Advocacy: Addressing Family Caregiving as a National Public Health Issue*,[16] which provides clear directives to caregiver advocates, health systems, and policymakers to encourage consideration of the caregiver role as an extension of the healthcare team. Further, the report emphasizes establishing public policies that sustain and support families and friends who provide health-related assistance to persons living with chronic disease and disability as a critical consideration to supporting population health.

For decades, the literature has underscored how most caregivers are ill-prepared for their role and provide care with little or no support.[17–19] A wide range of support services is needed to help cancer caregivers improve their caregiving skills and remain healthy and able to continue in their caregiving role.[20] Caregiver interventions should be targeted and tailored to effectively meet the needs of cancer caregivers throughout the caregiving trajectory, which even extends beyond their loved one's death.

It is imperative to develop effective caregiver interventions to reduce caregiver burden and improve QOL. In response to this need, ACS has strategically worked to design, develop, and implement relevant and accessible interventions to help caregivers manage their own emotional distress, find meaning in their caregiving experience, and find support in their day-to-day activities. While there continues to be a need for caregiver support and resources, we have taken important first steps. The ACS is committed to supporting the highest QOL for cancer caregivers, and we will continue to work relentlessly until that goal is achieved.

REFERENCES

1. American Cancer Society. *Cancer Treatment and Survivorship Facts and Figures 2016–2017*. Atlanta, GA: American Cancer Society; 2016.
2. Kim Y, Given BA. Quality of life of family caregivers of cancer survivors across the trajectory of the illness. *Cancer*. 2008;112(11)(suppl):2556–2568.
3. Brédart A, Kop JL, Beaudeau A, et al. Quality of care in the oncology outpatient setting from patients' perspective: a systematic review of questionnaires' content and psychometric performance. *Psychooncology*. 2014;24:382–394.
4. National Alliance for Caregiving in partnership with the National Cancer Institute and the Cancer Support Community. *Cancer Caregiving in the US*. Bethesda, MD: National Alliance for Caregiving; 2016.
5. Applebaum AJ, Breitbart W. Care for the cancer caregiver: a systematic review. *Palliat Support Care*. 2013;11:231–252.
6. Kent E, Rowland JH, Northouse L, et al. Caring for caregivers and patients: research and clinical priorities for informal cancer caregiving. *Cancer*. 2016;122:1987–1995.
7. Kim Y, Baker F, Spillers RL, et al. Psychological adjustment of cancer caregivers with multiple roles. *Psychooncology*. 2006;15:795–804.
8. Williams A. Cancer family caregivers: a new direction for interventions. *J Palliat Med*. 2012;15:775–783.
9. Shelby RA, Taylor KL, Kerner JF, et al. The role of community-based and philanthropic organizations in meeting cancer patient and caregiver needs. *CA Cancer J Clin*. 2002;52:229–246.
10. Kim Y, Spillers RL. Quality of life of family caregivers at 2 years after a relative's cancer diagnosis. *Psychooncology*. 2010;19:431–440.

11. Kim Y, Spillers RL, Hall DL. Quality of life of family caregivers 5 years after a relative's cancer diagnosis: follow-up of the National Quality of Life Survey for Caregivers. *Psychooncology*. 2012;21:273–281.

12. Kim Y, Shaffer KM, Carver CS, et al. Quality of life of family caregivers 8 years after a relative's cancer diagnosis: follow-up of the National Quality of Life Survey for Caregivers. *Psychooncology*. 2016;25:266–274.

13. Kim Y, Kashy DA, Spillers RL, et al. Needs assessment of family caregivers of cancer survivors: three cohorts comparison. *Psychooncology*. 2010;19:573–582.

14. National Alliance for Caregiving in collaboration with the AARP Public Policy Institute. *Caregiving in the US 2015*. Bethesda, MD: National Alliance for Caregiving; 2015.

15. Fallon BA, Driscoll D, Smith T, et al. The American Cancer Society Cancer Survivors Network: factors associated with continued engagement in an online community after registration. Poster presentation at the Biennial Cancer Survivorship Research Conference; Washington, DC; 2016.

16. National Alliance for Caregiving. *From Insight to Advocacy: Addressing Family Caregiving as a National Public Health Issue*. Bethesda, MD: National Alliance for Caregiving; 2018.

17. Given CW, Given B, Azzouz F, et al. Predictors of pain and fatigue in the year following diagnosis among elderly cancer patients. *J Pain Symptom Manage*. 2001;21:456–466.

18. Houts PS, Nezu AM, Nezu CM, et al. The prepared family caregiver: a problem-solving approach to family caregiver education. *Patient Educ Couns*. 1996;27:63–73.

19. Waldron EA, Janke EA, Bechtel CF, et al. A systematic review of psychosocial interventions to improve cancer caregiver quality of life. *Psychooncology*. 2013;22:1200–1207.

20. Northouse LL, Katapodi M, Song L, et al. Interventions with family caregivers of cancer patients: meta-analysis of randomized trials. *CA Cancer J Clin*. 2010;60:317–339.

CHAPTER 17

CancerCare
A Psychosocial Oncology Support
Organization

SARAH K. KELLY AND WILLIAM GOEREN

There are only four kinds of people in this world:
Those who have been caregivers;
Those who currently are caregivers;
Those who will be caregivers and
Those who will need caregivers.
> —Former US First Lady Rosalynn Carter,
> *Honorary Chair Speech, Last Acts, 1997*

INTRODUCTION

As the population in the United States continues to grow and life expectancy increases, the need for quality cancer care increases accordingly. In 2018, more than 1.7 million new cases of cancer are expected to be diagnosed,[1] and the estimated number of survivors, defined as any person with a history of cancer from the time of diagnosis through the remainder of their life, currently stands at more than 15.5 million.[2]

A cancer diagnosis and related treatments can significantly affect the quality of life of patients with cancer, including their physical, emotional, and spiritual well-being throughout the cancer trajectory. The trajectory itself is uniquely individual and may be experienced as short term or more chronic. Those who are post-treatment may also experience a recurrence of cancer, be diagnosed with a secondary cancer, or experience long-term side effects from the cancer or its treatment, all of which will further alter the

trajectory. Given these numerous changes, a cancer diagnosis may precip-
itate a complex crisis involving all aspects of the individual's functioning.[3]
For many patients, this crisis leads to acute distress requiring immediate,
supportive interventions. This distress is also often experienced more
chronically, with gradations of complexities as coping with cancer impacts
daily priorities, quality of life, and the anticipated and expected future of
hopes and plans.

The impact of the disease reaches well beyond that of the patient,
to affect all areas of the patient's life, including their support network.
CancerCare released a Patient Engagement Report in 2016 surveying patient needs. Respondents confirmed that their cancer diagnosis affects the
whole family and support systems. Additionally, patients' understanding
of "what is best for my family" influenced their preferences or treatment
goals.[4] Indeed, the patient's support network is an integral part of care,
deeply affected by all aspects of the cancer trajectory.

WHO ARE INFORMAL CANCER CAREGIVERS?

Informal cancer caregivers are unpaid spouses, partners, loved ones,
family, and friends who play an integral role in the management of cancer
throughout the illness trajectory. According to the 2015 National Alliance
for Caregiving and AARP study report, 7% of the general population are
caregivers of a loved one with cancer.[5] Their 2016 report examining cancer-
related data from 2015 indicated that this would mean that at least 2.8 million Americans were providing care to an adult family member or friend
due to a primary diagnosis of cancer.[6] These caregivers provide myriad support tasks for the person with cancer, including physical, emotional, and
practical assistance.[4] Caregivers may also assume multiple roles in addition
to their prescribed roles, requiring further adaptation. All of these factors
have a tremendous impact on caregivers and result in the psychological and
spiritual distress discussed in Section 1 of this textbook.

Given these challenges, the need for support services for this population is crucial. A state-of-the-science review in 2012 examined the effects
of caregiving on the health and well-being of caregivers and identified
basic interventions (Table 17.1) that can be implemented across practice
settings.[7] This review also recommended that clinicians refer caregivers and
patients to established organizations for comprehensive support services
and cited CancerCare as an essential organization to deliver these needed
interventions.[7]

Table 17.1 GUIDELINES FOR PROVIDING CARE TO CANCER CAREGIVERS IN PRACTICE SETTINGS

Assessment
  Willingness to provide care
    Who is available?
    Does caregiver live with patient?
    Is safe, affordable transportation available?
  Ability to provide care
    General health status
      Identify primary care provider (same provider for both caregiver and patient?)
      Assess comorbidities: physical and mental health
    Physical ability
      Evaluate for strength, range of motion, stamina, and vision
    Emotional stability
      Screen for anxiety, depression, and sleep disorders
      Assess coping skills
    Cognitive skills
      Evaluate for executive function (e.g., memory)
    Competing demands/time constraints
      Inquire about other responsibilities (i.e., work, household, other dependents such as children and disabled/elderly relatives)
  Knowledge and skill level
    Determine prior experiences with caregiving
    Evaluate understanding of patient's disease
    Assess knowledge of the required tasks
Education
  Caregiver tasks
    Personal care (bathing, eating, wound care, medications, and symptom management)
    Family care (communication and support)
    Instrumental tasks (finances and insurance reimbursement)
  Stress management
    Physical activity, meditation, guided imagery, and journaling
  Health promotion
    Nutrition, exercise, substance use, and respite care
  Disease prevention
    Health maintenance exams, screenings, and immunizations
Resources and services
  Inquire about current and needed resources
    Primary care provider and/or mental health provider
    Home care nursing
    Support group or social service agency
    Access to the Internet
    Availability of family/friends or other agency for respite care
    Financial ability to hire help
    Knowledge/use of family and medical leave benefit

Source: Guidelines for providing care to cancer caregivers. Reprinted from Psychosocial care for family caregivers of patients with cancer, by Northouse, L., Williams, A. L., Given, B., & McCorkle, R. *Journal of Clinical Oncology, 30*(11), 1227–1234. Reprinted with permission © 2012 American Society of Clinical Oncology. All rights reserved.

CANCER*CARE* MISSION

In response to the challenges of cancer, patients and caregivers often seek support or are referred for support beyond what may be provided by their primary medical team. Support is sought for a variety of reasons, including a general feeling of being overwhelmed and lost: "I am not sure why I am calling. My sister was diagnosed with breast cancer this morning. What do I do now?" (Cancer*Care* telephone client, March 2017).

Cancer*Care* was founded in 1944 in New York City by a group of oncologists to address the unmet needs of patients and caregivers, as well as begin the process of support by establishing a space to openly and honestly discuss living with cancer. The founding of Cancer*Care* was groundbreaking, setting a precedent counter to the established doctor-patient interaction at that time. These forward-thinking oncologists came to understand that their patients needed a quality of conversation about cancer that was foreign to their profession and contrary to their beliefs and what they were taught. It was normative at that time, and for many decades after, to minimize or withhold discussions with patients and caregivers about their cancer, including informing them of their diagnosis. A 1961 national survey of 219 physicians showed that 90% preferred not to disclose or discuss a cancer diagnosis with a patient, and this preference had no correlation to experience or age of the physician.[8] It was found that inconsistencies, steadfast belief in current medical opinion, and resistance to change and to research and personal judgment were determinants of physicians' decisions to withhold information.[8] It was not until the early 1970s that opinions and practice began to shift toward the direction of disclosure and discussions.[9] In addition to appropriately addressing the cancer diagnoses, Cancer*Care*'s founding oncologists also realized they were struggling with how to provide emotional and psychological support to their patients, just as their patients and their caregivers were struggling to understand and come to terms with the diagnosis. The parallel process was clear.

Today, Cancer*Care* is a leading national organization providing free, professional support services and information to help people manage the emotional, practical, and financial challenges of cancer. These programs and services helped 195,000 people affected by cancer, including caregivers, and we welcomed 2.1 million visits to the Cancer*Care* websites in 2017. Comprehensive services include counseling and support groups over the phone, online, and in person; educational workshops; publications; and financial and copayment assistance. All Cancer*Care* services are provided by oncology social workers and leading cancer experts. Cancer*Care* social workers provided emotional and practical support to 93,577 people through the Cancer*Care* Hopeline, individual counseling, support groups, and community programs in 2017 alone.

Cancer*Care* has, since its start in 1944, long determined three important themes focused on caregivers. First, Cancer*Care*'s counseling philosophy has always deemed that a cancer diagnosis is a family issue, however that family is constructed or designated. Second, Cancer*Care* considers that caregivers' experiences of distress can be of the same magnitude, or greater, than that of the patient and understands that the content of caregiver stress is often distinctly different from the distress of the patient. And, finally, a focus is that caregivers all have commonalities in caring for their loved one, but that multiple factors and circumstances—such as relationship between and ages of the patient and the caregiver, the patient's diagnosis and prognosis—can influence how they adapt and cope. With these three themes in mind, Cancer*Care* seeks to successfully address caregiver concerns through various modalities, as described in the sections that follows.

CANCER*CARE* HOPELINE

Cancer*Care* provides immediate support through the Cancer*Care* Hopeline, LUNGevity Line, and Triple Negative Breast Cancer Line. Oncology social workers on these telephone lines help clients manage the emotions surrounding cancer while also locating essential resources and providing assistance to navigate financial and practical challenges. Through comprehensive assessment, they also connect callers to appropriate Cancer*Care* services. These hopelines are the point of entry for all Cancer*Care*'s services.

Cancer*Care* Hopeline | 800-813-HOPE (4673). The Cancer*Care* Hopeline is available to people living in the United States with cancer, caregivers, or loved ones seeking support services. This year, Cancer*Care* answered 76,606 Hopeline calls.

LUNGevity Lung Cancer Helpline | 844-360-LUNG (5864). Launched by the nonprofit organization LUNGevity, the LUNGevity Lung Cancer Helpline is a free resource for people diagnosed with lung cancer and their caregivers. Callers are connected with Cancer*Care* oncology social workers, who can address their unique emotional, practical, and informational needs.

Triple Negative Breast Cancer Helpline | 877-880-TNBC (8622). In partnership with the Triple Negative Breast Cancer Foundation, the

Triple Negative Breast Cancer Helpline offers support to those who have been diagnosed with triple-negative breast cancer and their caregivers.

INDIVIDUAL COUNSELING

CancerCare's oncology social workers provide one-on-one counseling services in person and over the phone for patients, caregivers, and the bereaved; all these services are completely free of charge. CancerCare utilizes a short-term, strengths-based model consisting of 12 sessions for in-person counseling and 6 sessions for telephone counseling. CancerCare's telephone support services began at the founding of CancerCare in 1944 to address the needs of those who did not have access to or were physically unable to attend in-person counseling. Considering the numerous tasks of caregivers, financial and time constraints often inhibit their engaging in in-person support. Telephone counseling provides an opportunity for a broader group of caregivers to receive much needed services. Importantly, there have been numerous studies that indicate positive outcomes in evaluations of the impact of telehealth-based support for caregivers.[10] The success of CancerCare's telephone counseling program reflects this.

In the most recent Impact Report on CancerCare's Psychosocial Support Services among over 250 CancerCare clients, 20% of whom self-identified as caregivers, the following was reported: Before contacting CancerCare, only 15% of clients reported their emotional health/well-being as good or very good; the number of clients who said their emotional health/well-being was good or very good increased to 80% as a result of counseling sessions with a CancerCare social worker; and 98% of clients reported that they would recommend CancerCare's counseling services to another person in their situation.

CancerCare counseling services focus on the following client needs to reach the overall goal of improved quality of life:

- Improving understanding of cancer and its treatment
- Learning new ways to cope with cancer
- Managing emotions such as anxiety or sadness
- Improving communication with the healthcare team
- Better coping with the stress of caregiving
- Finding reliable information
- Talking to your support network about cancer
- Finding useful resources in your community

- Learning new ways to cope with grief
- Managing financial challenges
- Understanding patient rights and insurance information

CANCER*CARE* SUPPORT GROUPS

Cancer*Care* support groups offer support for patients, caregivers, and the bereaved and provide a space to connect with others who are facing similar challenges. Facilitated by oncology social workers, these specialized group environments allow attendees to both receive and offer support in a private, closed-group setting. In-person groups meet in weekly, regularly scheduled, 90-minute sessions and run for 12-week cycles. In 2017, Cancer*Care* hosted 27 in-person support groups for patients, caregivers, and the bereaved, including 12 groups for caregivers.

As with individual counseling, telephone support groups are also available for those interested in connecting with others who are coping with cancer in themselves or a loved one. The telephone support groups are offered nationally and bring people together from across the country. These groups also meet for 12 weekly, regularly scheduled 1-hour sessions. To ensure the utmost level of privacy and confidentiality, the groups meet on a password-protected, toll-free phone line and, as with all our services, are facilitated by oncology social workers. Cancer*Care* has hosted 15 telephone support groups for patients, caregivers, and the bereaved, including 3 groups for caregivers in 2017.

Cancer*Care*'s Online Support Group Program (OSGP) was started in 1996 to further expand the reach of support services as technology advanced. Group members can participate by posting in groups 24 hours a day, 7 days a week. Similar to the telephone support groups, the online support groups are password protected and are moderated by oncology social workers. Research on web-based interventions has shown that they can significantly improve psychological distress, including anxiety, stress, depression, and mood changes, and can significantly enhance coping skills.[11] Additionally, these interventions have the potential to reduce barriers to accessing support by offering a modality that is feasible and acceptable to users.[12] Traditional interventions may also be adapted to web-based interventions, which further address caregiver needs by reducing time constraints, financial constraints, and constraints related to geographic location.[13,14] Unlike other online support group models that may be peer moderated, Cancer*Care*'s groups are professionally moderated by oncology social workers. Results from a 2015 study looking at professionally moderated private groups highlighted their ability to reduce depression and improve quality of life for participants.[15] In 2017, CancerCare hosted 117 online support groups for patients, caregivers, and the bereaved, including 30 groups for caregivers. This support program is one of the most robust, and feedback from surveys has been positive. Following are several CancerCare OSGP participant responses to the latest survey:

- It allowed me to normalize what I was experiencing and made me feel less isolated. It gave me support and allowed me to be open with my thoughts and feelings. It was a safe place where I could broach any topic.
- Being able to share my experience helped me process it. The Moderator was very experienced and helpful and addressed me personally each time. It felt good to have people cheering me along.
- I met one wonderful friend out of this experience and we continue to support each other.
- People were friendly and supported one another. This helped tremendously, especially when I was feeling alone and depressed. It was also a great place to vent a little without being judged. The advice given was also very helpful and useful.
- Knowing there were others experiencing the same emotions and challenges was very comforting. Just knowing I wasn't the only one helped save my sanity a time or two as well.
- It is helpful to know there are others experiencing the same kind of isolation, frustrations, demands, and a whole host of emotions.
- Being able to "vent" and be "honest" about what was going on and what feelings people were having was wonderful. No one was being critical, but instead everyone was always supportive of each other.

CANCERCARE FINANCIAL ASSISTANCE

Financial burden, more pointedly described in recent literature as financial toxicity, is the measurable out-of-pocket expenses and the subjective emotional stress associated with the high cost of cancer care.[16] As the prevalence and impact of financial toxicity becomes more pronounced, a growing number of studies are being conducted to further determine the exact causes and solutions. For example, a study in 2011 found that the risk of high financial burden was significantly greater for patients with cancer compared with other chronically ill patients.[17] The study reported that 13.4% of patients with cancer spent more than 20% of their income on healthcare, as opposed to 9.7% among those with other chronic conditions. Another study in 2013 examined the link between cancer-related financial toxicity and the increased risk of bankruptcy and found that patients with cancer are nearly three times more likely to declare bankruptcy than those without cancer. Recent research is now suggesting a link between financial toxicity and greater risk of mortality, which highlights the significant impact of this domain of burden on emotional and physical health-related quality of life.[18]

CancerCare conducted a national survey of people with various types of cancer (N = 509) to determine patient needs. The survey reported that 33% of patients aged 21–64 and 20% of patients aged 65 and over had to give up basic needs, like transportation and groceries, in order to pay for their cancer treatment.[4] The same survey also reported that 21% of respondents aged 21–64 and 4% of those aged 65 and over could not pay at least one utility bill. Seventeen percent aged 21–64 and 4% aged 65 and over missed one rent or mortgage payment.[4] Last, 11% aged 21–64 and 4% aged 65 and over considered filing for bankruptcy, and 5% aged 21–64 and 2% aged 65 and over actually declared bankruptcy.[4] This financial burden significantly impacts caregivers, who often provide or supplement financial support. When financial toxicity prevents patients and caregivers from meeting their basic needs, it is more difficult for them to cope with the psychological impact of the diagnosis. When financial toxicity is identified and reduced, however, patients and their caregivers may more readily process the deeper meaning and impact of cancer on their lives.[19]

CancerCare has been addressing financial toxicity throughout its tenure, providing direct financial support to patients and caregivers. CancerCare recently conducted an extensive survey to better understand the financial challenges experienced by over 580 patients and caregivers and found that 75% of clients reported they were very distressed or extremely distressed about finances at the start of treatment. After contacting CancerCare, 93% of clients reported that CancerCare's financial assistance mitigated their distress.

CancerCare provides financial assistance for cancer-related costs, such as transportation, home care, and child care. The team of CancerCare oncology social workers is also dedicated to helping those they serve find additional resources to ease their financial burdens. Additionally, the CancerCare Co-Payment Assistance Foundation helps to cover the cost of chemotherapy and targeted treatments. During fiscal year 2017, CancerCare disbursed over $26.4 million in financial assistance to more than 24,516 people.

ONLINE HELPING HAND

While cancer is an expensive and difficult illness, there are many organizations that can provide assistance. In order to make these resources more easily accessible to patients and caregivers, CancerCare created the Online Helping Hand, a comprehensive online tool featuring the most up-to-date contact information and descriptions for hundreds of national and regional organizations offering financial help to people with cancer. In 2017, there were 20,000 searches conducted through CancerCare's Online Helping Hand. CancerCare believes that the ability of caregivers to understand medical and nonmedical costs is the first step to identifying solutions that can help them address these life-altering challenges.

CANCERCARE'S WEBSITES

CancerCare's websites are valuable resources for anyone affected by cancer. These comprehensive websites host a wealth of information on all of CancerCare services, as well as access to the Caregiver Portal, Connect Education Workshops, publications, and the Online Helping Hand. CancerCare websites welcomed 2.1 million visitors in 2017.

CAREGIVER-SPECIFIC ONLINE TOOLS

As caregivers juggle multiple tasks in addition to managing family, work, and other priorities in their own lives, it is an unnecessary added burden to navigate the process of seeking appropriate support. As a solution, CancerCare provides two caregiver-specific tools.

MyCancerCircle™ is a private support community created specifically for caregivers. Clients have found that this simple online tool helps to organize the community of people in their support network who are asking, "What can I do to help?" and more efficiently coordinates their efforts. Those in a caregiver's private community circle can post words of encouragement and support to one another, and the caregiver can post routine updates and information. MyCancerCircle web portal also contains CancerCare caregiver-specific resources. In 2017, MyCancerCircle served 40,089 active users in 3,019 active caregiving communities.

Help for Cancer Caregivers is an online tool to assist caregivers to create a private personal care guide to help them navigate the complex world of caregiving. Users answer six short questions based on how they have been coping in the past 7 days. A private personal care guide is instantly prepared based on the users' answers. The website also hosts a library of caregiver-specific literature, as well as a comprehensive list of resources from other organizations.

CONNECT EDUCATION WORKSHOPS

Cancer*Care*'s 1-hour educational cancer workshops directly connect attendees with leading oncology experts. These free workshops provide up-to-date information on the latest treatment options, coping techniques, and more. Registrants can listen live, over the phone, or online as a webcast. In 2017, leading experts in oncology led 69 Cancer*Care* Connect® Education Workshops, featuring 127 faculty members and 95 partner organizations, drawing 76,914 participants living in 39 different countries. Twenty-two of these workshops were created specifically for caregivers.

The following is a list of select Connect Education Workshops for Caregivers:

- For Caregivers: Care Coordination for Your Loved One Living with Cancer and Other Health Problems
- Helping Cancer Patients and Their Families Cope with the Stresses of Caregiving: A Workshop for Oncology Nurses and Social Workers, as well as Health Care Professionals, People Living with Cancer, and Their Caregivers
- Changing Roles and Responsibilities for Caregivers
- Stress Management for Caregivers: Taking Care of Yourself Physically and Emotionally
- Survivors Too: Family, Friends and Loved Ones—Managing the Fatigue of Caregiving
- For Caregivers: Coping with Holidays, Special Occasions and Birthdays, Throughout the Year
- Balancing Your Needs and Your Role as a Caregiver
- Coping with the Stresses of Caregiving When Your Loved One Has Triple Negative Breast Cancer
- When Your Loved One Has CML: How Caregivers Can Help Improve Adherence
- For Caregivers: Practical Tips to Cope with Your Loved One's Lung Cancer
- Getting Prepared: Knowing When to Ask for Help for Caregivers When Your Loved One Has Renal Cell Cancer

PUBLICATIONS

Cancer*Care*'s extensive library of easy-to-read booklets and fact sheets provides reliable information on cancer-related topics. Written by experts, we currently feature more than 275 educational titles with 21 titles specific to caregivers. These publications can be read instantly online, downloaded as PDFs, or mailed to the home. In 2017, there were 792,953 publications viewed online and distributed.

LEGALHEALTH CLINIC

In collaboration with the New York Legal Assistance Group (NYLAG), Cancer*Care* provides free, weekly on-site legal clinics for people affected by cancer, including caregivers. In 2017, the LegalHealth attorneys helped 104 individuals on 185 legal matters. These attorneys addressed legal concerns regarding government benefits, advance care planning, insurance concerns, employment, housing, and debt issues.

YOGA AND MEDITATION WORKSHOPS

Yoga and meditation can provide an outlet to calm and rejuvenate the mind and body for those affected by cancer. Cancer*Care*'s ongoing yoga and meditation workshops allow clients to come together in a quiet space, relax, and connect.

CASE EXAMPLE

The client story that follows exemplifies numerous issues caregivers may face and how Cancer*Care*'s services can assist with adaptation and coping

Steve, Caregiver, In-Person Group Member

Steve is a 74-year-old man whose only child, a 24-year-old daughter, was diagnosed with Stage 2 Hodgkin's lymphoma. Though Steve has a strong support network, including his wife, friends, and family, he found he was struggling to cope with the diagnosis:

> I freaked out when the doctors told my 24-year-old daughter, my wife and me that my daughter had cancer. I was dazed, numb and unbelieving. Cancer only happened to other people, not my only child. I didn't know what to do, what

to think—I was initially paralyzed. I felt helpless and was unable to express my feelings and my frustration. It took a week after the biopsy to get a full diagnosis. Every morning that week I cried my eyes out in the shower. I'm a glass half empty person and kept imaging the worst. I had constant morbid thoughts about my daughter's funeral.

My wife and I dealt with the situation clinically, facilitated my daughter's travel and her office visits and took care of the mounting medical bills. However, we were not dealing with the emotional toll. We did not discuss how we were feeling. I kept everything inside of me, was my stoic self but internal pressure and anxiety were building. I couldn't get rid of the negative thoughts and did not wish to express them at home because I did not want to bring my wife down or depress her.

Steve decided to seek support, and the hospital social worker referred him to CancerCare. Steve called the CancerCare Hopeline and spoke to an oncology social worker about his daughter's diagnosis and concerns as a caregiver. Steve and the CancerCare social worker explored concerns, and the social worker provided support and psychoeducation about caregiver-specific issues. In discussing which services would best meet Steve's needs, Steve registered for the in-person caregiver support group. This group met weekly for 12 weeks and consisted of eight caregivers from diverse backgrounds and in varying relationships to patients, who had varying cancer diagnoses, treatment plans, and prognoses.

When asked about the group experience, Steve stated: "I was never so depressed in my life. As the sessions went on I never felt so lucky in my life."

In the group, Steve was able to address the anxiety and fear he was experiencing, as well as learn new ways of coping as a caregiver. Additionally, he could provide support and help others who were struggling with their own caregiver-related concerns, which provided him with a sense of agency and purpose. Indeed, he learned from each of his group members.

At the end of the group, Steve said the following:

I soon realized that most caregivers need at least two things in order to cope and do the best for their loved one with cancer and themselves. First, the caregiver needs a break from the ongoing responsibilities which are physically and emotionally exhausting. They need to get out of the house, find some alone time . . . a trip to the movies or a walk in the park with a friend can rejuvenate someone. Second, and most importantly, they need someone to talk to, to express their anxieties, fears, hopes and dreams to, because they are emotionally involved. The CancerCare groups serve a meaningful purpose on both counts. We have this terrible thing in common that others, even close family friends, cannot really comprehend until it strikes home. We focused on the important things and we were there for each other in a way that very few others could be.

RESILIENCE AND HOPE

Despite the demands of caregiving and the physical and psychosocial burden it brings, cancer caregiving can also be a meaningful experience. Benefits of providing care may include increased self-esteem, greater sense of agency, meaning-making, spirituality, strengthened interpersonal relationships, and a sense of purpose.[13,20-26] Finding the benefit in difficult life experiences may also improve quality of life for caregivers and patients through survivorship.[27] Further, psychosocial support is directly linked to benefit-finding, which can improve overall quality of life.[28] By actively engaging caregivers, providing psychosocial support, and emphasizing strengths, oncology social workers are in a unique position to improve the quality of life of both the caregiver and the patient. This has always been the goal of CancerCare's services. As the caregiver population grows, CancerCare's oncology social workers, through numerous innovative services and modalities, will continue to help build resilience and inspire hope to improve physical and psychological well-being, reduce stress, and increase a sense of competence.

REFERENCES

1. American Cancer Society. (2017). *Cancer Facts and Figures 2018*. Atlanta, GA: American Cancer Society. https://www.cancer.org/content/dam/cancer-org/research/cancer-facts-and-statistics/annual-cancer-facts-and-figures/2018/cancer-facts-and-figures-2018.pdf
2. American Cancer Society. (2016). *Cancer Treatment & Survivorship Facts & Figures 2016–2017*. Atlanta, GA: American Cancer Society. https://www.cancer.org/content/dam/cancer-org/research/cancer-facts-and-statistics/cancer-treatment-and-survivorship-facts-and-figures/cancer-treatment-and-survivorship-facts-and-figures-2016-2017.pdf
3. Dégi, C. L. (2009). Non-disclosure of cancer diagnosis: an examination of personal, medical, and psychosocial factors. *Supportive Care in Cancer*, 17(8), 1101–1107.
4. CancerCare. (2016). *CancerCare Patient Access and Engagement Report*. New York, NY: CancerCare.
5. National Alliance for Caregiving and AARP. (2015). Caregiving in the US. http://www.caregiving.org/wp-content/uploads/2015/05/2015_CaregivingintheUS_Final-Report-June-4_WEB.pdf
6. National Alliance for Caregiving. (2016). Cancer caregiving in the US—an intense, episodic, and challenging care experience. http://www.caregiving.org/wp-content/uploads/2016/06/CancerCaregivingReport_FINAL_June-17-2016.pdf

7. Northouse, L., Williams, A. L., Given, B., & McCorkle, R. (2012). Psychosocial care for family caregivers of patients with cancer. *Journal of Clinical Oncology, 30*(11), 1227–1234.
8. Oken, D. (1961). What to tell cancer patients: a study of medical attitudes. *JAMA, 175*(13), 1120–1128. https://jamanetwork.com/journals/jama/article-abstract/330783
9. Figg, W. D., Smith, E. K., Price, D. K., et al. (2010). Disclosing a diagnosis of cancer: where and how does it occur? *Journal of Clinical Oncology, 28*(22), 3630.
10. Chi, N.-C., & Demiris, G. (2015). A systematic review of telehealth tools and interventions to support family caregivers. *Journal of Telemedicine and Telecare, 21*(1), 37–44. https://www.ncbi.nlm.nih.gov/pubmed/25475220
11. Tang, W. P., Chan, C. W., So, W. K., & Leung, D. Y. (2014). Web-based interventions for caregivers of cancer patients: a review of literatures. *Asia-Pacific Journal of Oncology Nursing, 1*(1), 9. https://www.ncbi.nlm.nih.gov/pmc/articles/PMC5123453/
12. DuBenske, L. L., Gustafson, D. H., Shaw, B. R., & Cleary, J. F. (2010). Web-based cancer communication and decision making systems: connecting patients, caregivers, and clinicians for improved health outcomes. *Medical Decision Making, 30*(6), 732–744. https://www.ncbi.nlm.nih.gov/pmc/articles/PMC3085247/
13. Applebaum, A. J., Buda, K. L., Schofield, E., et al. (2018). Exploring the cancer caregiver's journey through web-based meaning-centered psychotherapy. *Psycho-Oncology, 27*(3), 847–856.
14. Kaltenbaugh, D. J., Klem, M. L., Hu, L., Turi, E., Haines, A. J., & Lingler, J. H. (2015). Using web-based interventions to support caregivers of patients with cancer: a systematic review. *Oncology nursing forum, 42*(2), 156–164. https://pdfs.semanticscholar.org/143d/0b880b35602ad3c0689cd37e5691cf352771.pdf
15. Klemm, P. R., Hayes, E. R., Diefenbeck, C. A., & Milcarek, B. (2014). Online support for employed informal caregivers: psychosocial outcomes. *CIN: Computers, Informatics, Nursing, 32*(1), 10–20.http://vmcancercare.org/pdf/research/2014-Klemm.pdf
16. Zafar, S. Y., & Abernethy, A. P. (2013). Financial toxicity, part I: a new name for a growing problem. *Oncology (Williston Park), 27*(2), 80–81, 149.
17. Bernard, D. S., Farr, S. L., & Fang, Z. (2011). National estimates of out-of-pocket health care expenditure burdens among nonelderly adults with cancer: 2001 to 2008. *Journal of Clinical Oncology, 29*(20), 2821–2826. https://www.ncbi.nlm.nih.gov/pubmed/21632508.
18. Zafar, S. Y. (2015). Financial toxicity of cancer care: it's time to intervene. *JNCI: Journal of the National Cancer Institute, 108*(5), pii: djv370.
19. Chi, M. (2017). The hidden cost of cancer: helping clients cope with financial toxicity. *Clinical Social Work Journal.* https://doi.org/10.1007/s10615-017-0640-7
20. Adams, R. N., Mosher, C. E., Cannady, R. S., et al. (2014). Caregiving experiences predict changes in spiritual well-being among family caregivers of cancer patients. *Psycho-Oncology, 23*(10), 1184–1187.
21. Applebaum, A. J., Farran, C. J. Marilizano, A. M., et al. (2014). Preliminary study of themes of meaning and psychosocial service use among informal cancer caregivers. *Palliative and Supportive Care, 12*(2), 139–148.
22. Applebaum, A. J., Kulikowski, J. R., & Breitbart, W. (2015). Meaning-centered psychotherapy for cancer caregivers (MCP-C): rationale and overview. *Palliative and Supportive Care, 13*(6), 1631–1641.

23. Ellis, K. R., Janevic, M. R., Kershaw, T., et al. (2017). Meaning-based coping, chronic conditions and quality of life in advanced cancer & caregiving. *Psycho-Oncology, 26*(9), 1316–1323.
24. Farran, C. J., Keane-Hagerty, E., Salloway, S., et al. (1991). Finding meaning: an alternative paradigm for Alzheimer's disease family caregivers. *Gerontologist, 31*(4), 483–489.
25. Ferrell, B. R., & Baird, P. (2012). Deriving meaning and faith in caregiving. *Seminars in Oncology Nursing, 28*(4), 256–261.
26. Kim, Y., Schulz, R., & Carver, C. S. (2007). Benefit finding in the cancer caregiving experience. *Psychosomatic Medicine, 69*(3), 283–291. http://citeseerx.ist.psu.edu/viewdoc/download?doi=10.1.1.505.1502&rep=rep1&type=pdf
27. Given, B. A., Sherwood, P., & Given, C. W. (2011). Support for caregivers of cancer patients: transition after active treatment. *Cancer Epidemiology and Prevention Biomarkers, 20*(10), 2015–2021. https://pdfs.semanticscholar.org/0905/aa9a6cf2 5eb45935dce6f61ac2d11fa9effe.pdf
28. Brand, C., Barry, L., & Gallagher, S. (2016). Social support mediates the association between benefit finding and quality of life in caregivers. *Journal of Health Psychology, 21*(6), 1126–1136. http://journals.sagepub.com/doi/abs/10.1177/1359105314547244

SECTION 5

Future Directions

CHAPTER 18

Important Legal Concerns Faced by Informal Cancer Caregivers

DEBRA WOLF AND CRISTINA PEJOVES GORMAN

In addressing the often devastating consequences of a cancer diagnosis, attention is usually focused on the common legal issues faced by cancer patients. Such issues may include work accommodations, paid medical leave, access to medical care and the need for advanced planning. A combination of federal, state, and local laws governs each of these areas and provides rights, protections, and benefits to cancer patients and, in some circumstances, their families. More recently, attention has also been directed to the rights of caregivers, who may face work or financial implications when taking on the role of caregiver to a relative or friend diagnosed with cancer. When oncology, medical, and social work providers have a fundamental understanding of these legal issues and protections, they can better assist patient caregivers by helping them improve coping skills and expanding available patient services and resources.

This chapter explores the laws that offer various types of support to caregivers, as well as some of the conflicts faced by caregivers appointed as healthcare agents when making difficult medical decisions for their loved ones.

LEGAL CONCERNS

Federal Laws
Family Medical Leave Act

According to the Family Caregiver Alliance, the average age of a caregiver is 49.2 years, with 48% of caregivers falling between the ages of 18 and 49.[1] Parent care continues to be the primary caregiving situation for midlife caregivers, with 70% of the parent caregivers between the ages of 50 and 64.[2] As such, many caregivers struggle to balance jobs with their caregiving responsibilities. In addressing the workplace rights of caregivers, their relationship to the patient is critical. The principal law that offers job protection to caregivers is the Family Medical Leave Act of 1993 (FMLA),[3] a federal law that applies equally to all 50 states. To be covered under FMLA, an employee must work for an employer with 50 or more employees, and employees must have worked at their job for a minimum of 1 year, with at least 1,250 hours worked over the last 12-month period. Eligible employees are entitled to 12 weeks of job-protected leave per 12-month period to care for an immediate family member with a serious health condition. An immediate family member is defined as a spouse, minor child, adult disabled child, or parent with a serious health condition.

FMLA leave is unpaid, although a caregiver may be able to supplement time off with accrued sick or vacation time. The employer must maintain all employee benefits; however, the employee must continue to make any benefit contributions, including healthcare or other insurance premiums paid from his or her salary.

FMLA leave can be taken as a block of time for up to 12 weeks. FMLA also provides for intermittent leave when medically necessary, which allows the employee to take leave "in separate blocks of time for a single qualifying reason—or on a reduced leave schedule—reducing the employee's usual weekly or daily work schedule."[4] Thus, FMLA leave may be taken in periods of whole weeks, single days, hours, and in some cases even less than an hour. Intermittent FMLA may be useful if a caregiver plans to attend medical appointments and treatment while maintaining his or her job. An example where intermittent FMLA may benefit a caregiver includes the following:

Charlotte has been providing care to her father, Marcus, who has stage 4 lung cancer. Marcus has sufficient income to pay for home health aides during the hours that

Charlotte works. However, Charlotte must drive Marcus to his medical appointments and often sits with him during his chemotherapy. She always tries to schedule these appointments and treatment for the late afternoon to reduce the impact on her work schedule.

Charlotte has worked for a large advertising company with over 100 employees since 2011. Her employer offers generous sick time, but lately her supervisor has been commenting on the number of afternoons Charlotte has taken off. In order to understand her workplace rights prior to meeting with human resources, Charlotte consulted with an attorney, who advised her to apply for intermittent FMLA. Charlotte then met with her human resources representative and completed the paper work for FMLA, which required that Marcus's oncologist certify that he has a serious health issue. Charlotte requested FMLA intermittent leave for every other Thursday afternoon for Marcus's treatment, as well as other times on an "as needed" basis for any emergencies that may arise. Under FMLA, because Charlotte works full time, she will be covered for up to 480 hours of leave, calculated as 12 weeks times 40 hours per week.

The United States Department of Labor (DOL) has a website devoted to information on FMLA.[5] FMLA sets the minimum standard required by covered employers. Employers may choose to offer enhanced leave benefits, so it is critical that caregivers review their employee benefit plans regarding family medical leave. Employees who work in smaller offices of less than 50 employees do not have FMLA protection and should familiarize themselves with their employers' leave policies. State caregiver protection laws, discussed in material that follows, are inadequate or, in most states, nonexistent.

According to the DOL, only 15% of the workforce has paid family leave through employers.[6] Some states have recently enacted laws to offer paid or protected medical leave, although very few laws to date offer these protections to family caregivers.[7] Although various laws have been introduced, presently (2018) only Rhode Island, California, New Jersey, and New York have laws that offer paid leave to care for a family member with a serious illness. Washington State and the District of Columbia have similar laws that will be implemented in 2020. The leave time allowed varies, from 4 weeks (Rhode Island) to 8 weeks (New York). The amount of the benefit also varies and is generally a percentage of the employee's income, ranging from 50% to 70%, but each state also has a maximum benefit allowed. The benefits are limited and cannot be relied on to allow a caregiver to support themselves if they are planning to stop work for an extended period of time.

Americans With Disabilities Act

Another federal law, the 1990 Americans With Disabilities Act (ADA; amended in 2009) is often relied on by cancer patients for workplace protections.[8] The ADA prohibits employment discrimination based on disability and applies to employers with 15 or more employees. Although most of the protections of the ADA are for the benefit of the disabled employee, and caregivers are not considered a covered group under the law, the law does offer some protection to caregivers in that it prohibits "unlawful disparate treatment" of employees with caregiving responsibilities. The Equal Employment Opportunity Commission (EEOC), in their Enforcement Guidance on Unlawful Disparate Treatment of Workers With Caregiving Responsibilities, offers examples of disparate treatment, which include the following:

- Treating male caregivers more favorably than female caregivers;
- Reducing a female employee's workload after she assumes caregiving responsibilities based on the assumption that, as a female caregiver, she will not want to work overtime;
- Denying a male caregiver leave under such circumstances where such leave would be granted to a female;
- Stereotyping based on association with a person with a disability; for example, refusing to hire a worker who cares for someone with a disability based on the assumption his or her work will be unreliable; or
- Harassing caregiver workers based on the above criteria thus creating a hostile work environment.[9]

Recognize, Assist, Include, Support, and Engage Family Caregivers Act

In January 2018, the Recognize, Assist, Include, Support, and Engage (RAISE) Family Caregivers Act was signed into law. RAISE requires the Secretary of Health and Human Services to develop a strategy within a 3-year period to recognize and support family caregivers. The law also calls for the creation of an advisory council, which would include representatives from the private and public sectors, including family caregivers, veterans, providers of healthcare and long-term services and supports, employers, state and local officials, and others, to advise and make recommendations for communities, providers, government, and others.[10] They are likely to address topics affecting caregivers, such as workplace flexibility, education for navigating the healthcare system, and assessment and service planning, including care transitions and coordination.[11]

Patient Self-Determination Act

The Patient Self-Determination Act (PSDA; 42 U.S.C. Sec. 1395cc(f)(1) of 1990) requires most healthcare facilities to ask patients at the time of admission if they have advance directives; to provide written information about their healthcare decision-making rights under state law; to document in their medical records whether the patients have advance directives; to educate their staff about advance directives; and to never discriminate against patients based on whether they have advance directives. PSDA applies to hospitals, long-term care facilities, and home health agencies that receive Medicare and Medicaid reimbursement.[12] The completion of advance directives not only offers guidance to caregivers who may be forced to make critical decisions on behalf of the patient, but also minimizes family conflict surrounding treatment decisions.

State Laws

The Care Act

Caregivers take on responsibilities ranging from household tasks, such as shopping and handling finances; to nursing/medical tasks, like managing medications, providing wound care, and operating specialized medical equipment. In a survey of 1,677 family caregivers conducted by the AARP Public Policy Institute and the United Hospital Fund, many caregivers reported that they learned on their own how to manage many of the necessary medical tasks. Without proper training, however, caregivers justifiably feel anxious and fearful of making a mistake that could harm their family member.[13]

The AARP (formerly known as the American Association of Retired Persons) is the world's largest consumer advocacy organization, with nearly 38 million members age 50 and older. The AARP drafted model legislation that would standardize hospital procedures and help caregivers as their family members make the transition from the hospital back to home. The Caregiver Advise, Record, Enable (CARE) Act has three main provisions: First, it requires hospitals to record the name of the family caregiver on the medical record of his or her loved one who is admitted for treatment; second, the hospitals are required to inform the family caregiver when his or her loved one is to be transferred or discharged; and third, the hospitals must provide the family caregiver with education and instruction concerning the medical tasks he or she will need to perform for the patient at home. The AARP, recognizing the difficulty of passing federal legislation, has taken a state-by-state approach. To date, the CARE Act has been signed into law in 36 states, the District of Columbia, Puerto Rico, and the US Virgin Islands.[14] In 48 states, more than 90 AARP-backed laws, regulations, and rules have been adopted to help family caregivers.

Although many hospitals state that they have always done what the CARE Act requires, they also recognize that the Act is causing them to formalize procedures, in addition to contributing to a cultural shift whereby family caregivers are being recognized as partners in a patient's recovery and improved health outcomes. In 2017, the AARP conducted a national survey of hospitals in states that passed the CARE Act and found that the Act has given hospitals cause to rethink how they engage with patients and their families. Most hospitals had formed or were forming patient and family advisory councils, while others were including family caregivers in daily rounds. At least one hospital credited these changes with helping them to significantly reduce readmissions.[15]

The American Cancer Society Cancer Action Network has stated its support of the CARE Act, noting that "in particular, for older patients undergoing chemotherapy at home, patients and their designated caregivers need to understand the prescribed chemotherapy medications and any medications given to alleviate pain or nausea, as well as the signs and symptoms associated with adverse reactions. The CARE Act's focus on involving patients and their designated caregivers in discharge planning, and providing training for necessary after-care tasks such as managing medications, will help ensure that caregivers can help patients receive the necessary care at home."[16]

Palliative Care Laws

There has been a recent, albeit slowly forming, trend toward ensuring that patients who would benefit from palliative care are identified and assisted. Some of the recent state actions include the following:

New York passed the Palliative Care Information Act in 2011, which requires physicians and nurses to offer palliative care and end-of-life counseling to terminally ill patients. "The law is intended to ensure that patients are fully informed of the options available to them when they are faced with a terminal illness or condition, so that they are empowered to make choices consistent with their goals for care, and wishes and beliefs, and to optimize their quality of life."[17]

Massachusetts and Oregon both recently enacted laws that require medical facilities to identify patients who could benefit from palliative care and provide information regarding its availability.[18]

In a 2013 study based on California Assembly Bill AB487, which mandates physicians complete 12 hours of study in pain management and end-of-life care, 90% of physicians reported that they had changed their practices in specific ways to ensure the comfort of their patients. The law was designed to help patients maintain what they most desire at end of life: their dignity and to be free of pain. Studies showed that dying patients often receive inadequate pain relief.[19]

These laws and trends are important in the caregiving context as patient comfort relieves some of the emotional and physical burdens faced by caregivers, as discussed throughout this text.

FINANCIAL CONCERNS

Given the general lack of legal protections and pay continuation for caregivers, a common question concerns the rights of family members or friends to be compensated for their caregiving role. Under limited circumstances, it is possible for caregivers to be compensated or reimbursed for providing care at home for their loved ones.

Medicaid

All 50 states and Washington, DC, offer Medicaid waiver, self-directed, long-term care services and support programs that enable qualified individuals to manage their own care, which includes hiring their own caregivers. Eligibility and coverage under these programs varies state to state; for example, some programs will only pay care providers if they do not live in the same household as the care recipient. Other states, such as New York, permit the care recipients to hire a family member to provide their care. The next material is an example of how New York's program works.

To be eligible for New York's Consumer Directed Personal Assistance Program (CDPAP), a care recipient must have Medicaid, need home care, and be self-directing or have a representative that can direct care. In New York, for CDPAP reimbursement, children can provide care for their parents, parents can provide care for their adult children over 21, but a spouse cannot provide care for another spouse. A family member can live with the care recipient if the adult relative resides with them "because the amount of care the consumer requires makes such relative's presence necessary."[20]

Importantly, the care recipient must first qualify for Medicaid, which has strict income and asset requirements that differ state to state. Caregivers should contact their loved one's local Medicaid office to begin the process. If a care recipient needs home care but is over their state's Medicaid income and asset limits, the care recipient or his or her family member may benefit from contacting an attorney who can help with Medicaid planning.[21] Medicaid eligibility often has special programs or allows the use of certain trusts to enable both the elderly and disabled to access care even if over the income or resource limits.

Veterans

Veteran Directed Home and Community Based Care is available in 37 states; Washington, DC; and Puerto Rico for veterans of any age who are enrolled in the Veterans Health Administration standard medical benefits package and who need the high level of care a nursing home provides but want to live at home. The veteran can choose any physically and mentally capable caregiver, including a spouse, sibling, or grandchild. The veteran is given a flexible budget ($2,500 per month, on average) to choose goods and services they need, including a caregiver.

Aid and Attendance benefits are available to a smaller pool of veterans who meet specific requirements, including qualifying for VA pensions and serving a minimum of 90 days active duty and at least 1 day during a wartime period. This program helps supplement the VA pension to help pay the cost of a caregiver, who can be a family member. The veteran must also meet certain medical requirements, including being bedbound and needing help with activities of daily living.

Another program available to some veterans is the Program of Comprehensive Assistance for Family Caregivers, which offers needed services for primary caregivers of veterans who sustained a traumatic injury in the line of duty on or after September 11, 2001. Some of these benefits include a monthly stipend to the veteran's primary caregiver and coverage of lodging and travel expenses while travelling with veterans who are accessing care.

The VA also offers a Caregiver's Support line that is staffed by licensed professionals who can connect caregivers with VA services, a Caregiver Support Coordinator, or individuals who are just available to listen. The Department of Veterans Affairs website contains useful information about these and other programs and benefits for caregivers of veterans.[22]

Tax Credits and Deductions

Caregivers may be eligible for credits and deductions when they file their taxes. As many specific rules apply, caregivers should keep careful records and may want to consult with an accountant when they first assume their caregiving roles. Some examples include those discussed next.

The Internal Revenue Service (IRS) allows a family caregiver to claim as a dependent anyone related by blood, marriage, adoption, or even friends. If both parties meet the IRS requirements, the caregiver can claim the dependent deduction on their federal tax return.

Caregivers may be able to deduct the money they pay to cover their loved one's unreimbursed medical expenses if the medical expenses of everyone claimed on their taxes totals more than 10% of their adjusted gross income. Acceptable deductions include, but are not limited to, copays, deductibles, transportation, and hearing aids.

Caregivers may use their flexible spending accounts (FSAs) to pay for out-of-pocket medical expenses for dependents. If a caregiver uses an FSA, they cannot also take the deduction on their taxes.

The Child and Dependent Care Credit allows a caregiver who is paying for an adult day care program or a home health aide to claim a tax credit.[23]

Proposed Legislation

A national AARP study showed that family caregivers spend, on average, nearly $7,000 of their own funds annually on caregiving, which is almost 20% of their income.[24] The AARP has proposed legislation called the Credit for Caring Act, which would create a federal, nonrefundable tax credit of up to $3,000 for family caregivers who work while also financially supporting their loved ones.[25] This type of legislation would help alleviate the financial strain that many caregivers are facing.

HOW ADVANCE DIRECTIVES BENEFIT PATIENTS, CAREGIVERS, AND PROVIDERS

When first diagnosed, cancer patients should be encouraged to complete advance directives, written statements of a person's wishes regarding medical treatment that are prepared to ensure that his or her wishes are carried out should he or she lose capacity or the ability to effectively communicate with physicians. Advance directives are executed in advance and may become effective on incapacity to protect a person's right to decide what medical care he or she receives.

Although state law varies, the law generally presumes a person is competent and that a competent person has the right to consent to healthcare treatment as well as the right to refuse treatment. To make these medical decisions, the patient must be able to give "informed consent," meaning the individual understands the risks and benefits of a proposed treatment, any available alternative treatment, and who will provide the treatment.

The two most common advance directives are the healthcare proxy and living will. The healthcare proxy allows a person to choose an agent to make healthcare decisions should he or she become incapacitated and unable to communicate his or her wishes. Once a healthcare proxy is executed and doctors have determined that the patient no longer has capacity, the chosen agent becomes authorized to make health-related decisions for the patient. Healthcare proxy laws vary state by state, but, generally, an agent can make medical decisions, including end-of-life care, consult with doctors or request second opinions, and examine the patient's medical records.

The living will is a statement of one's wishes with respect to a number of potential end-of-life medical decisions. A living will may include a request to allow a person to maintain palliative care to ease pain, such as increased morphine, while requesting that measures such as cardiopulmonary resuscitation (CPR) or mechanical respiration, which will prolong life but not enhance quality of life, not be undertaken. Again, the legal requirements and recognition of a living will vary state by state.

Advance directives have been recognized in every state, although the forms and requirements vary.[26] They are relatively simple forms to complete without requiring an attorney. The American Bar Association has an online toolkit for advance planning that contains a link to state-specific advance directive forms.[27] Ensuring that the patient completes these documents early on is critical as the proper execution of advance directives requires that the patient have sufficient mental capacity to understand the purpose and implications of the document.

Caregivers are often viewed as partners with the medical team, and patients often rely on their caregiver's involvement in physician interaction. However, disputes can still arise that complicate decision-making for the care of the patient. Such conflicts may include the following:

- Disagreements between the caregiver and other members of the patient's family regarding the needs of the patient. These disputes may arise from many different concerns, ranging from ongoing medical care choices even to religious implications.

- Disagreements between the patient and family caregiver regarding a medical or treatment decision, including a caregiver's concern that they may not be able to meet the increased need of the patient or that the patient is making a poor treatment decision.
- Social work or physician concerns based on confidential discussions with the patient that the caregiver is not providing adequate support or meeting patient needs.

As a first step, in order to reduce the possibility of disputes or to minimize their impact, encourage patients to prepare advance directives. Along with an expression of the patient's wishes, advance directives offer guidance to caregivers, who may be forced to make critical decisions if the person they are caring for loses the capacity to make their own choices. They may also help to resolve family disputes that may arise when a relative is ill and requires care and assistance. Encouraging the preparation of advance directives can prevent exacerbating many of the family dynamics and resulting disputes, as the named agent is chosen by the patient and is legally authorized to make these decisions. One such example is illustrated next.

Case Example

George and Margaret have been married for 11 years, a second marriage for both. After spending time talking about their wishes for healthcare and end-of-life decisions, both executed healthcare proxies naming the other as their agent. Margaret was diagnosed with metastatic cancer and is now at end-stage illness. George has been her primary caregiver. Margaret has two adult daughters from her first marriage who have also been involved in assisting with her needs since she became ill. Margaret no longer has capacity, and, with her oncologist's recommendation, George has made a decision to discontinue treatment and provide increased palliative care. Margaret's daughters disagree and believe their mother should continue with her treatment, and the children have not been able to reach a resolution with George. A family meeting was scheduled to help George and his step-daughters find common ground on Margaret's care.

At the meeting, the hospital social worker prefaced the discussion by ensuring that the healthcare proxy was validly executed and thus a legally binding document. Should the family not reach agreement, George retained the legal right to make all healthcare decisions on Margaret's behalf.

If no healthcare agent has been named in advance, most states have surrogate decision-making laws that establish a priority list of family, or even good friends, that the medical team can look to for medical decision-making once a patient's capacity is lost. The American Bar Association has published a chart of states with surrogate consent statutes that can be useful in understanding the requirements of each state.[28] The surrogate laws also set forth any limitations on the agent's authority and a process for resolving disputes. For example, if, based on the priority list, the surrogates are the patient's adult children, it is possible that these adult siblings may disagree on decisions to be made for their parent.

The surrogate laws may be helpful when other matters arise that complicate the need for medical decisions for an incapacitated patient. For example, a caregiver named as agent may decide he or she no longer wants the responsibility of making medical decisions. Circumstances do arise when caregivers are either no longer interested in continuing this role or are unable to continue due to health or financial concerns of their own. Healthcare proxies do allow for the naming of an alternate surrogate, and these documents should always be examined to see if the patient has named an alternate. If not, the state's surrogate law will apply to designate someone with decision-making responsibilities.

Even with a healthcare agent named, the competent patient retains the sole right to make medical decisions. Continued discussions between the medical team and the patient are recommended.[29] Patients and caregivers or family members may disagree on a proposed treatment plan or decision to end treatment. Treatment decisions affect caregiving responsibilities, and social work intervention may be necessary to ensure not only that the patient's goals are met, but also that the impact on caregivers is acceptable and manageable.

Special consideration for the caregiver's role must also be made when discharge planning for hospitalized patients. Studies have shown that inadequate discharge planning not only impacts the patient's quality of life but also results in a lack of support for the caregiver.[30] Once palliative care is implemented, caregivers face added burdens, including meeting the needs of the patient, navigating the health systems, and ensuring financial obligations are met, while also coping with their own anticipatory grief. If a caregiver is unable to provide the needed care, it may be necessary to have a legal consult to determine if the patient qualifies for increased home care through the state Medicaid program as discussed previously.

Encourage the patient, if competent, to seek legal advice if family disputes are interfering with care or causing undue stress on the patient. For patients who may not be able to afford an attorney, the National Cancer Legal Services Network maintains a website with referrals for pro bono attorneys who provide legal guidance to cancer patients.[31] It may be necessary to engage with the hospital general counsel or risk management team if disputes cannot be resolved through a family meeting. Hospitals have developed strategies to address these conflicts and employ techniques that may include family meetings, social work intervention, and the use of the hospital ethics dispute resolution, which may range from informal to formal meetings.[32]

Note that it is also advisable for patients without caregivers, or who are "unbefriended," to complete advance directives. Without advance directives, these patients are at risk of receiving unwanted care, possibly at great expense. By identifying these patients while they retain sufficient mental capacity to execute advance directives, medical providers can help ensure that their patients' wishes are known, which benefits both the patients and the medical providers. Medical providers can help locate surrogate decision-makers or connect patients to community organizations that may serve as surrogates or who may petition for guardianship.

Other Advance Directives

The laws regarding do not resuscitate (DNR) orders vary from state to state and address both inpatient hospital and "nonhospital" DNR orders. DNR orders affect only CPR and are a request not to have CPR if the patient's heart stops or if he or she stops breathing. Every competent adult has the right to refuse life-sustaining treatment, such as CPR.

If there is a healthcare proxy, that agent has authority to decide about all medical treatment, including CPR, unless the proxy form states otherwise. The healthcare agent must decide in accordance with the patient's wishes or, if those wishes are not known, in accordance with the patient's best interests.

Some states also have surrogate decision laws for DNR issues only with a priority list of who can make these decisions. The surrogate is the person highest on the list if he or she is reasonably available, competent, and willing to make the decision. The surrogate must make decisions regarding CPR based on the patient's wishes (including the patient's religious and moral beliefs) or, if those wishes are not known, in accordance with the patient's best interests.

Physician Orders for Life-Sustaining Treatment

The Physician Orders for Life-Sustaining Treatment (POLST) form is an advance directive that also addresses medical care for people with life-threatening illnesses, such as cancer. While POLST forms can include a DNR order, they cover many additional types of medical treatments not included in a DNR, such as intubation, antibiotic use, and feeding tubes.

Unlike other advance directives, the POLST form must be signed by a doctor or other approved healthcare professional in order to be enforceable. The POLST addresses many types of medical treatment not contained in a DNR, such as intubation. The forms vary by state and often have different names, such as MOLST in New York and COLST in Vermont.

Power of Attorney

A power of attorney is an advance directive that allows an individual (known on the form as the "principal") to name an agent to handle their personal affairs during their lifetime, including banking, selling of real or personal property, and other financial matters. It is also useful for potential healthcare planning, particularly for Medicaid.

The most common version is called a durable power of attorney, with which the authority of the agent commences immediately on completion of the form. The durable power of attorney can be used regardless of the principal's capacity and may continue to be used even if the principal becomes incapacitated. A power of attorney is a vitally important advance directive because, without one, court-ordered guardianship may be the only way for a caregiver to access a patient's bank accounts or other financial resources that may be necessary to assist the patient in applying for Medicaid or to ensure their bills are paid. A power of attorney can also be "springing," which means the agent's authority only comes into effect if or when the principal becomes incapacitated and cannot manage his or her own affairs.

It is advised that an attorney assist with the completion of a power of attorney as the form must be completed correctly to be valid. Too often, a patient loses capacity and an error is subsequently discovered on the form. Given the sensitive nature of the agent's authority, including access to bank accounts, it is necessary to make sure the patient understands all of the implications of signing a power of attorney, as well as to ensure that he or she is choosing an agent who is trustworthy.

Both emotional and financial strain are commonly found among caregivers.[33] Encouraging the preparation of advanced directives can alleviate some of the burden in the following ways:

- Fostering a conversation among the patient, caregiver, and family regarding the patient's wishes for end-of-life care, as well as future treatment options.
- Avoiding or eliminating family conflict when the patient has legally designated a person to act as agent should the patient lose the ability to communicate wishes.
- Preparing family or other loved ones for difficult decisions they may have to make, including end-of-life decisions, and providing written guidance of the patient's wishes.
- Allowing the POLST, as well as living wills, to take the burden off the caregiver in making end-of-life decisions. They allow patients to express preferences that may incorporate religious beliefs and concerns about their quality of life and pain tolerance.[34]
- Using a power of attorney to alleviate financial stress by giving caregivers access to bank account funds to continue paying bills; talk to creditors such as credit card companies; sign a renewal lease to their apartment; interact with insurance companies should a medical claim problem arise; and plan for other potential nonmedical needs.

CONCLUSIONS

Cancer caregivers face unique challenges in meeting the needs of their loved ones. While dealing with their own grief, they must continue to provide medical, emotional, and often financial support to patients. Legal protections are limited and, due to their roles, caregivers often face employment implications, as well as family conflict. Caregivers play an integral role in the health and well-being of patients by taking on numerous responsibilities; therefore, an understanding of the legal landscape affecting caregivers will enable oncology medical and mental health providers to offer additional support and resources so that caregivers may better assist patients.

REFERENCES

1. Family Caregiver Alliance National Center on Caregiving. Caregiver statistics: demographics. https://www.caregiver.org/caregiver-statistics-demographics. Updated 2016. Accessed March 21, 2018.
2. Wagner, D., & Takagi, E. (2010). Health Affairs Blog: informal caregiving by and for older adults. https://www.healthaffairs.org/do/10.1377/hblog20100216.003722/full/. Published February 16, 2010. Accessed March 23, 2018.

3. 29 U.S. Code Chapter 28—Family and Medical Leave of 1993.

4. US Department of Labor, Wage and Hour Division. FMLA frequently asked questions. https://www.dol.gov/whd/fmla/fmla-faqs.htm. Accessed March 21, 2018.

5. US Department of Labor, Wage and Hour Division. Fact sheet #28: the Family and Medical Leave Act. https://www.dol.gov/whd/regs/compliance/whdfs28.htm. Updated 2012. Accessed March 21, 2018.

6. US Department of Labor. National compensation survey: employee benefits in the United States, March 2017, Table 32. https://www.bls.gov/ncs/ebs/benefits/2017/ebbl0061.pdf. Published September 2017. Accessed March 81, 2018.

7. National Council of State Legislatures. State family and medical leave laws. http://www.ncsl.org/research/labor-and-employment/state-family-and-medical-leave-laws.aspx. Updated July 19, 2016. Accessed March 21, 2018.

8. Americans With Disabilities Act of 1990, Pub. L. No. 101-336, 104 Stat. 328 (1990). Amended by ADA Amendments Act of 2008.

9. US Equal Employment Opportunity Commission. Questions and answers about EEOC's enforcement guidance on *Unlawful Disparate Treatment of Workers With Caregiving Responsibilities*. https://www.eeoc.gov/policy/docs/qanda_caregiving.html. Updated May 23, 2007. Accessed March 21, 2018.

10. AARP. Congress passes RAISE Family Caregiver Act. https://www.aarp.org/politics-society/advocacy/caregiving-advocacy/info-2015/raise-family-caregivers-act.html. Updated January 7, 2018. Accessed March 22, 2018.

11. Jefferson, R. S. Congress passes, Trump signs RAISE Family Caregivers Act "elevating caregiving to a priority." *Forbes*. https://www.forbes.com/sites/robinseatonjefferson/2018/01/24/congress-passes-trump-signs-raise-family-caregivers-act-elevating-caregiving-to-a-priority/#70262686331f. Published January 24, 2018. Accessed March 21, 2018.

12. American Bar Association. Law for older Americans. Healthcare advanced directives. What is the Patient Self Determination Act? https://www.americanbar.org/groups/public_education/resources/law_issues_for_consumers/patient_self_determination_act.html. Accessed March 22, 2018.

13. Reinhard, S., Levine, C., & Samis, S. Home alone: family caregivers providing complex chronic care. https://www.aarp.org/content/dam/aarp/research/public_policy_institute/health/home-alone-family-caregivers-providing-complex-chronic-care-rev-AARP-ppi-health.pdf. Published October 2012. Accessed March 23, 2018.

14. AARP. New state law to help family caregivers. https://www.aarp.org/politics-society/advocacy/caregiving-advocacy/info-2014/aarp-creates-model-state-bill.html Accessed March 21, 2018.

15. Mason, D. *JAMA* Forum: supporting family caregivers, one state at a time: the CARE Act. news@JAMA. https://newsatjama.jama.com/2017/12/13/jama-forum-supporting-family-caregivers-one-state-at-a-time-the-care-act/. Published December 13, 2017. Accessed March 22, 2018.

16. AARP. What caregiving experts are saying about the Care Act. https://www.aarp.org/politics-society/advocacy/caregiving-advocacy/info-2014/caregiving-experts-care-act.html. Accessed March 28, 2018.

17. New York State Department of Health. Palliative Care Information Act. https://www.health.ny.gov/professionals/patients/patient_rights/palliative_care/information_act.htm. Updated February 2011. Accessed March 23, 2018.

18. Sinclair, S., & Meier, D. Health Affairs Blog: end of life and serious illness. How states can expand access to palliative care. https://www.healthaffairs.org/do/10.1377/hblog20170130.058531/full/. Published January 30, 2017. Accessed March 23, 2018.

19. Leong, L., Ninnis, J., Slatkin, N., et al. Evaluating the impact of pain management (PM) education on physician practice patterns—a continuing education outcomes study. *J Cancer Educ.* 2010;25(2):224–228. https://www.ncbi.nlm.nih.gov/pmc/articles/PMC3751402/. Accessed March 30, 2018.

20. CDPAP by Edison Home Health Care. The ultimate guide to the Consumer Directed Personal Assistance Program (CPDAP). https://cdpapny.org. Accessed March 22, 2018.

21. AARP. Can I get paid to be a caregiver for a family member? https://www.aarp.org/caregiving/financial-legal/info-2017/you-can-get-paid-as-a-family-caregiver.html. Accessed March 22, 2018.

22. US Department of Veterans Affairs. VA Caregiver Support. https://www.caregiver.va.gov/. Accessed March 22, 2018.

23. AARP. Tax tips for caregivers. https://www.aarp.org/caregiving/financial-legal/info-2017/tax-tips-family-caregivers.html. Accessed March 22, 2018.

24. AARP. AARP: Family caregiver tax credit would provide critical help to NYS's middle class. https://states.aarp.org/aarp-family-caregiver-tax-credit-would-provide-critical-help-to-nyss-middle-class/. Accessed March 22, 2018.

25. AARP. The Credit for Caring Act. https://www.aarp.org/caregiving/financial-legal/info-2017/credit-for-caring-act.html. Accessed March 22, 2018.

26. Granter-Hunt, G., Mahoney, J., & Sieger, C. A comparison of state advance directive documents. *Gerontologist.* 2002;42(1):51–60. https://academic.oup.com/gerontologist/article/42/1/51/641490 Accessed March 23, 2018.

27. American Bar Association. Link to state-specific advance directive forms. https://www.americanbar.org/content/dam/aba/administrative/law_aging/2018-lnks-to-st-spcifc-advnc-drctv-frms.authcheckdam.pdf. Updated January 2018. Accessed March 28, 2018.

28. American Bar Association. Default surrogate consent laws. https://www.americanbar.org/content/dam/aba/administrative/law_aging/2014_default_surrogate_consent_statutes.authcheckdam.pdf. Updated January 1, 2018. Accessed March 22, 2018.

29. Mitnick, S., Leffler, C., & Hood, V. Family caregivers, patients and physicians: ethical guidance to optimize relationships. *J Geriatr Intern Med.* 2010;25(3):255–260.

30. Benzar, E., Hansen, L., Kneital, A., & Fromme, E. Discharge planning for palliative care patients: a qualitative analysis. *J Palliat Med.* 2011;14(1):65–69.

31. National Cancer Legal Service Network (NCLSN). Accessed March 23, 2018. http://www.nclsn.org/.

32. Baggish, D. The ethics consultation. *Quinnipiac Probate Law J.* 2010;23:432.

33. Tilden, V., Tolle, S., Drach, L., & Perrin, N. Out-of-hospital death: advance care planning. Decedent symptoms, and caregiver burden. *J Am Geriatr Soc.* 2004;23(4):532–539.

34. Family Caregiver Alliance. Advanced healthcare directives and POLST. https://www.caregiver.org/advance-health-care-directives-and-polst. Updated 2012. Accessed March 23, 2018.

CHAPTER 19
Conclusions and Future Directions

ALLISON J. APPLEBAUM

Cancer caregivers are an essential extension of the healthcare team. Today's shorter hospital stays and shift toward increased outpatient care has placed a significant burden of responsibility on caregivers, many of whom—as documented throughout the first section of this textbook—have little to no preparation for this role. Rapid advances in cancer care, including new drug and immunotherapies and more sophisticated diagnostic tools, have improved our ability to extend lives and enhance survival. Such good news is coupled with the reality that as patients are living longer and in many cases cancer is now a chronic, rather than an abruptly life-limiting, illness, the burden on caregivers and their needs has substantially increased. Indeed, the number of individuals currently providing care for patients with cancer (highlighted by Kent et al. in Chapter 1) is startling: recent US national estimates of cancer caregivers range from 2.8 million[1] to 6.1 million adult individuals,[2] with such caregivers providing care on average for 32.9 hours per week.[3] These demands come at a significant financial cost; time cost per year of informal cancer caregiving is as high as $73,000,[4] and approximately 25% of caregivers make extended employment changes to accommodate their caregiving responsibilities.[5]

Such demands, not surprisingly, are associated with severe personal disruptions and psychosocial impacts, which are explored in detail in Section 1 of this textbook. These chapters highlight the magnitude and multifaceted nature of caregiver burden (Chapters 1 and 2); the unique experience for caregivers at different life stages and with varying relationships to the patient (Chapter 3); distinct burdens placed by specific cancer and treatment types and patients' comorbid psychiatric conditions (Chapter 4); as well as the impact of the cultural context in which caregiving occurs (Chapter 5). It is evident that the impact of modern caregiver burden is vast and encompasses psychological, physical, spiritual, existential, and financial distress, all of which intensify if left untreated.

While no caregiver is immune to burden, as clearly indicated by the statistics on burden that are cited throughout Section 1, it is also clear that some caregivers, such as those who perceive the caregiving role as nonnormative (as discussed in Chapter 3) and those whose caregiving responsibilities and experiences are markedly impacted by unique aspects of the patient's illness or treatment (as discussed in Chapter 4), are at particular risk for negative outcomes. It is also clear that the experience of burden is largely culturally constructed and must be understood in the context of sociocultural factors, such as gender role socialization,[6,7] culturally embedded characteristics related to communalism and familial nurturance,[8] and ethnic group membership (e.g., for many African American, Asian, and Hispanic/Latino family caregivers compared with European American caregivers, providing care to a loved one with cancer is often done without question). Such factors have significant implications for caregivers' perceptions of their role and the associated burden they may eventually experience. Notably, data from the Cancer Support Community's Cancer Experience Registry (see Chapter 15) from over 1,000 caregiver registrants who were predominantly white (87%) showed that 68% reported having no choice in becoming a caregiver. This perspective implies feelings of powerlessness and likely varies from the experience of individuals from cultures that emphasize *familism*, a "strong identification and attachment of individuals with their families (nuclear and extended) and strong feelings of loyalty, reciprocity and solidarity among members of the same family" (p. 71) (in chapter 5, Sociocultural Investigation of Cancer Caregiving).[9]

In several previous editorials,[10–12] my colleagues and I highlighted the dearth of psychosocial interventions focused specifically on addressing the needs of cancer caregivers and noted that, generally, the state of the science of cancer caregiver intervention research was in its infancy. More recently, there has certainly been a burgeoning of research focusing on supporting caregivers across the care trajectory, as is evidenced by Sections 2 and 3 of this textbook. There is strong and growing evidence for the efficacy and effectiveness of empirically supported treatments, such as Psychoeducation (Chapter 7), Cognitive Behavioral Therapy (Chapter 9), and Problem-Solving Therapy (Chapter 10), to address various domains of caregiver burden and unmet needs. Such interventions have been shown to improve caregivers' skills, self-efficacy, and confidence in their role and to help them navigate the prolonged and often-intensifying challenges experienced across the caregiving trajectory. Indeed, short-term interventions such as the ENABLE program presented by Dionne-Odom and colleagues (Chapter 7) and the FOCUS program presented by Northouse and colleagues (Chapter 8) can afford caregivers the skills necessary to face the challenges of caregiving and protect them from the negative outcomes described in Section 1.

In Chapter 11, Schuler and colleagues present Family-Focused Grief Therapy (FFGT), an empirically supported, family-based approach that begins during palliative care and continues into bereavement. Through the promotion of family functioning, communication, cohesiveness, and conflict management, FFGT improves psychosocial outcomes among caregivers of patients with advanced and life-limiting cancers. The authors highlight several key points in their discussion of this powerful prophylactic approach that is targeted toward families at risk for poor psychosocial functioning. These include the effect of the family environment and functioning on family members' distress and the important recognition that the caregiving trajectory does not necessarily end when treatment is complete, but may persist long after a patient has died. A notable strength of this approach is the continuity of care for caregivers into bereavement, which serves as a critical reminder that our work is not complete at the time of a patient's death, but in many cases is just beginning.

Additionally, adaptations of empirically supported treatments show promise in addressing specific areas of caregiver distress and unmet needs. For example, Shaffer et al. (Chapter 12) highlight the caregiving context as a precipitating and perpetuating factor for insomnia and related distress and propose a tailored version of Cognitive Behavioral Therapy for Insomnia (CBT-I) to address insomnia in the context of caregiving. Insomnia among caregivers is one of the most distressing components of burden reported and is strongly associated with aggravated psychological and physical health. As CBT-I is recommended as a first-line treatment for insomnia,[13] the utility of this powerful, time-limited intervention for caregivers is clear.

In Chapter 13, Panjwani and colleagues describe an adaptation of Emotion Regulation Therapy (ERT) for cancer caregivers. ERT incorporates principles from CBT and experiential therapy to addresses the preservative negative thinking (e.g., worry, rumination) underlying anxiety and depression. As the caregiving trajectory often creates a prolonged period of uncertainty, this adaptation—Emotion Regulation Therapy for Cancer Caregivers (ERT-C)—shows significant promise in addressing anxious and depressive symptomatology through augmenting caregivers' emotion regulation skills and ability to flexibly attend to the challenges that arise in the caregiving context.

In Chapter 14, Meaning-Centered Psychotherapy for Cancer Caregivers (MCP-C) is described. Based on Meaning-Centered Psychotherapy (MCP), an empirically supported intervention developed originally to help patients at end-of-life (EOL) maintain a sense of meaning and purpose, MCP-C addresses existential distress by helping caregivers connect and reconnect to valued sources of meaning in their life. MCP-C assists caregivers in understanding how they can choose to face limitations endemic to caregiving, take responsibility for their lives in the context of caring for another, and recognize the sense of meaning and purpose that may be derived from the caregiving role.

While a significant portion of the research cited in Sections 2 and 3 was conducted in comprehensive cancer centers and academic institutions, we are very much reliant on community-based organizations to disseminate such interventions and establish their effectiveness. Indeed, the effectiveness of the FOCUS intervention described previously was established through partnership with the Cancer Support Community (CSC). Presented in Chapter 15, the CSC is an international nonprofit organization that provides patient and caregiver support, education, and programming and is involved in significant programs of research. Perhaps most notably, the CSC has developed and tested the CancerSupportSource—Caregiver®, a web-based distress screening program designed to identify caregiver needs and refer them to tailored support services. In the context of our already burdened healthcare system, the identification and routing of caregivers to appropriate support will be critical for overcoming treatment access barriers highlighted in Section 1 of the textbook.

Chapter 16 presents the American Cancer Society (ACS) Caregiver Support Program, which offers vast resources and supportive services for caregivers. In addition to their initiation of the largest quality-of-life study of cancer caregivers to date (the National Quality of Life Survey for Caregivers) and their comprehensive online and print education materials, the ACS serves as a leader in assisting families to navigate the significant financial and geographic barriers that prevent many patients from accessing care through their Hope Lodge and Hotel Partnership program, as well as their Road To Recovery and Transportation Program. Indeed, without these tremendous initiatives, one can imagine the multitude of families who would be unable to access necessary medical and psychosocial care.

In Chapter 17, the immense resources of CancerCare, a leading national organization providing free, professional support services and information to help people manage the emotional, practical, and financial challenges of cancer, is presented. The variety of psychosocial support that CancerCare delivers annually to assist caregivers during every stage of the caregiving trajectory is unparalleled. It is only through organizations such as CancerCare that reach thousands of caregivers annually that the true benefits of the interventions presented in Sections 2 and 3 may be fully realized.

The fifth and final section includes an essential chapter focused on important legal concerns faced by cancer caregivers and is written by two attorneys who work with a medical-legal partnership to provide free legal services in healthcare settings. Topics include laws that impact taking time off from work to provide care (e.g., Family Medical Leave Act, FMLA; Americans With Disabilities Act, ADA); financial concerns (e.g., securing Medicaid coverage to assist with maintaining loved ones at home); and the benefits of advance directives, including the Health Care Proxy, Living Will, Do-Not-Resuscitate (DNR) Orders, Physician Orders for Life Sustaining Treatment (POLST) and Power of Attorney. The authors also present an overview of relatively new legislations, including the Recognize, Assist, Include, Support, and Engage (RAISE) Family Caregivers Act and the Caregiver Advise, Record, Enable (CARE) Act, the latter of which requires hospitals to document the name of the family caregiver in the medical record of admitted patients, inform such caregivers when patients are to be transferred or discharged, and provide the family caregiver with education and instruction on the medical tasks he or she will need to perform for the patient at home. In effect, the CARE Act requires hospitals to recognize caregivers as formalized members of the healthcare team.

FUTURE DIRECTIONS

As I noted in the Preface to this volume, *Cancer Caregivers* reveals the depths of complexities inherent to caregiving that our field has been tirelessly exploring over the past decade and the open horizons that we have yet to understand. While there has been tremendous growth in the state of the science of research with cancer caregivers, there is much more work to be done. Several key areas of future growth are described here.

Distress Screening for Cancer Caregivers

Although distress screening has become a standard of care among cancer patients, routine and comprehensive distress screening for caregivers has yet to be implemented, despite their typically reporting higher distress than patients themselves.[14,15] There are several impediments to implementing routine distress screening for caregivers. The first, highlighted in Chapter 6, is a dearth of validated measures to identify unmet psychosocial needs of caregivers, or what I refer to as the *how* of distress screening. In fact, the CSC's CancerSupportSource—Caregiver (see Chapter 15) appears to be the only validated distress screening program designed to identify caregiver needs and refer caregivers to tailored support services. Data are needed on the utility and benefits of this tool across a wide variety of settings (e.g., inpatient, outpatient, community-based care, comprehensive medical center). The implementation of this measure and the development of other screening tools that can rapidly identify caregivers in need is a critical step for our field.

The establishment of validated distress screening measures is only the first challenge, however; the *when* and *where* of distress screening are equally important questions for us to address. Specifically, within oncological care, because they are not the identified patient, we face a much larger system-wide challenge to identify and screen for distress in caregivers. To date, despite repeated calls to integrate family-centered support services into cancer care,[16] most adult oncology practice settings have not established standardized processes to identify caregivers with emotional, social, and practical support needs. Assessing and addressing distress and psychosocial needs have been associated with important clinical benefits for patients, including fewer hospitalizations, emergency room visits, and number of prescriptions.[17] As such, the Institute of Medicine[18] and the National Comprehensive Cancer Network[19] have recognized that screening, referral, and follow-up for psychosocial concerns are critical to ensuring quality cancer care for the whole patient. However, extant distress screening programs primarily target patients alone. *This must be changed, now.* Caregiver-focused distress screening programs have the potential to improve the quality of care for all those affected by cancer. Beyond addressing the substantial mental and physical health burdens experienced by caregivers, such routine procedures may begin to shift caregivers' and healthcare systems' cultural norms around caring for caregivers—from the exception to the norm.

The CARE Act discussed in Chapter 18 offers one opportunity to identify and screen caregivers at the point of patient's hospitalization. Others must be identified and evaluated immediately. Additionally, we should more fully capitalize on individuals on the front lines: the various medical professionals who come into contact with families in inpatient and outpatient settings. These individuals should be trained to recognize the signs of caregiver burden and understand how to route caregivers to support in their unique systems.

In addition to improving our distress screening technology–the *how*, *when*, and *where* of distress screening referenced previously, several areas must be considered as we develop and implement screening processes for caregivers. For example, it is clear from Chapter 3 that caregivers at some life stages or in certain relationships to the patient may be at particular risk for burden and in need of support. It is also clear that the experience of caregiving is culturally constructed. Chapter 5 highlights the interaction between culture and caregiving and the need to examine multigenerational involvement in caregiving. However, the majority of work in this area to date has been conducted among non–cancer caregivers; there are only limited investigations of how cancer caregivers' ethnic and cultural backgrounds impact their experience of caregiving and burden; hence, this area remains critical for future study. The authors of Chapter 5 aptly note that in order to accomplish this, we need to engage in transdisciplinary and cross-cultural collaborations.

One additional area of burden that has received little (if any) comprehensive evaluation and that should be included in distress screening is the physical impact of engaging in caregiving tasks. Specifically, as is noted in Chapter 2, unintentional injuries such as muscle injuries, falls, cuts, scrapes, and bruises that result from care tasks (i.e., transferring patients from bed to wheelchair) have not been systematically studied in cancer caregivers and are likely more common among those who are overburdened and older, as has been found in studies of non–cancer caregiver populations. Such injuries exacerbate all elements of burden, create greater demands on caregiving networks, and often come with significant financial costs, as caregivers who are injured may not be able to assist the patient and must pay out of pocket for in-home skilled nursing aides. One can easily imagine the struggle experienced by a burdened caregiver who must choose between pushing themselves to a physical limit and emptying a bank account.

Intervention Development, Dissemination, and Implementation

Our field has made considerable progress in intervention development over the past decade. However, one area not explicitly addressed in these chapters but often implied is the need for improved communication between caregivers, patients, and healthcare professionals (HCPs). Effective communication between these three parties is the cornerstone of person-centered, family-oriented care. For example, in the setting of advanced cancer, discussions about advanced care planning (ACP), including prognosis and end-of-life (EOL) care, impact a number of critical patient, caregiver, and healthcare utilization outcomes, including prognostic awareness, psychopathology, timely hospice referral, and the use of unnecessary and aggressive treatments near death.[20–24] Caregivers, however, report often feeling unprepared or unwilling to engage in discussions with patients and physicians, and they are in need of skills that will allow them to feel confident as members of the healthcare team. Indeed, the 2016 AARP and National Alliance for Caregiving report[25] emphasized that the majority of caregivers do not have conversations with healthcare providers about their or the patients' needs. We therefore must examine the patient-caregiver-provider dynamics that promote or hinder caregiver well-being and discussions about goals of care. While it is critical that medical professionals assume a more-than-basic level of communication skills, training programs geared toward enhancing caregivers' communications skills specifically will enhance their ability to navigate the complicated waters of our healthcare system. Interventions that address communication between patients and caregivers exist[26,27] but have primarily been in service of enhancing social support.[28–35] Innovations aimed at improving the effectiveness of caregiver communication skills therefore represent a vital frontier to address this lingering gap.

Moving forward, much of our efforts should also focus on dissemination and implementation. Such research will allow us to understand why some interventions may be appropriate for some caregivers versus others and which interventions may be appropriate for caregivers based on factors such as life stage, relationship to the patient, cultural background, and coping capacity. This work will help us to further adapt and tailor our interventions to enhance outcomes and meet the needs of this incredibly vulnerable population. We must also continue to capitalize on the rapidly advancing telehealth technologies to deliver interventions to diverse groups of caregivers across the country and the world. In effect, this work will move us toward accomplishing precision and individualized medicine for cancer caregivers.

Public Policy and the Cancer Caregiving Landscape

In addition to efforts focused on distress screening and the dissemination and implementation of empirically supported treatments for caregivers, it is equally important for our field to (1) understand how the changing public policy landscape will impact cancer caregivers and (2) push for additional policies that will improve the capacity of caregivers to serve in this crucial role. For example, the CARE Act requires hospitals to formalize the procedures by which they identify and document the existence of caregivers, which represents a cultural shift where caregivers are being recognized as partners in a patient's recovery and improved health outcomes. According to AARP, by 2017, most hospitals evaluated had formed or were forming patient and family advisory councils, while others were including family caregivers in daily rounds.[36] As of June 2018, the CARE Act was approved by 37 states, but we still have a ways to go. And once approved, additional steps are needed to ensure that the CARE Act is implemented. The documentation of caregivers in the patient's medical record brings to focus the role of caregivers in the healthcare team and their involvement as healthcare proxies and individuals intimately involved in the patient's care. Surely, the process of documenting a caregiver may be an opportunity not only for distress screening, but also for the initiation of engaging in important—albeit difficult—conversations with HCPs and patients about EOL and goals of care.

Second, we must make it a priority to address the financial toxicity of caregiving. According to AARP, caregivers spend, on average, nearly $7,000 of their own funds annually on caregiving, which is almost 20% of their income.[37] As was noted in Chapter 3, from a policy perspective, the recognition of caregiving as a life course issue is essential for maximizing the impact of caregiving resources. Specifically, some available support is tied to the age of the caregiver or patient or the patient's health condition(s), such as the National Family Caregiver Support Program, which provides services to caregivers who are 55 years of age or older themselves or who are caring for someone 60 years of age or older (or someone with dementia, regardless of age).[38] Other programs such as Medicare and Medicaid (explored in Chapter 18) provide additional mechanisms of financial support based on life stage (e.g., eligible individuals in receipt of Medicare are age 65 or older, or in the case of Medicaid, those who are elderly or permanently disabled may qualify even if they do not meet the income restrictions). These programs, therefore, exclude younger and middle-adulthood caregivers who may be, due to competing demands of caregiving and child care, in significant need of financial support but ineligible to receive such support because of their age. We must systematically examine groups of caregivers who fall through these financial support cracks and create new ways to support them, which likely will include changes in policy. Toward this end, the AARP has proposed legislation called the Credit for Caring Act, which would create a federal, nonrefundable tax credit of up to $3,000 for family caregivers who work while also financially supporting their loved ones.[39] This type of legislation would help alleviate the financial strain that many caregivers face.

Finally, future research is needed to understand if—and to what extent—existing and developing public policies may shape the experience of sexual and gender minority (SGM) caregiver-patient dyads. A growing body of research indicates that the SGM experience is characterized by actual and anticipated prejudice within health and social services.[40] Importantly, as SGM may be more likely than majority group members to identify nonblood or legally partnered individuals as family,[41] efforts are needed to ensure that all policies and programs that impact caregivers (e.g., Family and Medical Leave Act, Consumer Directed Personal Assistance Program [CDPAP]) are nondiscriminatory and recognize the broad definition of family and the wide range of shapes that families take.

CONCLUSIONS

I am a scientist-practitioner and clinical psychologist. My practice focuses on supporting cancer caregivers throughout all stages of the caregiving trajectory. When I began working in this field, one of my first caregiver patients said to me, "What I'm doing for my Mom is just as important as her chemotherapy." And, in so many ways, I agree. Informal caregivers have become the backbone of our healthcare system, concurrently playing the role of partner/parent/child/sibling/friend and physician, nurse, social worker, lawyer, and patient navigator. Without a doubt, the presence of a caregiver who is dressed in invisible armor, ready to advocate (fight) on behalf of patients, negotiate our complicated healthcare system, and attempt clear and productive communication with medical, administrative, and legal professionals, is not only optimal, but also essential to the well-being of patients today.

As clearly delineated throughout the comprehensive literature reviews, analyses, and narrative descriptions in this volume, we must, as professionals engaged in supporting cancer caregivers, press strongly and advocate for policies that broadly acknowledge caregiver burden as a national healthcare issue. This perspective—assisted by the foundations of facts and felt human experience—will greatly assist with the implementation and legitimization of strategies to support caregivers. To that end, caregivers must be considered a critical part of the patient care unit by cancer care professionals, and we must continue to advocate for a paradigm shift from patient-centered to family-centered care.

REFERENCES

1. Hunt GG, Longacre ML, Kent, E. E., Weber-Raley L. *Cancer Caregiving in the US: An Intense, Episodic, and Challenging Experience.* Bethesda, MD: National Alliance for Caregiving; 2016.
2. National Cancer Institute. *Health Information National Trends Survey V, Cycle 1.* Bethesda, MD: National Cancer Institute; 2017.
3. National Alliance for Caregiving. *Cancer Caregiving in the US: An Intense, Episodic, and Challenging Care Experience.* Bethesda, MD: National Alliance for Caregiving; 2016.
4. Yabroff KR, Kim Y. Time costs associated with informal caregiving for cancer survivors. *Cancer.* 2009;115(18)(suppl):4362–4373.
5. de Moor JS, Dowling EC, Ekwueme DU, et al. Employment implications of informal cancer caregiving. *Journal of Cancer Survivorship.* 2017;11(1):48–57.
6. Barusch AS, Spaid WM. Gender differences in caregiving: why do wives report greater burden? *Gerontologist.* 1989;29(5):667–676.
7. Gilligan C. *In a Different Voice: Psychological Theory and Women's Development.* Cambridge, MA: Harvard University Press; 1982.
8. Schofield T, Connell RW, Walker L, Wood JF, Butland DL. Understanding men's health and illness: a gender-relations approach to policy, research, and practice. *Journal of American College Health.* 2000;48(6):247–256.
9. Sabogal F, Marín G, Otero-Sabogal R, Marín BV, Perez-Stable EJ. Hispanic familism and acculturation: what changes and what doesn't? *Hispanic Journal of Behavioral Sciences.* 1987;9(4):397–412.
10. Applebaum, A. Isolated, invisible, and in-need: there should be no "I" in caregiver. Guest Editorial. *Palliative and Supportive Care, 13,* 415–416.
11. Applebaum A. (2017). Survival of the fittest . . . caregiver? *Palliative and Supportive Care.* 2017;15(1):1–2.
12. Deshields TL Applebaum AJ. The time is now: assessing and addressing the needs of cancer caregivers. Invited editorial. *Cancer.* 2015;121(9):1344–1346.
13. Schutte-Rodin S, Broch L, Buysse D, Dorsey C, Sateia M. Clinical guideline for the evaluation and management of chronic insomnia in adults. *Journal of Clinical Sleep Medicine.* 2008;4(5):487–504.
14. Lambert SD, Jones BL, Girgis A, et al. Distressed partners and caregivers do not recover easily: adjustment trajectories among partners and caregivers of cancer survivors. Annals of Behavioral Medicine. 2012;44(2):225–235.
15. Kim Y, Shaffer KM, Carver CS, et al. Prevalence and predictors of depressive symptoms among cancer caregivers 5 years after the relative's cancer diagnosis. Journal of Consulting and Clinical Psychology. 2014;82(1):1.
16. Kent EE, Rowland JH, Northouse L, et al. Caring for caregivers and patients: research and clinical priorities for informal cancer caregiving. Cancer. 2016;122(13):1987–1995.
17. Badr H, Herbert K, Reckson B, et al. Unmet needs and relationship challenges of head and neck cancer patients and their spouses. *Journal of Psychosocial Oncology.* 2016;34(4):336–346.
18. Adler NE, Page AEK, eds. *Cancer Care for the Whole Patient: Meeting Psychosocial Health Needs.* Washington, DC: National Academies Press; 2008.
19. National Comprehensive Cancer Network. Distress management clinical practice guidelines. *Journal of the National Comprehensive Cancer Network.* 2003;1:344–374.

20. Nilsson ME, Maciejewski PK, Zhang B, et al. Mental health, treatment preferences, advance care planning, location, and quality of death in advanced cancer patients with dependent children. *Cancer*. 2009;115(2):399–409.

21. Wright AA, Mack JW, Kritek PA, et al. Influence of patients' preferences and treatment site on cancer patients' end-of-life care. *Cancer*. 2010;116(19):4656–4663.

22. Detering KM, Hancock AD, Reade MC, Silvester W. The impact of advance care planning on end of life care in elderly patients: randomised controlled trial. *British Medical Journal*. 2010;340:c1345.

23. Temel JS, Greer JA, Muzikansky A, et al. Early palliative care for patients with metastatic non–small-cell lung cancer. *New England Journal of Medicine*. 2010;363(8):733–742.

24. Heyland DK, Barwich D, Pichora D, et al. Failure to engage hospitalized elderly patients and their families in advance care planning. *JAMA Internal Medicine*, 2013;173(9):778–787.

25. Hunt GG, Longacre MLK, Kent EE, Weber- Raley L. *Cancer Caregiving in the US: An Intense, Episodic, and Challenging Experience*. Bethesda, MD: National Alliance for Caregiving; 2016.

26. Northouse LL, Katapodi MC, Song L, Zhang L, Mood DW. Interventions with family caregivers of cancer patients: meta-analysis of randomized trials. *CA: A Cancer Journal for Clinicians*. 2010;60(5):317–339.

27. Applebaum AJ, Breitbart W. Care for the cancer caregiver: a systematic review. *Palliative and Supportive Care*. 2013;11(3):231–252.

28. Scott JL, Halford WK, Ward BG. United we stand? The effects of a couple-coping intervention on adjustment to early stage breast or gynecological cancer. Journal of Consulting and Clinical Psychology. 2004;72(6):1122.

29. Northouse L, Kershaw T, Mood D, Schafenacker A. Effects of a family intervention on the quality of life of women with recurrent breast cancer and their family caregivers. *Psycho-Oncology*. 2005;14(6):478–491.

30. Budin WC, Hoskins CN, Haber J, et al. Breast cancer: education, counseling, and adjustment among patients and partners: a randomized clinical trial. *Nursing Research*. 2008;57(3):199–213.

31. Campbell LC, Keefe FJ, Scipio C, et al. Facilitating research participation and improving quality of life for African American prostate cancer survivors and their intimate partners. *Cancer*. 2007;109(S2):414–424.

32. Baucom DH, Porter LS, Kirby JS, et al. A couple-based intervention for female breast cancer. *Psycho-Oncology*. 2009;18(3):276–283.

33. Given B, Given CW, Sikorskii A, Jeon S, Sherwood P, Rahbar M. The impact of providing symptom management assistance on caregiver reaction: results of a randomized trial. *Journal of Pain and Symptom Management*. 2006;32(5):433–443.

34. Lyon ME, Jacobs S, Briggs L, Cheng YI, Wang J. A longitudinal, randomized, controlled trial of advance care planning for teens with cancer: anxiety, depression, quality of life, advance directives, spirituality. *Journal of Adolescent Health*. 2014;54(6):710–717.

35. Bernacki R, Hutchings M, Vick J, et al. Development of the Serious Illness Care Program: a randomised controlled trial of a palliative care communication intervention. *BMJ Open*. 2015;5(10):e009032.

36. Mason D. JAMA Forum: supporting family caregivers, one state at a time: the CARE Act. news@JAMA. December 13, 2017. https://newsatjama.jama.com/2017/12/13/jama-forum-supporting-family-caregivers-one-state-at-a-time-the-care-act/. Accessed March 22, 2018.

37. Kriss E. Family caregiver tax credit would provide critical help to NYS's middle class. https://states.aarp.org/aarp-family-caregiver-tax-credit-would-provide-critical-help-to-nyss-middle-class/. Published December 6, 2017. Accessed March 22, 2018.

38. Administration for Community Living. National Family Caregiver Support Program. 2017; https://www.acl.gov/programs/support-caregivers/national-family-caregiver-support-program. Last modified December 13, 2017. Accessed March 7, 2018.

39. AARP. The Credit for Caring Act. https://www.aarp.org/caregiving/financial-legal/info-2017/credit-for-caring-act.html. Accessed March 22, 2018.

40. Washington KT, McElroy J, Albright D, et al. Experiences of sexual and gender minorities caring for adults with non-AIDS-related chronic illness. *Social Work Research*. 2015;39:71–82.

41. Muraco A, Fredriksen-Goldsen KI. "That's what friends do": informal caregiving for chronically ill midlife and older lesbian, gay, and bisexual adults. *Journal of Social and Personal Relationships*. 2011;28:1073–1092.

INDEX